Coping with Chronic Illness
and Disability

M000311690

Coping with Chronic Illness and Disability

Theoretical, Empirical, and Clinical Aspects

Edited by

Erin Martz
University of Memphis
Memphis, Tennessee, USA

Hanoch Livneh
Portland State University
Portland, Oregon, USA

Foreword by Beatrice A. Wright

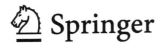 Springer

Erin Martz
University of Memphis
Memphis, Tennessee 38152
USA
emartz@memphis.edu

Hanoch Livneh
Portland State University
Portland, Oregon 97207-0751
USA
Livnehh@pdx.edu

ISBN   978-1-4419-4308-8   e-ISBN   978-0-387-48670-3

Printed on acid-free paper.

9 8 7 6 5 4 3 2 1

springer.com

The Uninvited Guest

It's there every
day, every hour,
every minute,
begging you for attention
like a hungry child,
demanding your thoughts
like an expectant teacher,
draining your energy
like an air-conditioner
on a monsoon day.
It's permanently there,
like a deep scar, a tattoo,
like a traumatic memory,
like the stars in a Hawaiian sky,
like the soft, clingy Bahraini sands,
like the bubbling Arkansas hot springs,
like the friend who forgives your mistakes.
Disability permeates the wrinkles of our lives
and can blossom into new growth,
as we shed the shame and pain
that usher in its arrival.

– Erin Martz

Contents

Part II

Foreword

A volume that deals in depth with a coping approach to chronic illness and disability (CID), based on theory, research and clinical aspects, holds much promise to improve the lives of people directly affected. But such a volume, with its many contributors and wide scope, may also harbor minefields along the way that undermine the actual individuals who are trying to cope with their condition. The reader, therefore, needs carefully to think through the implications of the particular content of each chapter, in order to detect and thereby avoid prejudicial consequences. This foreword concerns flawed human perception and corrective perspectives, not statistical issues.

To alert the reader, a variety of factors commonly involved in how we, as humans, perceive people, are briefly described – factors that unconsciously interfere with the promise of coping well or even adequately with adversity. This is followed by a set of counteracting strategies. An elaboration of the concepts involved, together with supporting research, may be found in Wright (1983, 1991).

One interfering factor is the **Fundamental Negative Bias**. It states that when something stands out as negative, and when the context lacks positives to control the negative spread, the mind goes negative; i.e., the train of thought on the part of the perceiver, be it oneself or another person, is forced onto a negative track of inferences concerning causes and effects of the troubling situation. Coping possibilities have then to break through the grip of overwhelming negatives.

The **Potency of Negatives** is another powerful force reinforcing the negative thrust. It refers to the tendency to give more weight to negatives than to positives. This tendency steers the perceiver away from coping possibilities which, after all, require taking advantage of whatever is positive and potentially helpful.

A third factor is known as the **Just World Phenomenon** (Lerner, 1980). It refers to the belief that suffering and punishments, like joys and rewards, should be deserved. By aligning the existing reality with what is right and ought to be, the danger is that the mind unconsciously slips into blaming the victim, be it oneself or someone else, for the distress – a force that clearly has to be reckoned with in encouraging a coping approach to difficulties.

Still another formidable factor obscuring coping possibilities is the strong tendency toward the **Eclipse of the Environment** when the target of concern is a person. Essentially, this is a figure-ground problem. To recognize that the *realities of the environment* need to be included in assessment and rehabilitation procedures would appear to be axiomatic, because behavior is always a function of both the person and the environment (Lewin, 1935). And yet, because it is the person who comes in for treatment, not the environment, the environment remains ignored in the murky background. Special effort is thus required to bring the un-illuminated environment into focus.

Fortunately, there are a number of perspectives that serve to counter the factors that interfere with the best coping efforts. One important perspective is that of the **Insider vs. Outsider** (Dembo, 1964). The insider is the person directly experiencing CID, whereas the outsider is the observer or evaluator of the condition. Frequently, it is the insider who is more attuned to the immediate environment, in which one's own behavior must take place. To take full advantage of the insider's personal understanding of the situation, including what is helpful and harmful, the insider's involvement in assessing it should be sought and encouraged. Furthermore, to maximize potential, the person with CID can well serve as **co-manager** in the rehabilitation process whenever feasible.

Another significant perspective is provided by the **Coping vs. Succumbing Frameworks.** These two frameworks orient the person in opposite directions. In considering their essential differences presented below, bear in mind that whenever "the person" is referred to, it is the person who is perceiving the situation, that is, oneself or an outsider, such as a professional, stranger, friend, and so on as the case may be.

The significance of the two contrasting frameworks may best be clarified by highlighting the striking *qualitative differences* regarding their positive and negative emphases. The succumbing focus is on the difficulties and heartbreak of the condition, not on the challenge of meaningful adaptation and change. Attention is placed on what the person cannot do, on what the person cannot enjoy. The condition is seen as central, overriding everything else about the person. *The person as an individual, with a highly unique personality, is lost.*

The coping framework, on the other hand, represents a constructive view of life with CID. It orients the perceiver to appreciate the person (self or other) as having abilities of *intrinsic value*. People with CID are regarded as *active participants* in their own lives and community, not as devastated, passive victims. Managing difficulties has a double focus. One focus is on *environmental change* – that is, changing those alterable conditions that add to the person's limitations, such as architectural barriers, lack of employment opportunities, discriminatory practices, family problems, and inadequate health care, education, housing and transportation. The second focus is directed toward *change in the person* through medical, psychological, and other health-care approaches, through education and training that lead to new skills, and through *value changes* that reinforce self-respect.

With regard to the suffering connected to some aspects of disability, the coping framework is oriented toward seeking solutions and discovering satisfaction in living. It recognizes the illness or disability as only one aspect of a multi-faceted life that includes abilities as well as disabilities, gratifications as well as frustration. To move toward accomplishing these diverse and ideal goals obviously requires the work of many people over time. Note that the coping framework applies not only to the person with a CID, but also to the outsider, including the wider society, in helping to improve the situation.

Keeping in mind the significance of the main qualitative differences between the two frameworks, we can briefly summarize the essence of the coping framework in the following statement: *What is at stake is replacing the negative cognitive-affective focus by consciously deciding to discover those resources in both the person and the environment that need to be accessed to cope effectively with the negative barriers of the total situation.*

We need to be aware, however, that not all coping efforts can be regarded as positive. For example, consider the case of coping with stigma that ends up in social withdrawal and unnecessary isolation. We also need to be aware that there are times when it is better for the person experiencing an illness or disability to temporarily withhold the coping framework by acknowledging the frustration and suffering, rather than to dismiss these feelings in pursuing change and adaptation. Furthermore, we need to realize that coping is not a uniform process. There may be down times when the person is unmotivated, needs "time out," or even is in despair, having succumbed to the negatives. With the sensitive support of others, however, time is on the side of the person who generally rallies to become re-engaged in the coping process. As for professionals, because the negative flaws of human perception are so powerful, it is incumbent to deliberately search for and marshal those constructive forces in the person and resources in the environment that can energize this progress.

Finally, there is the crucial role played by **Values** undergirding theory, research, and clinical approaches. For example, it makes a difference if the professional values the *uniqueness* of the individual and situation in order to avoid a generic approach, and instead, takes into account the special needs of the person and the particular issues in the social and physical environment. It makes a difference if the professional believes that the active participation of the person in the planning and execution of the rehabilitation program is to be sought as fully as possible. It behooves professionals to self-monitor their efforts in order to detect possible violations of their own values. Twenty elaborated value-laden beliefs and principles are available, for the reader to review, in the preface of Wright (1983).

In conclusion, sensitization to the pitfalls of flawed human perception allows the professional to shift to a viable coping approach. The goals, to reduce limitations and suffering and to improve the quality of life of the individual, are best served by drawing upon the insider's perspective and active participation, with the support of underlying values. Keeping the caveats in mind, the reader will be in a better position to separate the wheat from the chaff in harvesting a rich store of ideas for theory, research, and clinical applications that will enable people to live constructively with CID.

Beatrice A. Wright, Ph.D.
University of Kansas

References

Dembo, T. (1964). Sensitivity of one person to another. *Rehabilitation Literature, 25*(8), 231–235.

Lerner, M. J. (1980). *The belief in a just world: A fundamental delusion.* New York: Plenum Press.

Lewin, K. A. (1935). *Dynamic theory of personality.* New York: McGraw Hill.

Wright, B. A. (1983). *Physical disability: A psychosocial approach* (2nd ed.). New York: Harper and Row.

Wright, B. A. (1991). Labeling: The need for greater person-environment individuation. In C. R. Snyder & D. R. Forsyth (Eds.), *The handbook of social and clinical psychology: The health perspective* (pp. 469–487). New York: Pergamon Press.

Quoted from p. 195 in Wright, B. A. (1983). *Physical disability—a psychosocial approach* (2nd ed.). New York: HarperCollins Publishers.

Coping	Succumbing
1. The emphasis is on what the person *can do.*	1. The emphasis is on what a person *cannot do.*
2. Areas of life in which the person can participate are seen as worthwhile.	2. Little weight is given to the areas of life in which the person can participate.
3. The person is perceived as playing an *active role* in molding his or her life constructively.	3. The person in seen as *passive,* as a victim of *misfortune.*
4. The accomplishments of the person are appreciated in terms of their benefits to the person and others (asset evaluation), and not evaluated because they fall short of some irrelevant standard.	4. The person's accomplishments are minimized by highlighting their shortcomings (comparative–status evaluation, usually measured in terms of "normal" standards).
5. The negative aspects of the person's life, such as the pain that is suffered or difficulties that exist, are felt to be manageable. They are limited because satisfactory aspects of the person's life are recognized.	5. The negative aspects of a person's life, such as the pain that is suffered or difficulties that exist, are kept in the forefront of attention. They are emphasized and exaggerated and even seen to usurp all of life (spread).
6. Managing difficulties mean reducing limitations route changes in the social and physical environment as well as in the person. Examples are: a. eliminating barriers b. environmental accommodations c. medical procedures d. prostheses and other assistive devices e. learning new skills	6. Prevention and cure are the only valid solutions to the problem of disability.
7. Managing difficulties also means *living on satisfactory terms* with one's limitations (although the disability may be regarded as a nuisance and sometimes a burden). This involves an important *value changes.*	7. The only way to live with the disability is to resign oneself or to act as if the disability does not exist.
8. The fact that individuals with disabilities can live meaningful lives is indicated by their participation in valued activities and by their sharing in the satisfaction of living.	8. The person with a disability is pitied and his or her life essentially devaluated.

Preface

Far from a digression in the stream of existence, trauma intensified existence, bringing forth elements of experience too easily clouded over by the seductive predictability of day-to-day, so-called "normal" life. From the beginning, disability taught that life could be reinvented.

John Hockenberry (1995, p. 79)

The purpose of this book is to study human coping following the onset of, and the ongoing stressor of, a chronic illness or disability (CID). Theories and empirical studies about coping will be examined about individuals who have faced the challenge of CID and who have coped with CID in different ways. It is hoped that the multifaceted aspects of this book will spark new research and clinical work, which in turn, may encourage individuals with CID to explore better ways of coping and of appreciating the time-limited phenomenon called life.

Stress Related to Chronic Illness and Disability

Most people consider the *onset* of a CID as a *negative* event (e.g., for some, it is a time of psychological "darkness"). This is evident not only by individuals' reactions (e.g., anxiety, anger, depression) when a CID occurs, but also by the reactions (e.g., frustration, anxiety, confusion, avoidance) of family members and friends. Even if an individual with a CID has accepted the bodily or mental changes, and family and friends have become accustomed to these changes, psychological reverberations of the CID can still be experienced in a person's social environment (i.e., employment, leisure, or other public settings), due to strangers' reactions of fear, curiosity, avoidance, prejudice, or other types of stereotypical perceptions and discriminatory practices. Social attitudes toward people with CID often have negative under-tones and, as a consequence, may cause additional stress for the individual with CID.

The view that the onset of CID is a *negative occurrence* (i.e., a distressing event) is ubiquitous: Who would hold celebratory parties or congratulate someone after it happened? Yet, ironically, sometimes the diagnosis of a CID can literally *save* a person's life, if followed by appropriate treatment (e.g., the diagnosis of insulin-dependent diabetes or cancer). Further, sometimes a CID is a conse-quence of a sudden event (e.g., loss of a limb due to stepping on a mine, paralysis from a severe motor vehicle accident) that could have resulted in a much more serious outcome, including death. Despite experiencing "lesser trauma" than what could have occurred, it may be difficult for individuals with CID (or their family and friends) to appreciate the fact that *one is still alive,* especially when life following some CID is so different from the life that was anticipated or imagined, and when that life requires alterations in personal habits, modes of functioning, and even self-perceptions. The affected individual may dwell on the perceived tragedy of the CID, instead of emphasizing existing and new potentials that ensue from continued life, though radically altered, or focusing on the abilities that were preserved and the possibilities that still remain.

The Battle with Oneself

Living with CID is often challenging. Some people, such as those who have active disease-processes, may feel as if their bodies or minds are a war-zone on a microcosmic level (e.g., neurobiological levels that fluctuate danger-ously outside of normal levels, viruses or cancers that wage war against one's own body and the immune system). Daily living may be a focus on a life-or-death survival within one's own microcosm, and thus may be perceived as dangerous, uncontrollable, and unpredictable. Life can take on a different kind of meaning and value when a person fights daily to live, or when they have come close to death. The existential awareness of life and death can lead to heightened appreciation of life, relationships, and what is still possible.

In cultures that emphasize physical strength, beauty, self-control, and certain ideals and idolizations of "perfection," individuals with a CID may battle with themselves and their conditions, bodies, or minds, and their lack of control in certain areas. They may battle feelings of anger and self-hatred, because they resent their appearance and physical or mental functioning, or because their expectations about their own ability to lead "normal" lives do not match the reality they experience. So how can people with CID learn to successfully cope with their CID? How do they find successful ways of managing their changed or changing selves, and their often oppressive physical and social environments?

The Battle with Environmental Influences

Because of their conditions, individuals with CID may encounter a wide range of responses from the environment, some negatively tainted (e.g., stigmatization, discrimination) and some positive (e.g., compassion, needed assistance). The reactions from the social environment may create a negative feedback loop, in which societal negative attitudes toward people with CID may feed into one's own battling with the perceived negative experience of CID. Similarly, because of these attitudinal and physical barriers, individuals with CID may experience all sorts of continuous environmental battles (e.g., on architectural, attitudinal, and financial levels).

Family, friends, or acquaintances may provide a balance to negative environmental influences by their positive messages and empathic support. Because CID often involves a long, if not life-long, journey, which will require a wide range of coping strategies for numerous life challenges, the question, "How can I help you cope?" may be an effective expression of support to an individual with a newly-acquired CID. Such a question permits an individual with CID to state if help is indeed required and what kind of help is needed, and also sends the implicit message that the person has the ability to cope (with or without support). It also allows people in the individual's social network to assuage CID-related feelings of anxiety and helplessness, and to replace those feelings with tangible, active measures that are in harmony with the wishes of the person with CID.

Coping with CID

Coping can take many forms. It may be growth-oriented (e.g., problem-solving of issues impeding one's functioning, thinking positively about the possibilities available in the future) or negatively weighted (e.g., avoiding certain situations, catastrophizing), or it can encompass both forms simultaneously. Some coping strategies can help individuals restore a holistic equilibrium, while others can cause them to spiral into stressful and dissatisfying lives.

Despite the sometimes enormous challenges created by CID, many people have reported the development, over time, of positive perspectives and experiences in their lives (e.g., a greater appreciation for life, relationships, their own strengths; newly found meanings in life). Even with positive personal views and supportive physical, social, and emotional environments, CID can still be a constant hassle. How can people learn to minimize the ever-present ramifications of a CID, to view their conditions as only one component of multiple aspects of their lives, and to integrate the CID into their daily lives, as one of many challenges?

The theories and research that are examined in this book will hopefully help answer some of the aforementioned questions. Coping strategies may offer a means by which the impact of a CID is minimized, and may help a person arrive at the psychological place in which the undeniable presence of a CID no longer dominates the person's mental and emotional landscapes, but becomes a part of an individual's cognitive-affective background, permitting positively-valenced perceptions, thoughts, feelings, and activities to take primary importance.

Contents of the Book

This book focuses on understanding the multifaceted processes of how people struggle and cope with the irreversible presence of CID in their lives. Although every individual will experience a unique mixture of life events, processes, outcomes, and successes in their coping with CID, this book surveys trends that clinicians and researchers have observed. This book also examines empirical findings, because patterns noted among individuals with specific types of CID may provide clinicians with valuable information on those coping styles and strategies, which may help to alter or bolster one's coping with CID-generated, stressful life-events.

This book contains two parts. Part I discusses a range of theoretical and conceptual perspectives on coping, including selected applications of coping with CID. Part II contains chapters that focus on coping with 12 specific types of CID. Most of the chapters in Part II follow a rather standardized format, although this format is applied flexibly, in view of the expansive research in specific areas (e.g., newly developed therapeutic modalities, randomized clinical intervention studies). The format of the Part II chapters includes the following components: Etiology and description of the CID, typical medical regimens, the empirical literature on coping with the specific CID, physical and psychosocial/ behavioral interventions, and finally, when applicable, vocational and social implications of the CID.

A Note about CID and Employment

Some chapters include discussions about vocational rehabilitation. This topic is included, because employment may be one of the most effective means of social integration for individuals with disabilities. Employment not only provides financial independence, but it often provides needed health insurance, a regained meaning in life, personal independence, a place to learn new skills, and social interaction with a diverse group of people. Thus, sections on employment-related issues are included in several of the chapters of this book, as adaptive coping often increases vocational functioning and successful integration into the community.

References

Hockenberry, J. (1995). *Moving violations: War zones, wheelchairs, and declarations of independence.* New York: Hyperion.

Acknowledgments

The editors would like to thank two people, who provided feedback on two of the chapters: Dr. Federico Montero (Coordinator of the Disability and Rehabilitation Team, World Health Organization, Geneva) and Michael Bricker (Counseling psychology doctoral student, University of Memphis).

Erin Martz would like to thank Dr. Aric Rimmerman (University of Haifa, Israel) for helping her to begin conceptualizing a book on coping with CID. She would also like to thank Dr. Hanoch Livneh for his continuous support for and insightful feedback about her work, and for almost a decade of collaboration, which evolved into a fascinating research-related journey.

Hanoch Livneh would like to thank Dr. Richard Antonak, with whom he has collaborated for the past 20 years, for his professional insights and long-term friendship. The editors would also like to thank Carol Bischoff (executive editor) and Amanda Breccia (editorial assistant) at Springer for their support and feedback during the preparation of this book.

Erin Martz
Hanoch Livneh

About the Contributors

Chase A. Allen, M.R.C., C.R.C., is a Ph.D. candidate in the Department of Rehabilitation Psychology and Special Education, University of Wisconsin-Madison and a research assistant in the Charles Matthews Laboratory of Neuropsychology, Department of Neurology, University of Wisconsin-Madison. His research interests include psychosocial aspects of disability, adaptation to disability, evidenced-based practice, and neuropsychological progression in new onset epilepsy.

Kymberley K. Bennett, Ph.D. is an assistant professor in the Department of Psychology at Indiana State University. Her research interests include the effect of social cognition on physical and mental health and the role played by causal attributions in recovery efforts among individuals with cardiovascular disease.

Malachy Bishop, Ph.D., C.R.C. is an associate professor with the Rehabilitation Counseling Program at the University of Kentucky. His research interests include quality of life, adaptation to chronic illness and disability, and the psychological and social aspects of chronic neurological conditions, including multiple sclerosis and epilepsy.

Jennifer L. Boothby, Ph.D. is an associate professor in the Psychology Department at Indiana State University. Her research interests include chronic pain, mental health and physical health problems among offenders, and health services in correctional institutions.

Melissa G. Bresnick, B.S. is a research associate for the Johns Hopkins Burn Center at the Johns Hopkins Bayview Medical Center, where she manages the research activities of the Burn Injury Rehabilitation Model System. Her research interests include investigating the psychological repercussions of burn injury, and determining effective prevention and treatment methods for injury complications.

Fong Chan, Ph.D., C.R.C. is a licensed psychologist, professor, and the director of clinical training (doctoral program), Rehabilitation Psychology Program, Department of Rehabilitation Psychology and Special Education, University of

Wisconsin. His research interests include multicultural counseling, computer applications, outcome measurements, and psychosocial aspects of disabilities.

Julie Chronister, Ph.D. is an assistant professor in the Counseling Department, College of Health and Human Services at San Francisco State University. Her research interests include the role of social support and coping in rehabilitation.

Laura Cramer-Berness, Ph.D. is an assistant professor of Psychology at William Paterson University. Her research interests include developing non-pharmacological ways to alleviate pain and exploring how individuals cope with medical illnesses that affect themselves and/or their families.

Jeanne Dalen, M.S. is a clinical psychology graduate student specializing in behavioral medicine at the University of New Mexico. She is currently a project coordinator for the Oregon Research Institute and is working on her dissertation involving the use of complementary medicine among women with cervical cancer.

Kim E. Dixon, Ph.D., M.B.A., is a clinical assistant professor in the Department of Psychiatric Medicine, Brody School of Medicine, East Carolina University, Greenville, North Carolina. Her research interests include examining psychosocial aspects of chronic pain.

James A. Fauerbach, Ph.D. is chief psychologist for the Johns Hopkins Burn Center at the Johns Hopkins Hospital (pediatrics) and the Johns Hopkins Bayview Medical Center (adults), and Director of Cognitive Behavioral Training for psychiatry residents in the Anxiety Disorders Clinic at Johns Hopkins Hospital. He is an associate professor in the Department of Psychiatry and Behavioral Sciences at Johns Hopkins University School of Medicine and holds a joint appointment in the Department of Physical Medicine and Rehabilitation. His research interests include investigating emotional factors mediating physical and psychological health and functional outcomes following serious illness or injury.

Joseph H. Hinkebein, Ph.D. is a clinical associate professor in the Department of Health Psychology at the University of Missouri-Columbia and a licensed psychologist specializing in the provision of psychological services to individuals with brain injury. He holds a Diplomate in Rehabilitation Psychology and is an APA Fellow in the Division of Rehabilitation Psychology. His research interests include neurobehavioral adjustment following traumatic brain injury, spiritual contributors to coping with disability, and the traumatically-induced alteration of smell (anosmia).

Charles J. Holahan, Ph.D. is a faculty member at the University of Texas at Austin and has been a visiting faculty member at the Center for Health Care Evaluation at the Stanford University School of Medicine. His research involves stress, coping, and health, with an emphasis on stress resistance.

John F. Kosciulek, Ph.D., C.R.C. is a professor and director of the MA Program in Rehabilitation Counseling at Michigan State University. Dr. Kosciulek is a former National Institute on Disability and Rehabilitation Research Switzer Fellow, and is currently co-editor of the professional journal *Rehabilitation Education*. His research interests include research methodology, family adaptation to brain injury, consumer direction in rehabilitation, and the transition from school to adult life of youth with disabilities.

Shlomo Kravetz, Ph.D. is a professor in the clinical rehabilitation program in the Department of Psychology at Bar-Ilan University, Israel. His research interests include psychiatric rehabilitation, the interface between qualitative and quantitative research in psychiatric rehabilitation, the neuropsychology of severe mental illness, and the link between theories of motivation and the assessment of outcomes in rehabilitation.

Hanoch Livneh, Ph.D., C.R.C., is a professor and coordinator of the Rehabilitation Counseling program at Portland State University. He is an APA Fellow in the division of Rehabilitation Psychology. His research interests include coping with and adaptation to chronic illness and disability, attitudes toward people with disability, and the measurement of outcomes in rehabilitation.

Sharon L. Manne, Ph.D. is a Senior Member in the Population Science Division at the Fox Chase Cancer Center and Clinical Professor in the College of Health Professions at Temple University. She is an APA Fellow in the Divisions of Health Psychology and Pediatric Psychology. Her primary research interests include examining the role of the marital relationship in adaptation to cancer, as well as evaluating methods of improving quality of life for individuals with cancer and their family members.

Erin Martz, Ph.D., C.R.C. is an assistant professor and coordinator of the Rehabilitation Counseling program at the University of Memphis. She has been a U.S. Department of State Fulbright Fellow (Russia) and a Switzer Merit Fellow (National Institute on Disability and Rehabilitation Research). Her research interests include psychosocial adaptation to and coping with chronic illness and disability, posttraumatic stress reactions following disability, disability-related employment issues, attitudes toward disability, and international rehabilitation.

Kristy McNulty, M.S., C.R.C., is a doctoral candidate in Educational Leadership (Special Education and Counselor Education specialization) at Portland State University. Her primary research interests include issues that influence coping, adaptation, and life quality among people with multiple sclerosis.

Rudolf H. Moos, Ph.D. is a Senior Research Career Scientist at the Department of Veterans Affairs Health Care System and a professor in the Department of Psychiatry and Behavioral Sciences at Stanford University in Palo Alto, California. He has written about concepts and measures of coping, coping with health conditions, the association between coping and the outcome of treatment, and how effective adaptation to life stressors can lead to personal growth.

Robert A. Neimeyer, Ph.D., is director of psychotherapy in the Department of Psychology, University of Memphis, where he has published 20 books. He serves as editor of the journal *Death Studies* and the *Journal of Constructivist Psychology*. Dr. Neimeyer has been granted the Distinguished Research Award, the Distinguished Teaching Award, and the Eminent Faculty Award by University of Memphis. He is an APA Fellow in Division 12 (Clinical Psychology), and a recipient of the Research Recognition Award by the Association for Death Education and Counseling.

Cynthia L. Radnitz, Ph.D. is a professor in the School of Psychology at Fairleigh Dickinson University in Teaneck New Jersey, and a staff psychologist at the Department of Veterans Affairs Medical Center, Bronx, New York. She has conducted research in several areas of health psychology, including chronic headache, irritable bowel syndrome, and spinal cord injury, and published a book on cognitive-behavioral therapy for persons with disabilities. More recently, she has become interested in research on vegetarian diets and health.

David Roe, Ph.D. is a clinical psychologist, associate professor, and chair of the Department of Community Mental Health in the Faculty of Social Welfare and Health Studies at University of Haifa, Israel. His primary research interests focus on exploring factors related to recovery from serious mental illness and their clinical, policy, and legal implications.

Susan Roos, Ph.D., LCSW works in private practice. She serves as adjunct faculty for The Union Institute and University, is an instructor in the Professional Development Program, University of Texas at Arlington Graduate School of Social Work, and consults on doctoral committees regarding research on chronic sorrow. She authored a book on chronic sorrow. She is president of the Dallas Society for Psychoanalytic Psychology.

Bruce W. Smith, Ph.D. is an assistant professor in the Department of Psychology at the University of New Mexico. He is the director of the Health Psychology program. His research interests focus on the relationship between emotion and health. He is currently using neuroimaging, psychophysiological, and behavioral methods to examine resilience in people with chronic pain.

Michael T. Smith, Ph.D. is a clinical psychologist and assistant professor of Psychiatry at Johns Hopkins School of Medicine. He is certified in Behavioral Sleep Medicine and conducts clinical research on the neurobehavioral causes, consequences, and treatments of insomnia and sleep loss. His research investigates the impact of sleep disturbance on central pain-processing mechanisms in both healthy subjects and patients with chronic pain syndromes.

Renee C. Stucky, Ph.D. is a clinical assistant professor in the Department of Health Psychology, University of Missouri, and is the director of the Inpatient Rehabilitation Psychology service at Rusk Rehabilitation Center in Columbia, Missouri.

Howard Tennen, Ph.D. is a Board of Trustees Distinguished Professor at the University of Connecticut and editor of the *Journal of Personality*. His teaching focuses on the application of social cognitive theory to coping with threatening events. His research applies daily process methods to examine stress, coping, and adjustment in the context of chronic illness and in everyday life.

Beverly E. Thorn, Ph.D. is professor of Psychology, director of the Ph.D. program in Clinical Psychology at the University of Alabama, and editor of the *Journal of Clinical Psychology*. Her research focuses on assessing and treating non-adaptive beliefs and cognitions regarding chronic pain.

Lana Tiersky, Ph.D. is an associate professor of Psychology at Fairleigh Dickinson University. Her research interests include chronic illness and disease, chronic fatigue syndrome, Gulf War illness, and mild traumatic brain injury.

Julie Wagner, Ph.D. is assistant professor in the Division of Behavioral Sciences and Community Health at the University of Connecticut Health Center and is a licensed clinical health psychologist. Her program of research explores psychosocial contributors to cardiovascular complications of diabetes in women and minorities. Her studies investigate diabetes health behaviors, the relationship between mood disturbance and diabetes complications, and psychophysiological mechanisms of stress in diabetes.

Jamie Walkup, Ph.D. is a clinical psychologist on the faculty of Rutgers University. He teaches in the Graduate School of Applied and Professional Psychology, and is affiliated with the Institute for Health, Health Care Policy, and Aging Research. His research interests include severe mental illness, HIV, and health-care policy.

Beatrice A. Wright, Ph.D. is an Emerita professor of Psychology, University of Kansas, is a founder of the Division on Rehabilitation Psychology of the American Psychological Association (APA), and is an author of numerous articles and books. APA selected two of her books using a psychosocial approach to disability issues for inclusion in the canon of distinguished and classic books in psychology.

Part I

1
An Introduction to Coping Theory and Research

Hanoch Livneh and Erin Martz

The literature on coping with chronic illness and disability (CID) has grown exponentially during the past 40 years. The reasons for this growth are manifold. First, as people of industrialized societies live longer, the probability of their encountering the experience of CID increases dramatically. Indeed, with the life expectancy in the U.S. now averaging 77.6 years (Centers for Disease Control [CDC], 2006b), medical conditions, such as gradual sensory losses, cancers, cardiovascular diseases, orthopedic impairments, and neurological disorders, have become more common in the general population. The CDC (2006a) reports that there are 34.3 million people, or 12% of the population in the U.S., who have one or more limitations in their usual activities due to chronic conditions. The American Community Survey (2003) indicates that there are 45.5 million people with disabilities between the ages of 16–64 in the U.S., with an additional 28.2 million people with disabilities who are 65 years or older.

Estimates of the prevalence of disability world-wide suggest that 500 million people have disabilities, and that in most countries, 10% of the population has some kind of physical, mental or sensory impairment (United Nations, 2006). The rise in numbers of people with disabilities throughout the world can be attributed to many different causes, according to the United Nations (2006), which include: Wars, poverty, and epidemics; overcrowded and unhealthy living conditions and pollution in the environment; low literacy levels and the related lack of knowledge about health measures or services, as well as inaccurate understanding about the cause and treatment of disability and the range of possibilities in life when having a disability; lack of health-care infrastructures; lack of access to available health-care resources; low priority in social and economic development for activities related to equalization of opportunities, disability prevention and rehabilitation; an increase in industrial and motor-vehicle accidents; and the psychosocial stress related to transitioning a modern society.

At the other end of the age spectrum, many congenital disabilities, which decades ago were considered high mortality risks to most of these affected (e.g., spina bifida, cystic fibrosis, AIDS, heart abnormalities), no longer spell

3

a "death sentence" and have been gradually transformed into a progressively higher rate of prolonged lives. These lives, however, are often accompanied by increased number of physical, sensory, cognitive, and neurological disabilities. This "death-to-life" transformation is the product of successful advances in genetic screening, post-conception intrauterine preventive measures, and modern medical and surgical procedures (Bowe, 2000; Keith & Aronow, 2005). As the prospects of living with severe and life-threatening medical conditions increased, researchers and clinicians gradually broadened their interests and began to explore the quality of life associated with these conditions. Coping efforts to overcome CID-linked functional limitations were viewed by many as one of the cardinal links between condition-related factors (severity, duration, time, and manner of onset) and quality of life (Livneh, 2001; Maes, Leventhal, & de Ridder, 1996; Moos & Schaefer, 1984).

A second reason for the growth of coping research was spawned by advances within the larger field of psychosocial adaptation to CID. With the increase in life-sustainable chronic illnesses, survival following traumatic injuries, and living with severe and chronic disabilities, the interest in the psychosocial consequences of these conditions also grew. Accounts of how individuals, who had almost incomprehensible odds against survival, managed to not only survive but also adjust successfully to their "new worlds," captured the imagination of lay persons and professionals alike. Consequently, the study of the types of internal (e.g., coping modes and skills) and external (e.g., social networks, tangible goods) resources, which are required to bolster life with severe, debilitating medical conditions (many of which were also caused by military combat and work-related injuries), increased in popularity. Research examining the effectiveness of these resources gradually began to consume much of the interest of theoreticians and clinicians, who focused their energies on studying coping with stress and life crises.

A third reason for the growing interest in coping can be traced to the emergence of the field of positive psychology during the 1980s and 1990s (Dunn & Dougherty, 2005; Seligman & Csikszentmihalyi, 2000; Tedeschi & Calhoun, 1995). As the interest in positive psychology grew in its popularity, the now-established field of coping found itself an ideal traveling companion. The term coping, despite its inherent dissociation from the outcomes produced (i.e., mental health, environmental mastery, quality of life), has traditionally been regarded as reflective of a broad adaptive orientation toward reducing life stresses, regulating distressing emotions, and gaining control of one's immediate environment (Haan, 1977; Moos & Schaefer, 1984; Vaillant, 1977). As such, the common themes between positive psychology and adaptive coping have been stressed in the extant literature and have also been examined in empirical studies, most of which conceptualized coping efforts as important mediators and moderators between the nature, type, duration, prognosis, perception, and severity of these CIDs, and psychosocial outcomes (Helgeson, 1992; Livneh & Wilson, 2003; Martz, Livneh, Priebe, Wuermser, & Ottomanelli, 2005; see discussions in Aldwin & Yancura, 2004; Maes et al., 1996; Mishel & Sorenson, 1991).

Yet, interest in coping in the rehabilitation field preceded the expansion of the positive psychology field during the 1980s and 1990s. This is evident in the writings of Beatrice Wright (see the Foreword of this book), who was a pioneer in the effort to define coping in relation to CID. She posited a "coping versus succumbing" framework, which delineated philosophical differences in perspectives of individuals with CID ("insiders"), as well as members of one's social network and professionals ("outsiders"). The "coping" world-view stressed those positive aspects, qualities, and abilities inherent in an individual, whereas the "succumbing" framework focused on the impairment, pathology, or insufficiency in one's mind or body (Wright, 1983).

Finally, interest in coping research expanded with the advent of rigorous and sophisticated statistical procedures (e.g., growth modeling or growth curve analysis, confirmatory factor analysis, structural equation modeling). Such statistics permitted analyses of the complex relationships among sets of psychological, social, vocational, medical, and environmental variables, coping strategies, and psychosocial outcomes, allowing these associations to be more comprehensively and fruitfully investigated. The very essence of coping is an intricate, dynamic and process-like nature. In order to study the coping process, multi-factorial longitudinal research designs have been successfully employed over the past 20 years, which have assessed the impact of coping strategies, at different time periods post-injury or following initial diagnosis of severe and chronic illnesses, on a large set of psychosocial outcome measures.

Before addressing the evolving conceptualization of coping styles and strategies, their nature, functions, structure, and other inherent characteristics, several terms must first be clarified, which are essential to this book and will be encountered frequently throughout the various chapters. In this introductory chapter, first an array of definitions of chronic illness, disability, stress, and coping will be presented, followed by a brief historical overview of the concept of coping. This chapter will end with a discussion of the various facets of coping, including the functions, structure and resources of coping and finally, the nature of adaptive coping, its temporal aspects, and measurement considerations.

Definitions

In this section, a brief overview will be provided about four central concepts to this book, namely, chronic illness, disability, stress, and coping. The goal here is not to offer new definitions of these concepts, but rather to review existing ones.

Chronic Illness

There are a range of definitions of chronic illness. Burish and Bradley (1983) distinguished between acute, infectious diseases and chronic illnesses on four primary dimensions: (a) *The cause*, for which acute illnesses are a result of infectious agents, while chronic illnesses often are a result of lifestyle choices; (b) *time-line*, for which acute illnesses are brief and last a somewhat predictable period of time, while chronic illnesses "have a slow, insidious onset and endure over a long and indefinite period" (p. 4); (c) *identity*, for which the individual has an idea of what is wrong and is able to readily identify the symptoms that are connected to specific causes, whereas chronic illnesses may not have a single, specific cause and may not manifest obvious symptoms until the illness is in an advanced stage (e.g., cancer or heart disease); and (d) *outcomes*, for which acute illnesses will be cured over time with proper treatment, while chronic illnesses will continue to exist (despite treatment), for the remainder of a person's life.

Other definitions of chronic illness include the following: MedicineNet (2006b) described a chronic illness as "an illness that has persisted for a long period of time. It is a continuing disease process." The U.S. National Center for Health Statistics defines a chronic illness as one with "a duration of three months or longer" (MedicineNet, 2006a). The Chronic Illness Alliance (2006) defines chronic illness as "an illness that is permanent or lasts a long time. It may get slowly worse over time. It may lead to death, or it may finally go away. It may cause permanent changes to the body. It will certainly affect the person's quality of life." Sperry (2006) summarized distinctions, made by researchers and clinicians, between chronic disease and chronic illness. Chronic disease is viewed as an objective and definable process "marked by periods of exacerbation and remission as well as progressive degeneration" (p. 6). Chronic illness is viewed as a subjective experience of a chronic disease. Further, Sperry (2006) delineated four types of chronic illnesses, noting that each type tends to require different types of multi-aspected (i.e., biopsychosocial) counseling and therapy: (a) Life-threatening diseases; (b) non-life-threatening chronic diseases, which are often manageable; (c) progressively severe diseases; and (d) diseases that fluctuate in symptoms, but are not life-threatening.

Disability

Disability, according to the International Classification of Impairments, Disabilities, and Handicaps (IDICH) system by the World Health Organization (WHO, 1980), is defined as a restriction or limitation of activity that results from an impairment (the latter is viewed as a loss, deficiency, abnormality, at an organ level or any of the body system). The WHO (2001) revised their classification system to focus more on the components of health, rather than the consequences of diseases. Their new system, called the International Classification of Functioning (ICF), makes a distinction between disability and functioning. According to the new WHO definition, disability denotes a form of an activity limitation or restriction in participation, while functioning indicates whether an impairment or problem exists in body function or structure. Contextual factors, such as those from oneself or one's environment, also influence the impact of disability and functioning (see WHO, 2006).

Although the WHO's definition of disability as a functional limitation is the most commonly used in the fields of disability studies and rehabilitation, other definitions are also noteworthy. According to the U.S.'s Social Security Administration (2006), disability is defined the lack of ability to do any substantial work because of a physical or mental impairment and this impairment must have lasted or can be expected to last at least 1 year or result in the individual's death. Keith and Aronow (2005) defined disability as an "inability to complete a meaningful task" (p. 16).

Stress

Because this book focuses on coping with CID, and because coping models are said to play a central role in managing stress (Holahan, Moos, & Schaefer, 1996; Lazarus & Folkman, 1984) the concept of stress must first be discussed and clarified. Stress has been viewed by Lazarus and his colleagues (Lazarus, 1966; Lazarus & Folkman, 1984; Lazarus & Launier, 1978) as a set of, or rubric of, interacting personal and environmental characteristics and processes. Within this context, Lazarus and colleagues consider three broad definitional orientations of stress. These include:

1. *Stimulus definitions.* Here, stress stimuli are conceived as acting on the organism from either internal (e.g., hunger, lack of sleep, sexual arousal) or external (i.e., the environment) sources. They can be further classified by their durations and frequency as (a) acute, time-limited (e.g., surgery, hospitalization); (b) chronic intermittent (e.g., role strains, daily hassles); (c) chronic (CID, prolonged social isolation); and (d) sequential stressors (stresses resulting from job loss, bereavement, etc.) (Elliott & Eisdorfer, 1982).
2. *Response definitions.* This category regards stress as a response state of the individual; that is, feeling distressed or experiencing distress. The more common stressful reactions are indicated by bodily (i.e., physiological, systemic) reactions that include, among others, increased heart rate, elevated blood pressure, increased perspiration, and heightened muscle tension.
3. *Relational definitions.* These definitions offer the most comprehensive outlook and posit psychosocial stress to be "a particular relationship between the person and the environment that is appraised by the person as *taxing* or *exceeding* his or her resources and endangering his or her well-being" (Lazarus & Folkman, 1984, p. 19). This relational definition has laid the ground to Lazarus' highly influential paradigm, in which cognitive appraisal and coping processes indicate the relationship among the person, his or her environment (i.e., the person-environment fit), and the resultant psychosocial outcome.

Hans Selye, one of the founding fathers of stress research during the 1950s and 1960s, defined stress as "the non-specific (that is, common) result of any demand upon the body, be the effect mental or somatic" (Selye, 1982, p. 7). He further argued that stress ensues when existing coping modes and available external resources are inadequate in dissipating increased tension.

Katkin, Dermit, and Wine (1993) viewed stress as these "environmental stimuli that impinge on the organism" (p. 142). Such stress may be chronic (e.g., poverty), transitory (e.g., noise), or highly idiosyncratic (e.g., a bad relationship with a significant other). Katkin et al. also indicated that stress is used to describe *responses* of the organism (e.g., high blood pressure).

Aldwin (1994) regarded stress as "that quality of experience, produced through a person-environmental transaction, that, through either over-arousal or under-arousal results in psychological or physiological distress" (p. 22). She further suggested that stress is composed of three components, namely: (a) Strain, an internal stressful state, which is comprised of both physiological (e.g., sympathetic activation, parasympathetic suppression) and emotional (i.e., negative affect) reactions; (b) stressor, an external event that includes both the type of stress (e.g., trauma, negative life event) and a temporal dimension (e.g., duration); and (c) a transaction component that is made of cognitive appraisals (e.g., harm, threat) and intensity (weak, strong). The latter component, as also reflected in the work of Lazarus and his colleagues, provides an integrative framework to the study of stress, as it pays homage to both the internal characteristics of the individual and the influence of the external environment.

Kaplan (1996), in focusing on the psychological and social ingredients of stress, argued that "*psychological* stress refers to the socially derived, conditioned, and situated psychological processes that stimulate any or all of the many manifestations of dysphoric affect falling under the rubric of objective distress" (pp. 3–4). Wheaton (1997) defined (social) stressors as those "threats, demands, or structural constraints that, by the very fact of their occurrences or existence, call into question the operating integrity of the organism" (p. 46). Taylor (1999) saw stress as "the consequence of a person's appraisal processes: the assessment of whether personal resources are sufficient to meet demands or the environment" (p. 169).

The above views on the nature of stress seem to recognize the person's inherent ability to be aware of the experiences of stress; that is, an individual's gaining awareness of both overtaxed internal (physiological, cognitive, affective, and motivational processes), as well as the stifling (or, in contrast, accommodating) nature of the external environment. The experience of stress, therefore, is a subjective dynamic, unfolding, only partially controllable, often unpredictable, and a typically negatively-valenced experience that is triggered by an intricate interaction of internal and external conditions and that disrupt the existing equilibrium. Or, to use Haan's (1993) pragmatic and succinct definition, stress is "whatever stresses people" (p. 259).

The Nature of Coping

Definitions

Prior to outlining the history of coping, its structural components, and its inherent functions and processes, various definitions of coping will be reviewed. In one of the earlier attempts to differentiate coping from similar constructs (e.g., mastery, defense), White (1974) regarded coping as "adaptation under relatively difficult conditions" (p. 49). According to White, coping efforts are situationally determined and are focused on ongoing adaptive maneuvers under difficult and unusual circumstances. Defense, in contrast, is a safety mechanism that focuses on protection from anxiety and danger. Finally, mastery refers to behaviors emanating from successfully implemented adaptive efforts that result in the completion of tasks.

In her now classical treatise, Haan (1977) argued for a tripartite model of coping, defense, and fragmentation (for a full discussion of her work, see Chronister and Chan's chapter in this book). Haan posited that coping, unlike the other two sets of processes, is distinguished by its (a) flexible and purposeful behaviors; (b) future-orientation, combined with a recognition of the present; (c) reality orientation; (d) integration of conscious and preconscious elements; (e) "metered" processing of distressing affect; and (f) affect expenditure in an ordered and tempered fashion. She further maintained that the following processes – objectivity, empathy, sublimation, concentration, and substitution – are the hallmarks of coping efforts. For an excellent and comprehensive review of the differences between defense mechanisms and coping strategies, the reader is referred to Cramer (1998).

Probably the most influential contributor to the study of coping, Richard Lazarus (Lazarus, 1966, 1991, 1993; Lazarus & Folkman, 1984; Lazarus & Launier, 1978) defined coping as "constantly changing cognitive and behavioral efforts to manage specific external and/or internal demands that are appraised as taxing or exceeding the resources of the person" (Lazarus & Folkman, 1984, p. 141). In defining coping in this way, Lazarus and Folkman argued that coping (a) is *process-oriented* (rather than trait-based), (b) should not be confounded with *outcomes* of these efforts to manage stress, and (c) should not be confounded with successful environmental mastery, because it focuses mostly on those *attempts* to master the environment.

Moos and his colleagues (Moos & Schaefer, 1984, 1986; Holahan et al., 1996) offered another comprehensive definition of coping. They viewed coping as "a stabilizing factor that can help individuals maintain psychosocial adaptation during stressful periods. It encompasses cognitive and behavioral efforts to reduce or eliminate stressful conditions and associated emotional distress" (Holahan et al., 1996, p. 25).

Finally, Snyder and Dinoff (1999) defined coping as "a response aimed at diminishing the physical, emotional, and psychological burden that is linked to stressful life events and daily hassles" (p. 5). They further maintained that the effectiveness of coping modes is linked to their dual ability to reduce psychosocial distress and, ultimately, to foster long-term psychological well-being.

In summary, definitions of coping regard the following elements as essential to understanding the concept:

1. Coping is a broader construct than defending. Whereas most defense mechanisms are inherently rigid, somewhat automatically engaged, intra-psychic efforts that focus on thwarting anxiety and impending danger, coping

strategies may be viewed as mostly flexible, integrated, and environmentally-attuned efforts that are concerned with both internal and external demands and available resources.

2. Although coping is viewed by some as a global personality trait (i.e., disposition), it is by no means an inflexible, trans-situational psychological construct. In fact, coping efforts and behaviors are very much influenced by state (i.e., situational) factors such as the nature, severity, and duration of the encountered crisis, trauma, or loss.

3. Coping efforts encompass a wide range of cognitive, emotional, and behavioral strategies directed at both external (i.e., environmental) stressors and internal demands and needs.

4. Combining both stable characteristics and process-oriented aspects, coping efforts should not be confused with psychosocial outcomes. Indeed, coping efforts should be viewed as moderators of these outcomes and mediators between initially existing environmental or internal conditions (e.g., crises, losses, disabling conditions, cognitive schemata) and the psychosocial end product they seek to influence (e.g., decrease in psychological distress, removal of noxious environmental conditions, increase of mastery, and re-establishing a psychological homeostasis).

Coping: A Historical Overview

A comprehensive review of the historical developments of coping (and defensive modalities) is beyond the scope of this chapter. Readers, however, may find the contributions of Haan (1993), Lazarus (1993), Lazarus and Folkman (1984, 1991), Parker and Endler (1996), and Gottleib (1997), to be most satisfying in this respect. In this section, accordingly, a succinct historical overview will be provided of the concept of coping as it unfolded over the past 80 years.

The early study of coping and defending, as ego-initiated processes, could be traced to the seminal work of Sigmund Freud during the 1920s and early 1930s. In discussing the human struggle against suffering, Freud (1930/1961) recognized the following methods as contributory to thwarting human suffering and bolstering pleasure: (a) Intoxication (i.e., the use of chemical substances), (b) displacement and sublimation (of libidinal urges) that serve to circumvent frustrations emanating from the external world, (c) use of illusions that arise from unleashing imaginary wishes at the expense of loosening links to reality, and (d) total withdrawal from the real world when facing a reality that is too painful. Freud was also the first to recognize the notion of an overtaxed ego – combining both stressors and threats that stem from the external world, as well as excessive demands and pressures that are triggered internally and continuously impinge upon the individual's psyche (1940/1969). It was left to Anna Freud (1936/1966) to further elucidate the concept of the ego's defense mechanisms and the modalities by which the ego seeks to defuse anxiety and exercise control over negative emotions and distressing impulses. These early psychodynamic (i.e., psychoanalytic and ego psychology) approaches to the study of defending and coping posited that coping with stress was primarily determined by stable personality attributes and perceptual styles.

Within the two decades that followed the work of Sigmund and Anna Freud, person-based approaches to the study of defending and coping shifted their emphasis by gradually focusing on the hierarchical structure inherent in human coping with stress (Haan, 1969, 1977; Kroeber, 1963; Menninger, 1963; Vaillant, 1977). Accordingly, upon recognizing that there were different levels of coping effectiveness toward stressful life situations, the following trends emerged:

- Defense mechanisms were ordered along a continuum of "adaptation" (or level of maturity), ranging from those viewed primarily as immature, primitive, indeed even psychotic (e.g., delusional projection, distortion) to those seen as mature and successful (e.g., sublimation, humor) (Vaillant, 1977).
- Defending and coping (along with fragmentation) were further trichotomized into distinct categories of ego processes, ranging from the more dysfunctional group of fragmentary processes (e.g., delusional, concreteness, depersonalization), to the more "neurotic" class of defensive processes (e.g., isolation, regression, displacement), and to the more functional category of coping modalities (e.g., logical analysis, sublimation, substitution) (Haan, 1977).

For an extensive review of Haan's and other psychodynamic models of coping the reader is referred to the chapter by Radnitz and Tiersky in this book.

The work of Haan, Vaillant, and Menninger during the 1960s and 1970s paved the way to the gradual appreciation of the inherently more successful, adaptive, reality-oriented, consciously driven, and environmentally cognizant processes, now referred to as coping modes and strategies (Lazarus, 1966; Lazarus & Launier, 1978). Along with this shift toward studying the "healthier," more positive approaches to coping with life stresses, theoreticians, clinicians, and researchers also came to recognize the central role played by the environment and, more specifically, the individual's appraisal of the situation in which stress is experienced (Lazarus, 1966; Lazarus & Launier, 1978). Coping was, therefore, perceived as a cognitive approach and a product of situational appraisal. With this shift to viewing coping as situationally determined, coping responses were perceived as influenced *less* by stable, rigid, personality dispositions and *more* as fluid processes determined by the context of the situation. Following an initial appraisal that the situation is indeed stressful or problematic (i.e., constraining one's abilities or available resources), the individual proceeds to select from several available coping strategies. These coping strategies were seen by Lazarus and his colleagues as belonging to two broad categories, namely, problem- (or task-) focused (focusing on the external environment) and emotion-focused (focusing on one's affective domain) strategies. Additionally, a third broad coping mode was identified by others and was labeled avoidance coping (Billings & Moos, 1981; Feifel, Strack, & Nagy, 1987; Roth & Cohen, 1986).

Following the pioneering work of Lazarus and his colleagues (Folkman & Lazarus, 1980; Lazarus & Folkman, 1984; Lazarus & Launier, 1978), researchers continued to further explore and elaborate upon the structure of coping, leading to more refined and contextually-based models of coping. Among the more notable contributions were: (a) Pearlin and Schooler's (1978) sociological model, (b) Moos and colleagues' integrative (biopsychosocial) model (Billings & Moos, 1981, 1984; Moos & Schaefer, 1984), and (c) Endler and Parker's (Endler, 1983, 1997; Endler & Parker, 1990) interactive model.

Pearlin and Schooler's (1978) model examined the efficiency of coping behaviors within several social contexts, such as marriage, parenting, household activities, and occupational settings. Their model highlighted the nature of social role-strain in each of these contexts. In addition, it contributed to the understanding of how coping patterns differed under role-specific demands.

Moos and his colleagues (Billings & Moos, 1984; Holahan et al., 1996; Moos & Schaefer, 1986, 1993) have continued to refine their model of coping with chronic illness and physical disabilities over the past 25 years (for Moos' most recent view, see the chapter he co-authored with Holahan in this book). Briefly, their comprehensive model, which paid tribute to the importance of the environmental context, also incorporated the following primary processes and components: (a) An environmental system (social and economic resources, life stressors triggered by the illness); (b) a personal system (socio-demographic and personality resources); (c) cognitive, appraisal, and coping responses; (d) event-related factors (the specific crises and transitions experienced by the individual); and (e) health and well-being outcomes. These components (i.e., panels, as referred to by Moos and his colleagues) provide for an integrative conceptual framework through which coping with life crises, and coping with CID more specifically, could be understood.

Endler and Parker's (Endler, 1983, 1997; Endler & Parker, 1990, 1994) multidimensional interactive model sought to explore the complex relationships among personality, anxiety, stress, and coping. In their model, Endler and Parker were concerned with how one's personality both impacted and was influenced by situational/environmental and behavioral factors. They focused on those cognitive, motivational, physiological, and content-based variables that affected the processing of information, paying particular emphasis to a subset of the interactive model of personality, namely trait and state anxiety. For Endler and Parker, person variables (such as trait anxiety, cognitive style, and level of emotionality) interacted with stressor situations (such as life events, crises, and traumas) and activated perceptions of danger (i.e., threat). These perceptions, in turn, led to changes in state anxiety, necessitating reactions to these changes in state anxiety. These reactions to state anxiety were viewed as coping responses (and psychological defenses). [For the interested reader, other models of coping with crises, life transitions, and CID, can be found in the works of Schlossberg (1981), Maes et al. (1996), and Livneh (2001).]

A thoughtful historical review of the psychosocial investigation of coping and its relationship to stress and life crises may be found in Suls, David, and

Harvey (1996). These authors suggested that coping theory and research could most usefully be viewed as progressing through three major phases (or "generations," as they termed the phases). The first phase was best captured by early psychoanalytic and ego psychology contributions and ranged from the early decades of the 20th century up until the 1960s. It was most notably influenced by the works of Sigmund and Anna Freud, Haan, and Vaillant. The second phase focused on the transactional perspective of coping, emerging in the 1960s, and emphasized the combined influences of situational and cognitive factors, while viewing coping as a dynamic process rather than a stable personality disposition. This phase is most heavily recognized by the works of Lazarus and Folkman, and Moos and his colleagues, among others. Finally, the third phase, emerging mostly during the 1980s, is represented by renewed efforts to better understand the role of personality in generating, maintaining, and directing coping. At the same time, researchers of this current, third "generation" also seek adherence to "strong operational distinctions among coping, personality, appraisal, and adaptational outcomes" (Suls et al., 1996, p. 711).

The Functions of Coping

Over the past 30 years there have been various efforts to elucidate the functions (occasionally referred to as goals) of coping (Cohen & Lazarus, 1979; Janis & Mann, 1977; Mechanic, 1974; Pearlin & Schooler, 1978; White, 1974; Zeidner & Saklofske, 1996). These authors cited the following functions (goals) as paramount to understanding the operational bases of coping:

1. Securing accurate information about the demands imposed by the external (i.e., social and physical) environment.
2. Maintaining adequate internal mechanisms to process incoming information and initiating action.
3. Creating a stable psychological (emotional) equilibrium that successfully directs energy and skilled behaviors to meet external demands.
4. Making decisions following a search and evaluation of the obtained information.
5. Reducing, and if possible, eliminating harmful environmental conditions.
6. Maintaining a positive self-image and psychological well-being.
7. Increasing tolerance of negative events and situations or changing those situations that trigger stressful experiences.
8. Controlling the meaning of the stressful experiences, so as to thwart their deleterious nature.
9. Reducing existing psychological stress, or conflict, while it is being experienced.
10. Maximizing the probability of returning to pre-stress activities.

Lazarus and Folkman (1984) attempted to summarize these functions into two overarching functional categories of problem-focused and emotion-focused coping. Problem-focused coping has been regarded as reflective of those strategies directed at modifying the problem that lies at the root of the distress. It is therefore *alloplastic* in nature, as it seeks to alter the external environment to decrease situation-triggered stress (Perrez & Reicherts, 1992). In contrast, emotion-focused coping focuses on regulating emotions after an initial appraisal was made that the threatening environmental conditions are un-modifiable. In this case, the coping is *autoplastic*, because the efforts are directed at adopting, or accommodating oneself, to the existing stressful environment (Perrez & Reicherts, 1992).

In a recent comprehensive analysis and integration of the literature on the functions and structure of coping, Skinner, Edge, Altman, and Sherwood (2003) maintained that the global adaptive functions of coping can be categorized into 12 distinct groups. These groups were further collapsed into three functionally derived adaptive processes, namely: (a) Coordination of environmental actions and contingencies (e.g., adjusting actions to be effective, finding additional contingencies); (b) coordination of available social resources (e.g., using available social resources, withdrawing from unsupportive contexts); and (c) coordination of preferences and available options (e.g., finding new options, removing constraints). Skinner et al. further argued that each of these coping dimensions serves to assist the individual in adapting successfully to his or her stress-triggering environment.

The Structure of Coping

Efforts to examine the structural components of coping have been typically classified according to their level of inclusiveness, ranging from macro-analytic to micro-analytic (Krohne, 1993, 1996) [See also Chronister and Chan in this book]. At the macro-analytic level (Level 1 according to Krohne), coping is conceptualized as mostly a stable personality construct or dimension. At this level of abstraction, coping has been dichotomized into such operating, and often contrasting, dimensions as: repression vs. sensitization, engagement vs. disengagement, approach vs. avoidance, vigilance vs. avoidance, attention vs. rejection, monitoring vs. blunting, emotion-focused vs. problem-focused, coping vs. succumbing, adaptive vs. non-adaptive, and successful (noted by its competence, mastery, hope, and personal growth) vs. unsuccessful (noted by its withdrawal, passive, angry, self- or other-blaming, and hopeless tendencies) (Kleinke, 1998; Krohne, 1996; Moos & Schaefer, 1993). Included in this level of broad coping categories is also the cognitive (i.e., appraisal), emotional, and behavioral (i.e., problem-focused) trichotomy of Moos and Schaefer (1986), Feifel et al. (1987), and Pearlin and Schooler (1978), as well as the basic categories of coping processes advocated by Moos and Schaefer (1993, 1996) namely: (a) Cognitive approach (e.g., positive reappraisal), (b) behavioral approach (e.g., problem-solving), (c) cognitive avoidance (e.g., resigned acceptance), and (d) behavioral avoidance (e.g., emotional discharge).

At a middle level of abstraction (Level 2 according to Krohne, 1993, 1996), coping is viewed as a set of strategies or modalities focusing on conceptually coherent classes of coping efforts. A review of the literature suggests that up to 30 coping strategies have been considered (Parker & Endler, 1992; Schwarzer & Schwarzer, 1996); they parallel coping scales, as measured by such instruments as the Ways of Coping Questionnaire (Folkman & Lazarus, 1988) COPE (Carver, Scheier, & Weintraub, 1989), the Coping Strategies Inventory (Tobin, Holroyd, Reynolds, & Wigal, 1989), the Coping Inventory for Stressful Situations (Endler & Parker, 1990), and the Coping Strategy Indicator (Amirkhan, 1990) to name just a few. Typically listed strategies (i.e., scales) include cooperative coping, seeking social support, planful problem-solving, denial, wishful thinking, cognitive reappraisal, acceptance and venting emotions.

Finally, at the micro-analytic level (Level 3, according to Krohne, 1993, 1996), the focus is upon specific coping behaviors, acts, and reactions. At this level, coping is viewed as a state-like, situationally specific behavior that is determined by the nature, severity, timing, and level of the stress encountered. The many and diverse items listed by the various coping scales best represent this level of abstraction.

In their analysis of the structure of coping, Skinner et al. (2003) suggested a somewhat similar hierarchical system for the classification of coping strategies. Their system posits dimensions or modes of coping (referred to by these authors as "families" of coping) as the highest order (superordinate) categories, followed by mid-level coping strategies (termed "ways of coping"). At the lowest order (subordinate) level, Skinner and her colleagues propose the category of coping instances (i.e., situation-specific responses to stress).

Perrez and Reicherts (1992) offered a different view on the relationship between stressful situations and coping behaviors. First, their model distinguishes between objective and subjective dimensions of the encountered situation. Both, however, are assessed along similar characteristics that include valence, controllability, changeability, ambiguity, and reoccurrence characteristics of the situation (e.g., valence as an objective property relates to the inherent stressfulness of the situation, while valence as a subjective property refers to the personal meaning attached to the situation). Following this observation, Perrez and Reicherts presented a taxonomy of coping behaviors that included:

1. Situation-oriented coping that seeks to modify internal or external stressors. It includes: (a) Actively approaching the stressful situation, (b) evasion or withdrawal, and (c) passivity.
2. Representation-oriented coping that focuses on changing the cognitive representation of the stressor. It includes: (a) Searching for information about the situation, and (b) suppressing information.
3. Evaluation-oriented coping, which aims to alter goals and intentions. It includes: (a) Changing personal goals and intentions associated with uncontrollable or unchangeable situations, and (b) re-evaluating the situation.

Coping Resources

Coping resources are normally classified into internal and external types of resources (Hobfoll, 1998; Kaplan, 1996; Moos & Schaefer, 1993). Internal resources refer to certain personal (i.e., personality) traits or dispositions that were found to predict better psychosocial adaptation to stress, including stress engendered by CID. They include self-mastery, hardiness, positive self-esteem, sense of coherence, increased energy, self-efficacy, personal control, hopeful disposition, optimistic outlook, problem-solving skills, and interpersonal skills. In contrast, certain personality factors (perceived as diluting personal resources) were found to be associated with poorer psychosocial outcomes and include neuroticism, feelings of hopelessness, pessimistic outlook, and low self-concept.

External resources refer to social and material goods such as existing social networks (both quality and size of support groups), financial resources, standard of living, availability of time, and the presence (or lack thereof) of other life stressors. [For further discussion of the social context of coping, and the role of adaptive tasks within social and physical contexts, the reader is referred to the chapters by Kosciulek, and Moos and Holahan in this book, respectively.]

Adaptive vs. Non-Adaptive Coping

As mentioned earlier in this chapter, several, and often inconsistent efforts have been advanced in the coping literature regarding the level of successful psychosocial adaptation triggered by the various coping strategies. Earlier efforts by Haan (1977) and Valliant (1977) posited a dichotomy (or a dichotomy-like distinction) between mature and immature defenses (Valliant) and between coping and defending (Haan). In a similar view, Carver and his colleagues (Carver et al., 1993; Carver et al., 1989), Tobin et al. (1989), and Endler and Parker (1994) reported findings indicating that the use of certain coping strategies, typically termed "disengagement" coping (e.g., reducing efforts to deal with the stressor, daydreaming, attempting to escape stressful situation by resorting to age-regressive activities, waiting for a miracle to happen) was associated with poor psychosocial outcomes, while the use of strategies termed "engagement" coping, which reflect goal-or target-oriented coping (e.g., actively seeking to remove or deal with the stressor, planning steps to successfully handle the stressful situation, consulting others on how to solve the problem, reappraising the situation) was associated with salutary outcomes. Indeed, in a recent study, Victorson, Farmer, Burnett, Quellette, and Barocas (2005) reported that, in a sample of recently injured adults, coping strategies of behavioral disengagement, emotional venting, self-blaming, and substance abuse were related to higher levels of injury-related distress experienced among participants.

Other researchers (e.g., Lazarus & Folkman, 1984; Moos & Schaefer, 1984; Pearlin & Schooler, 1978) paid greater attention to the context within which coping takes place, emphasizing that successful psychosocial outcomes (or the effectiveness of coping strategies) should be viewed in relative terms and considered as situation-specific. Indeed, Zeidner and Saklofske (1996) argued that "coping effectiveness must be examined in the context in which problems occur" (p. 509), and that coping efforts are designed and targeted to reach certain goals and address specific problems. Therefore, although problem-focused efforts are typically necessitated to directly manage the stressful or problematic events and thus, can be, regarded as adaptive, their usefulness is limited and may even be detrimental under conditions where the situation is unchangeable (Zeidner & Saklofske, 1996). In a similar vein, emotion-focused and avoidance-coping modes that have been widely viewed as non-adaptive, because they are unable to eliminate the problem, could, in fact, be beneficial when they help to maintain emotional balance (i.e., emotional regulation) under conditions that are beyond personal control or that may be unchangeable (Aldwin, 1994; Mattlin, Wethington & Kessler, 1990; Taylor, 1999; Zeidner & Saklofske, 1996). Indeed, Stanton and colleagues (Stanton et al., 2000; Stanton, Danoff-Burg, Cameron, & Ellis, 1994) have argued that emotion-focused coping, especially when involving active processing and expression of emotions, is a highly useful coping mode when dealing with severe and chronic medical conditions. Avoidance-coping, which includes strategies such as denial, mental or behavioral disengagement, and wishful thinking could, indeed, be helpful when negotiating short-term stressors. Perhaps the single coping strategy that has been universally associated with (a) non-adaptive efforts to manage stress, (b) the co-occurrence of other non-adaptive coping strategies, and (c) poor psychosocial outcomes is that of alcohol and drug use (Carver et al., 1989; Wills & Hirky, 1996).

The Temporality Aspects of Coping

Another dimension of coping, which has been only sporadically addressed in the literature, is that of the temporal context of coping. Several distinct phases of the coping experience have been suggested (Aspinwall & Taylor, 1997; Auerbach, 1992; Folkman & Moskowitz, 2004; Schwarzer & Knoll, 2003). Although this classification of phases is primarily descriptive and remains silent on any functional or explanatory properties of coping, it merits mention. Folkman and Moskowitz suggested that research is needed specifically on future-oriented coping, especially in intervention research, because of the benefits of reducing stress related to potential adverse events in one's future. The suggested temporal phases of coping include:

- Preventive or proactive coping that occurs *long before* stress (a) is experienced or (b) might even occur; this is referred to as distal anticipatory coping. Examples include planned retirement and age-related illness.
- Anticipatory coping that occurs when stress is *being anticipated* to occur in the immediate future (pending threat); this is referred to as proximal anticipatory coping. Examples include waiting for a doctor appointment and preparing for an important exam.
- Dynamic (or present) coping that is being employed while stress is *ongoing* (i.e., while stress is being experienced). Examples include experiencing a severe marital discord and dealing with acute pain.

- Reactive coping that occurs *after stress* has been experienced, typically in the immediate past. Examples include recent loss of a job and dealing with the aftermath of an automobile accident.
- Residual coping that occurs *long after* stress has been experienced and when the person deals with the long-term effects of the stress. Examples include living with an early life-onset CID and mourning the loss of a parent.

The Measurement of Coping

Coping researchers have made numerous efforts to measure coping styles and strategies since the 1980s. Although earlier attempts to measure defense mechanisms should be recognized (e.g., Gleser & Ihilevich, 1969; Haan, 1965; Joffe & Naditch, 1977), it was the groundbreaking work of Folkman and Lazarus (1980, 1988), with the development of the Ways of Coping Checklist (WOC) and its revised version, the Ways of Coping Questionnaire (WOQ), that set the stage for the development of psychometrically-sound coping measures. It is beyond the scope of this chapter to provide a just review of these existing measures. The interested reader is invited to consult the excellent reviews on coping assessment provided by Parker and Endler (1992), Endler, Parker, and Summerfeldt (1993), Aldwin (1994), Schwarzer and Schwarzer (1996), and de Ridder (1997), among others. Readers can also find a brief description of the most commonly used coping measures in the appendix of this book.

Despite the proliferation of coping scales (mostly of a self-report style), and the gradual improvement of their conceptual, substantive, structural, and psychometric aspects, many inadequacies still remain. A review of existing coping scales reveals that, in many instances, different coping styles, modes, and strategies are being measured (Aldwin, 1994; Parker & Endler, 1992; Skinner et al., 2003). Indeed, those identified and measured coping dimensions range from 2 to 28, often using different terminologies and item content (Parker & Endler, 1992; Schwarzer & Schwarzer, 1996). This heterogeneity of coping types and nomenclature makes it virtually impossible to compare findings across studies and to generalize these findings across contexts and populations.

A related problem stems from the inconsistencies inherent in the definition and conceptualization of coping. Obviously, dispositional (or trait-like) and situational (process or state-like) views of coping result in two disparate types of assessment tools. Carver and Scheier (1994) and Porter and Stone (1996), among others, have reported findings suggesting that coping dispositions and coping processes (e.g., daily measured coping) are indeed only weakly associated with one another. Dispositional-based measures seek to address the respondent's habitual (i.e., stylistic) use of coping, typically across different types of contexts and time periods. These are, then, measures of coping with stress that are regarded as trans-situational and trans-temporal. Accordingly, these inter-individual approaches to coping measurement view coping efforts as only minimally affected by situational or temporal contingencies. They are best typified by Carver et al.'s (1989) COPE and Endler and Parker's (1994) Coping Inventory for Stressful Situations (CISS) measures.

In contrast, proponents of context-specific coping view coping efforts as determined by idiosyncratic situations. In this view, coping is regarded as a dynamic process where coping behaviors are applied selectively across and within stressful situations, problems, and time points (Aldwin, 1994; Endler et al., 1993, Schwarzer & Schwarzer, 1996). It is further argued, that if human adaptation to crises and traumatic events indeed proceeds through some sort of broad psychosocial sequence of phases, then it is rather likely that different coping modalities may be adopted to meet specific temporal demands and needs (Aldwin, 1994). The intra-individual approach to coping assessment is best exemplified by Folkman and Lazarus's (1988) WOC questionnaire and Billings and Moos's (1981) set of coping scales.

Schwarzer and Schwarzer (1996) have raised another conceptual issue associated with coping scales and their use as clinical or research instruments. These authors pointed to a lack of clarity found in some coping scales' directions, as to whether the scales measure efforts expended by the respondent (coping process) or successful acts (coping outcomes). Moreover, they maintain that it is often unclear whether these measured efforts focus on respondents' expressed behaviors or merely cognitive appraisals.

Another substantive concern relates to the dimensionality, or level of abstractness, tapped by the various coping scales. When measured at its broadest (typically dichotomous) level (e.g., approach vs. avoidance coping, problem- vs. emotion-focused coping), this categorization is not only dangerously simplistic, but could also result in inaccurate generalizations. For example, some strategies within the broader emotion-focused coping may be subsumed under approach, while others under avoidance coping (Aldwin, 1994; Schwarzer & Schwarzer, 1996).

A final substantive problem centers on event-referencing. Whereas some coping measures direct the respondents to imagine hypothetical stress-producing events (i.e., generic stress), others require them to report coping efforts within the context of personally experienced life event(s). Aldwin (1994) further argues that the reliance on a single, even if recent, stressful episode is problematic for self-reported coping, because even such a single episode typically triggers "diversity in the types of problems that evoke the (coping) behavior" (p. 113), and consequently, a diversity in the coping responses.

Several of the reported findings on the relationships between coping and a host of other variables, such as personality factors, indices of mental health and quality of life, psychological distress, and indicators of daily functioning, are further hampered by psychometric inadequacies of the coping scales used (de Ridder, 1997; Parker & Endler, 1992; Skinner et al., 2003). These include: (a) An unstable and poorly justified factor structure that results in conceptually fuzzy factors; (b) overlapping factor-item patterns, which make it impossible to determine if uniquely derived factors correspond to homogeneous, functional categories of coping efforts; (c) failure to meet acceptable criteria of conceptual clarity (i.e., poor construct validity); and (d) inappropriate reliability estimates that often stem from a failure to address the extent to which the coping measure taps an ostensibly stable construct or a temporally fluid behavior.

In sum, then, although the conceptual and psychometric sophistication has advanced appreciably over the past quarter of century, extant coping scales are still burdened by many unresolved issues that future reseach efforts must address.

Coping: Tentative Conclusions

Based on the research findings and review papers of Moos (1984; Moos & Schaefer, 1986), Lazarus and Folkman (1984), Lazarus (1993), Carver et al. (1993), Zeidner and Saklofske (1996), the following tentative conclusions about coping are offered:

1. Coping strategies vary both within (they change over time) and between (they are person-specific) individuals. When they change over time, they are typically used to manage the effects of both short-term and long-term stressful situations.
2. Specific coping strategies are differentially effective (or adaptive), depending on the type of stressor (e.g., entrance vs. exit events), severity, duration (acute vs. chronic), and context of the experienced stress.
3. Coping effectiveness demands a good balance (or fit) between the person-environment transaction and the coping strategies adopted to manage the stressful situation.
4. Adaptive, or successful, coping requires a flexible and versatile repertoire of coping strategies, and the combined use of both problem-focused and emotion-focused efforts. That is, problem-focused coping may be more adaptive under changeable and controllable conditions, while emotion-focused coping may be more adaptive under unchangeable and uncontrollable situations.
5. Regardless of their level of effectiveness, coping strategies may be viewed as a mediating factor between stressful encounters and the ultimate psychosocial outcomes.

Summary

The study of coping has attracted a growing number of theoreticians, clinicians, and researchers for almost an entire century. Historically, coping (or more accurately, psychological defense) emerged largely as part of an emphasis on viewing human functioning within a pathological context, which typically included the terms mental illnesses, abnormal behaviors, maladaptive functioning, and impaired psychological structures and processes. It is only more recently that coping research has undergone a metamorphosis and has begun to focus more fully on coping modalities that seek to link psychological processes, operating in the aftermath of crises and traumatic events, with efforts that are reflective of searching for meaning, making sense of the loss, positive reappraisal, and benefit-finding. This growing trend has resulted in a substantive body of work that is strongly indicative of the benefits accrued from these, and related, coping strategies in fostering positive emotions, personal strengths, mental health, and successful human adaptation to stressful life events, personal losses, and traumatic experiences (Davis, Nolen-Hoeksema, & Larson, 1998; Folkman & Moskowitz, 2000, 2004; Holahan & Moos, 1991; Tennen & Affleck, 1999).

The study of coping has indeed evolved from its original focus on intra-individual, trait-like, psychodynamic defense processes to include a more inter-active view of coping as a process, which inevitably includes an individual's perception of events, as well as "extra-individual" influences, such as social support and environmental factors. While a dynamic model of coping explains that coping is differentially utilized according to circumstances, this view compli-cates efforts to research aspects of coping. Fortunately, multivariate statistical techniques are available to test the more sophisticated coping models and allow scientists to map common responses to challenging and traumatic events, such as those involving CID.

Because the consequences of CID involve long-term stressors, a book that focused on the theoretical and empirical aspects of coping with CID is urgently needed to better understand how coping is differentially and effectively used with the myriad of challenges created by CID. Sharoff (2004) stated, in his insightful book about coping with chronic and terminal illnesses, that coping requires skills, which are often unknown to the person with a new CID and that:

Disease and treatment invariably cause some degree of suffering, discomfort, bitterness, deprivation, helplessness, uncertainty, and rejection of the patient, but if appropriate coping abilities are present, these problems or situations will cause less harm and far less psychological pain (p. 4).

As theory and research on coping with CID expands, hopefully the clinical applications (Guterman, 2006; Sharoff, 2004; Sperry, 2006; also see Devins & Binik, 1996, Table 27.1 for a summary of coping interventions for various CID) will also increase in quantity and effectiveness. Clinical interventions, and research on what works with whom, will help to provide knowledge about how individuals with CID find ways to cope and to develop positive meaning from unexpected, traumatic life-events, such as the onset of CID.

References

Aldwin, C. M. (1994). *Stress, coping, and development: An integrative approach.* New York: Guilford.

Aldwin, C. M., & Yancura, L. A. (2004). Coping and health: A comparison of the stress and trauma literatures. In P. P. Schnurr & B. L. Green (Eds.), *Trauma and health: Physical health consequences of exposure to extreme stress* (pp. 99–125). Washington, DC: American Psychological Association.

American Community Survey (2003). *Table P058.* Retrieved on April 16, 2006, from *http://factfinder.census.gov/servlet/DTTable?_bm=y&-geo_id=04000US03&-ds_name =ACS_2003_EST_G00_&-redoLog=false&-mt_name=ACS_2003_EST_G2000_P058*

Amirkhan, J. H. (1990). A factor analytically derived measure of coping: The coping strategy indicator. *Journal of Personality and Social Psychology, 59*, 1066–1074.

Aspinwall, L. G., & Taylor, S. E. (1997). A stitch in time: Self-regulation and proactive coping. *Psychological Bulletin, 121*, 417–436.

Auerbach, S. M. (1992). Temporal factors in stress and coping: Intervention implications. In B. N. Carpenter (Ed.), *Personal coping: Theory, research, and application* (pp. 133–147). Westport, CT: Praeger.

Billings, A. G., & Moos, R. H. (1981). The role of coping responses and social resources in attenuating the stress of life events. *Journal of Behavioral Medicine, 4*, 139–157.

Billings, A. G., & Moos, R. H. (1984). Coping stress, and social resources among adults with unipolar depression. *Journal of Personality and Social Psychology, 46*, 877–891.

Bowe, F. (2000). *Physical, sensory, and health disabilities: An introduction.* Upper Saddle River, NJ: Merrill.

Burish, T. G., & Bradley, L. A. (1983). Coping with chronic disease: Definitions and issues. In T. G. Burish & L. A. Bradley (Eds.), *Coping with chronic disease: Research and applications* (pp. 3–12). New York: Academic Press.

Carver, C. S., Scheier, M. F., & Weintraub, J. K. (1989). Assessing coping strategies: A theoretically based approach. *Journal of Personality and Social Psychology, 56*, 267–283.

Carver, C. S., Pozo, C., Harris, S. D., Noriega, V., Scheier, M. F., Robinson, D. S., Ketcham, A. S., Moffat, F. L., & Clark, K. C. (1993). How coping mediates the effect of optimism on distress: A study of women with early stage breast cancer. *Journal of Personality and Social Psychology, 65*, 375–390.

Carver, C. S., & Scheier, M. F. (1994). Situational coping and coping dispositions in a stressful transaction. *Journal of Personality and Social Psychology, 66*, 184–199.

Centers for Disease Control. (2006a). *Disability.* Retrieved on April 15, 2006, from *http://www.cdc.gov/nchs/fastats/disable.htm.*

Centers for Disease Control. (2006b). *Life expectancy.* Retrieved on April 15, 2006, from *http://www.cdc.gov/nchs/fastats/lifexpec.htm.*

Chronic Illness Alliance. (2006). *Chronic illness alliance website.* Retrieved on April 11, 2006, from *http://www.chronicillness.org.au/.*

Cohen, F., & Lazarus, R. S. (1979). Coping with stresses of illness. In G. C. Stone, F. Cohen, & N. E. Adler (Eds.), *Health Psychology* (pp. 217–254). San Francisco: Jossey-Bass.

Cramer, P. (1998). Coping and defense mechanisms: What's the difference? *Journal of Personality, 66*, 919–946.

Davis, C. G., Nolen-Hoeksema, S., & Larson, J. (1998). Making sense of loss and benefiting from the experience: Two constructs of meaning. *Journal of Personality and Social Psychology, 75*, 561–574.

de Ridder, D. (1997). What is wrong with coping assessment? A review of conceptual and methodological issues. *Psychology and Health, 12*, 417–431.

Devins, G. M., & Binik, Y. M. (1996). Facilitating coping with chronic physical illness. In M. Zeidner & N. S. Endler (Eds.), *Handbook of coping: Theory, research, applications* (pp. 24–43). New York: John Wiley & Sons.

Dunn, D. S., & Dougherty, S. B. (2005). Prospects for positive psychology of rehabilitation. *Rehabilitation Psychology, 50*, 305–311.

Elliott, G. R., & Eisdorfer, C. (1982). *Stress and human health.* New York: Springer.

Endler, N. S. (1983). Interactionism: A personality model, but not yet a theory. In M. M. Page (Ed.), *Nebraska symposium on motivation 1982: Personality-current theory and research* (pp. 155–200). Lincoln, NE: University of Nebraska Press.

Endler, N. S. (1997). Stress, anxiety, and coping: The multidimensional interaction model. *Canadian Psychologist, 38*, 136–153.

Endler, N. S., & Parker, J. D. (1990). Multidimensional assessment of coping: A critical evaluation. *Journal of Personality and Social Psychology, 58*, 844–854.

Endler, N. S., & Parker, J. D. (1994). Assessment of multidimensional coping: Task, emotion, and avoidance strategies. *Psychological Assessment, 6*, 50–60.

Endler, N. S., Parker, J. D., & Summerfeldt, L. J. (1993). Coping with health problems: Conceptual and methodological issues. *Canadian Journal of Behavioral Science, 25*, 384–399.

Feifel, H., Strack, S., & Nagy, V. T. (1987). Degree of life-threat and differential use of coping modes. *Journal of Psychosomatic Research, 31*, 91–99.

Folkman, S., & Lazarus, R. S. (1980). An analysis of coping in a middle-aged community sample. *Journal of Health and Social Behavior, 21*, 219–239.

Folkman, S., & Lazarus, R. S. (1988). *Manual for the ways of coping questionnaire*. Palo Alto, CA: Consulting Psychologist Press.

Folkman, S., & Moskowitz, J. T. (2000). Positive affect and the other side of coping. *American Psychologist, 55*, 647–654.

Folkman, S., & Moskowitz, J. T. (2004). Coping: Pitfalls and promise. *Annual Review of Psychology, 55*, 745–774.

Freud, A. (1936/1966). *The ego and the mechanisms of defense* (Rev. ed.). New York: International Universities Press.

Freud, S. (1930/1961). *Civilization and its discontents*. New York: W. W. Norton & Co.

Freud, S. (1940/1969). *An outline of psycho-analysis*. New York: W. W. Norton & Co.

Gleser, G. C., & Ihilevich, D. (1969). An objective instrument for measuring defense mechanisms. *Journal of Consulting and Clinical Psychology, 33*, 51–60.

Gottlieb, B. H. (1997). *Coping with chronic stress*. New York: Plenum Press.

Guterman, J. T. (2006). *Mastering the art of solution-focused counseling*. Alexandria, VA: American Counseling Association.

Haan, N. (1965). Coping and defense mechanisms related to personality inventories. *Journal of Consulting Psychology, 29*, 373–378.

Haan, N. (1969). A tripartite model of ego functioning values and clinical and research applications. *Journal of Nervous and Mental Disease, 148*, 14–30.

Haan, N. (1977). *Coping and defending: Processes of self-environment organization*. New York: Academic Press.

Haan, N. (1993). The assessment of coping, defense, and stress. In L. Goldberger & S. Breznitz (Eds.), *Handbook of stress: Theoretical and clinical aspects* (2nd ed., pp. 258–273). New York: Free Press.

Helgeson, V. S. (1992). Moderators of the relation between perceived control and adjustment to chronic illness. *Journal of Personality and social Psychology, 63*, 656–666.

Hobfoll, S. E. (1998). *Stress, culture, and community: The psychology and philosophy of stress*. New York: Plenum Press.

Holahan, C. J., & Moos, R. H. (1991). Life stressors, personal and social resources, and depression: A 4-year structural model. *Journal of Abnormal Psychology, 100*, 31–38.

Holahan, C. J., Moos, R. H., & Schaefer, J. A. (1996). Coping, stress resistance, and growth: Conceptualizing adaptive functioning. In M. Zeidner & N. S. Endler (Eds.),

Handbook of coping: Theory, research, applications (pp. 24–43). New York: John Wiley & Sons.

Janis, I. L., & Mann, L. (1977). *Decision making.* New York: The Free Press.

Joffe, P., & Naditch, M. P. (1977). Paper and pencil measures of coping and defense processes. In N. Haan (Ed.), *Coping and defending* (pp. 280–297). New York: Academic Press.

Kaplan, A. B. (Ed.) (1996). *Psychological stress: Perspectives on structure, theory, life-course, and methods.* New York: Academic Press.

Katkin, E. S., Dermit, S., & Wine, S. K. (1993). Psychological assessment of stress. In L. Goldberger & S. Breznitz (Eds.), *Handbook of stress: Theoretical and clinical aspects* (2nd ed., pp. 142–157). New York: The Free Press.

Keith, R. A., & Aronow, H. U. (2005). Comprehensive rehabilitation: Themes, models, and issues. In H. H. Zaretsky, E. F. Richter, & M. G. Eisenberg (Eds.), *Medical aspects of disability* (3rd ed., pp. 3–29). New York: Springer.

Kleinke, C. L. (1998). *Coping with life challenges* (2nd ed.). Prospect Heights, IL: Waveland Press.

Kroeber, T. C. (1963). The coping functions of the ego mechanisms. In R. White (Ed.), *The study of lives* (pp. 179–198). New York: Atherton Press.

Krohne, H. W. (1993). Vigilance and cognitive avoidance as concepts in coping research. In H. W. Krohne (Ed.), *Attention and avoidance: Strategies in coping with aversiveness* (pp. 19–50). Seattle, WA: Hogrefe & Huber.

Krohne, H. W. (1996). Individual differences in coping. In M. Zeidner & N. S. Endler (Eds.), *Handbook of coping: Theory, research, applications* (pp. 381–409). New York: John Wiley & Sons.

Lazarus, R. S. (1966). *Psychological stress and the coping process.* New York: McGraw-Hill.

Lazarus, R. S. (1991). *Emotion and adaptation.* New York: Oxford.

Lazarus, R. S. (1993). Coping theory and research: Past, present, and future. *Psychosomatic Medicine, 155,* 234–247.

Lazarus, R. S., & Folkman, S. (1984). *Stress, appraisal, and coping.* New York: Springer.

Lazarus, R. S., & Launier, R. (1978). Stress-related transactions between person and environment. In L. A. Pervin & M. Lewis (Eds.), *Perspectives in interactional psychology* (pp. 287–327). New York: Plenum.

Livneh, H. (2001). Psychosocial adaptation to chronic illness and disability. *Rehabilitation Counseling Bulletin, 44,* 151–160.

Livneh, H., & Wilson, L. M. (2003). Coping strategies as predictors and mediators of disability-related variables and psychosocial adaptation: An exploratory investigation. *Rehabilitation Counseling Bulletin, 46*(4), 194–208.

Maes, S., Leventhal, H., & de Ridder, D. T. (1996). Coping with chronic diseases. In M. Zeidner & N. S. Endler (Eds.), *Handbook of coping: Theory, research and applications* (pp. 221–251). New York: John Wiley & Sons.

Martz, E., Livneh, H., Priebe, M., Wuermser, L., & Ottomanelli, L. (2005). Predictors of psychosocial adaptation among individuals with spinal cord injury/disorder. *Archives of Physical Medicine and Rehabilitation, 86,* 1182–1192.

Mattlin, J. A., Wethington, E., & Kessler, R. C. (1990). Situational determinants of coping and coping effectiveness. *Journal of Health and Social Behavior, 31,* 103–122.

Mechanic, D. (1974). Social structure and personal adaptation: Some neglected dimensions. In G. V. Coelho, D. A. Hamburg, & J. E. Adams (Eds.), *Coping and adaptation* (pp. 32–44). New York: Basic Books.

MedicineNet (2006a). *Definition of chronic illness*. Retrieved on April 15, 2006, from *http://www.medterms.com/script/main/art.asp?articlekey=2731*.

MedicineNet (2006b). *Definition of illness, chronic*. Retrieved on April 15, 2006, from *http://www.medterms.com/script/main/art.asp?articlekey=3903*.

Menninger, K. A. (1963). *The vital balance: The life process in mental health and illness*. New York: Viking.

Mishel, M. H., & Sorenson, D. S. (1991). Uncertainty in gynecological cancer: A test of the mediating functions of mastery and coping. *Nursing Research, 40*, 167–171.

Moos, R. H. (Ed.) (1984). *Coping with physical illness 2: New perspectives*. New York: Plenum Press.

Moos, R. H., & Schaefer, J. A. (1984). The crisis of physical illness. In R. H. Moos (Ed.), *Coping with physical illness. Volume 2: New Perspectives* (pp. 3–31). New York: Plenum Press.

Moos, R. H., & Schaefer, J. A. (1986). Overview and perspective. In R. H. Moos (Ed.), *Coping with life crises: An integrated approach* (pp. 3–28). New York: Plenum Press.

Moos, R. H., & Schaefer, J. A. (1993). Coping resources and processes: Current concepts and measures. In L. Goldberger & S. Breznitz (Eds.), *Handbook of stress: Theoretical and clinical aspects* (2nd ed., pp. 234–257). New York: The Free Press.

Parker, J. D., & Endler, N. S. (1992). Coping with coping assessment: A critical review. *European Journal of Personality, 6*, 321–344.

Parker, J. D., & Endler, N. S. (1996). Coping and defense: A historical overview. In M. Zeidner & N. Endler (Eds.), *Handbook of coping: Theory, research, applications* (pp. 3–13). New York: John Wiley and Sons.

Pearlin, L. I., & Schooler, C. (1978). The structure of coping. *Journal of Health and Social Behavior, 19*, 2–21.

Perrez, M., & Reicherts, M. (1992). *Stress, coping, and health: A situation-behavior approach, theory, methods, applications*. Seattle, WA: Hogrefe & Huber.

Porter, L. S., & Stone, A. A. (1996). An approach to assessing daily coping. In M. Zeidner & N. S. Endler (Eds.), *Handbook of coping: Theory, research, applications* (pp. 133–150). New York: John Wiley and Sons.

Roth, S., & Cohen, L. J. (1986). Approach, avoidance, and coping with stress. *American Psychologist, 41*, 813–819.

Schlossberg, N. K. (1981). A model for analyzing human adaptation to transition. *The Counseling Psychologist, 9*, 2–18.

Schwarzer, R., & Knoll, N. (2003). Positive coping: Mastering demands and searching for meaning. In S. J. Lopez & C. R. Snyder (Eds.), *Positive psychological assessment: A handbook of models and measures* (pp. 393–609). Washington, DC: American Psychological Association.

Schwarzer, R., & Schwarzer, C. (1996). A critical survey of coping instruments. In M. Zeidner & N. S. Endler (Eds.), *Handbook of coping: Theory, research, applications* (pp. 107–132). New York: John Wiley and Sons.

Seligman, M. E. P., & Csikszentmihalyi, M. (Eds.) (2000). Positive psychology [Special issue]. *American Psychologist, 55*(1), 1–183.

Selye, H. (1982). History and present status of the stress concept. In L. Goldberger & S. Breznitz (Eds.), *Handbook of stress: Theoretical and clinical aspects* (pp. 7–17). New York; The Free Press.

Sharoff, K. (2004). *Coping skills therapy for managing chronic and terminal illness*. New York: Springer Publishing Co.

Skinner, E. A., Edge, K., Altman, J., & Sherwood, H. (2003). Searching for the structure of coping: A review and critique of category systems for classifying ways of coping. *Psychological Bulletin, 129*, 216–269.

Snyder, C. R., & Dinoff, B. L. (1999). Coping: Where have we been? In C. R. Snyder (Ed.), *Coping: The psychology of what works* (pp. 3–19). New York: Oxford University Press.

Social Security Administration (2006). *How does social security decide if I am disabled?* Retrieved on April 17, 2006, from *http://www.ssa.gov/disability/disability_starter_kits_adult_factsheet.htm#disability*.

Sperry, L. (2006). *Psychological treatment of chronic illness: The biopsychosocial therapy approach.* Washington, DC: American Psychological Association.

Stanton, A. L., Danoff-Burg, S., Cameron, C. L., Bishop, M., & Collins, C. A., Kirk, S. B., Sworowski, L. A., & Twillman, R. (2000). Emotionally expressive coping predicts psychological and physical adjustment to breast cancer. *Journal of Consulting and Clinical Psychology, 68*, 875–882.

Stanton, A. L., Danoff-Burg, S., Cameron, C. L., & Ellis, A. P. (1994). Coping through emotional approach: Problems of conceptualization and confounding. *Journal of Personality and Social Psychology, 66*, 350–362.

Suls, J., David, J. P., & Harvey, J. H. (1996). Personality and coping: Three generations of research. *Journal of Personality, 64*, 711–735.

Taylor, S. E. (1999). *Health psychology* (4th ed.). New York: McGraw-Hill.

Tedeschi, R. G., & Calhoun, L. G. (1995). *Trauma and transformation: Growing in the aftermath of suffering.* Thousand Oaks, CA: Sage.

Tennen, H., & Affleck, G. (1999). Finding benefits in adversity. In C. R. Snyder (Ed.), *Coping: The psychology of what works* (pp. 279–304). New York: Oxford University Press.

Tobin, D. L., Holroyd, K. A., Reynolds, R. V., & Wigal, J. K. (1989). The hierarchical factor structure of the coping strategies inventory. *Cognitive therapy and research, 13*, 343–361.

United Nations. (2006). *General description.* Retrieved on April 16, 2006, from *http://www.un.org/esa/socdev/enable/diswpa04.htm*.

Vaillant, G. E. (1977). *Adaptation to life.* Boston: Little, Brown & Co.

Victorson, D., Farmer, L., Burnett, K., Quellette, A., & Barocas, J. (2005). Maladaptive coping strategies and injury-related distress following traumatic physical injury. *Rehabilitation Psychology, 50*, 408–415.

Wheaton, B. (1997). The nature of chronic stress. In B. H. Gottlieb (Ed.), *Coping with chronic stress* (pp. 43–73). New York: Plenum Press.

White, R. W. (1974). Strategies of adaptation: An attempt at systematic description. In G. V. Coelho, D. A. Hamburg, & J. E. Adams (Eds.), *Coping and adaptation* (pp. 47–68). New York: Basic Books.

Wills, T. A., & Hirky, A. E. (1996). Coping and substance abuse: A theoretical model and review of the evidence. In M. Zeidner & N. S. Endler (Eds.), *Handbook of coping: Theory, research, applications* (pp. 279–302). New York: John Wiley and Sons.

World Health Organization. (1980). *International classification of impairments, disabilities, and handicaps.* Geneva, Switzerland: Author.

World Health Organization. (2001). *International classification of functioning.* Geneva, Switzerland: Author.

World Health Organization. (2006). *International classification of functioning.* Retrieved on April 17, 2006, from *http://www.who.int/classifications/icf/en/*

Wright, B. A. (1983). *Physical disability: A psychosocial approach* (2nd ed.). New York: Harper and Row.

Zeidner, M., & Saklofske, D. (1996). Adaptive and maladaptive coping. In M. Zeidner & N. S. Endler (Eds.), *Handbook of coping: Theory, research, applications* (pp. 505–531). New York: John Wiley & Sons.

2
Psychodynamic and Cognitive Theories of Coping

Cynthia L. Radnitz and Lana Tiersky

During the 20th century, the theories of coping that came to predominance arose from two traditions: psychodynamic thought and cognitive psychology (Folkman & Lazarus, 1991). Although other work had described an animal model of coping, which focused on animal behavior serving a survival function in dangerous situations (Miller, 1980; Selye, 1976; Ursin, 1980), the inadequacy of this model to explain the complexity of human coping was recognized (Folkman & Lazarus, 1991; Shapiro, 1998), and consequently, the model has, for the most part, been abandoned.

Psychodynamic models of coping emphasize the role of ego defenses (Menninger, 1954; Vaillant, 1992) and typically specify a hierarchy of mature and primitive coping responses. One such model (Haan, 1977) describes such a hierarchy of ego functions, their development, and their relation to affect (including stress). Cognitive theories of coping (e.g., Pretzer, Beck, & Newman, 2002; Stroebe & Schut, 1999, 2001) are distinguished by their emphasis on cognitive processes that are intermediary between the external stressor(s) and the individual's emotional and behavioral responses. Prominent among these cognitive coping theories is the theory proposed by Folkman and Lazarus (Lazarus, 1966; Lazarus & Folkman, 1984), which specifies an intricate relationship between cognition, coping, emotion, and the person-environment fit.

Haan's Model of Coping, Defense, and Fragmentation

The Ego Processes: Coping, Defense, and Fragmentation

One psychodynamically-oriented author who has studied a broad range of human adjustment is Norma Haan (1969). She proposed a tripartite model of ego processes that includes coping, defense, and fragmentation. In her model, an "ego process" is a basic strategy used to solve significant, as well as mundane, problems in daily living (Haan, 1977). Ultimately, these ego processes help maintain a consistent sense of self and a realistic connection to the environment.

For the sake of clarity, it is important to define the terms coping, defense, and fragmentation before proceeding with a more complete explication of Haan's theory. *Coping* is defined as "... an attempt to overcome difficulties on equal terms; it is an encounter wherein people reach out and within themselves for resources to come to terms with difficulties" (Haan, 1993, p. 260). *Defense* is a method of adaptation or self protection that involves "unyielding fortification" (Haan, 1993, p. 260) of beliefs and/or behaviors. Finally, *fragmentation* is a form of adaptive "failure." Psychotic behavior, for example is considered fragmented. Optimally, the individual copes with adversity and maintains self-consistency. Less optimally, the individual defends against internal and external threats to self-integration. And, in times of extreme stress when the maintenance of self-consistency is precarious, fragmentation ensues.

Haan (1965) argues that an individual "constructs" a response to the environment, rather than "reacting" to it. Moreover, as cognitive development proceeds, the individual is able to respond to internal and external stresses in an increasingly sophisticated and adaptive manner. Coping becomes a more predominant means of adaptation as cognitive functions mature. Thus, the adult can control his or her behavior, can choose how to do so, and can cope with the consequences (Haan, 1977).

The Haan vs. Freudian Model of Ego Functioning

Haan's (1977) model differs considerably from the classical Freudian model of ego functioning (A. Freud, 1936; S. Freud, 1936). One central difference between the two models is that, according to classical Freudian thinking, defenses operate on an unconscious level (Freud, 1923). Alternatively, Haan (1977) suggests that defenses operate on a preconscious level and are not inherently conscious or unconscious in nature. A second difference between the two models is that, for Haan, the individual is an active and rational agent in constructing his or her response to the environment. She notes that several ego functions represent rational processes (e.g. objectivity, intellectuality, logical analysis, concentration, tolerance of ambiguity, empathy, and regression in service of the ego). Classical Freudian theory places more emphasis on impulses and wishes in shaping behavior (Freud, 1923). Individuals are inherently irrational; rationality is only achieved through the psychoanalytic process (Brenner, 1982).

A third major departure from classical theory is Haan's view of the motivation for behavior. According to Freudian theory, two drives – one sexual and the other aggressive – motivate behavior. All behaviors stem from these motivating forces. According to Haan (1977), however, individuals are motivated by a need for self-consistency. Ego functions, then, serve to help realize this basic striving.

Finally, another primary difference between Haan's theory and classic Freudian theory is the role the ego functions play in mediating between internal and external conflict. According to classical theory, defensive functions help an individual master intrapsychic conflict (Nersessian & Kopff, 1996). Coping behaviors, on the other hand, help mediate between an individual's conflicts and the external environment (A. Freud, 1936). According to Haan's (1993) model however, defense and coping mechanisms help mediate between both intrapersonal and interpersonal conflicts. This shift in thinking suggests that an individual has more resources available to manage both internal and external conflicts. Intrapersonal stresses can be dealt with using rational and flexible coping responses.

The Tripartite Model

Properties of the Ego Functions

According to Haan (1969) the three basic modes of ego functioning (coping, defense, and fragmentation) differ from one another only in their basic properties. In an earlier paper, Haan (1963) notes that defensive functions and coping mechanisms are identical in their "mental processes," (p. 1) or how they operate, but not in their basic properties. Moreover, although the basic properties that govern the three modes of ego processing are different, they are parallel in operation (see Table 2.1).

Essentially, *coping* involves problem-solving in a way that is purposeful and flexible. Affects are appropriately expressed and contained, while objective reality is recognized. An individual who is "coping" with a newly diagnosed chronic illness might acknowledge the psychological and physical implications

TABLE 2.1. Properties of the ego processes.

Coping processes	Defensive process	Fragmentary process
Behaviors are open, individually determined, and resolute	Behaviors are rigid and inflexible	Behaviors are ritualistic and automated
Guided by future interests and take into account current wants	Compelled by the past	Functioning in a manner that is wholly self-absorbed
Interpersonal reality remains intact and is not distorted	Distorting of interpersonal reality	Interpersonal reality is violated
Thinking is differentiated and includes conscious/pre-conscious elements	Predominantly undifferentiated thinking that is symbolic in nature and includes unconscious aspects	Affects govern thinking and behavior
Affects are modulated	Filled with "magical thinking" with respect to the alleviation of disturbing affects	Affects are not modulated
Balanced affective gratification	Indirect in allowance of affective gratification	Intensive affective gratification is allowed in some situations

Source: Adapted from Haan, 1977.

of the disease and seek external support and new information. On the other hand, *defensive* behavior is bound and rigid. Defensive processes do not effectively modulate affect, but instead distort interpersonal reality. An individual who is defensive with regard to a newly diagnosed chronic illness might deny any change has occurred in his or her life and, consequently, might not seek treatment or support. *Fragmentation* involves behavior that is ritualistic and automated. Interpersonal reality is negated and affect dominates thought and behavior. The individual who fragments following a diagnosis of chronic illness may withdraw into a fantasy world and become non-communicative.

The Four Categories of Ego Functions

According to Haan (1977), there are 10 generic or basic ego functions, each of which has three possible expressive modes of coping, defense, or fragmentation. These 10 generic ego processes are then divided into the following four categories based on function: (a) cognitive, (b) reflexive-intraceptive, (c) attention-focusing, and (d) affective-impulse regulating (see Table 2.2). These four categories were created for conceptual convenience. Each is not mutually exclusive; one category may share many similar features with several others.

TABLE 2.2. Haan's 10 basic ego functions by category and mode.

	Modes		
Generic ego process	Coping	Defense	Fragentation
Cognitive			
1. Discrimination	Objectivity	Isolation	Concretism
2. Detachment	Intellectuality	Intellectualizing	Word salad, neologisms
3. Means-ends	Symbolization	Logical analysis, rationalization	Confabulation
Reflexive-intraceptive			
4. Delayed response	Tolerance of doubt	Immobilization	Ambiguity
5. Sensitivity	Empathy	Projection	Delusion
6. Time reversion	Regression	Ego regression	Decomposition
Attention-focusing			
7. Selective awareness	Concentration	Denial	Distraction, fixation
Affective-impulse regulating			
8. Diversion	Sublimation	Displacement	Affective preoccupation
9. Transformation	Substitution	Reaction-formation	Unstable alternation
10. Restraint	Suppression	Repression	Depersonalization

Source: Adapted from Haan, 1977.

Cognitive Functions. The three ego processes that are part of this category include discrimination, detachment, and means-end symbolization. They all involve active and externally directed attempts to problem-solve. Cognitive processes also facilitate adaptation by helping the individual accommodate to the environment.

Reflexive-Intraceptive Functions. The three generic ego functions that fall into this category include delayed response, sensitivity, and time reversion (e.g., regression). These ego processes help maintain self-reflective capacities (Aldwin, 1994). Moreover, all three reflect the extent of absorption with inner thoughts and desires.

Attention-Focusing Functions. The generic process that falls into this category is selective awareness. The defensive function, denial, is an extreme form of selective awareness; in this process, aversive realities are selectively ignored and non-aversive realities are attended to.

Affective-Impulse Regulating Functions. The three generic ego processes included in this category are diversion, restraint, and transformation. All three serve to help manage affect. In addition, the management of anxiety is fundamental to these mechanisms. Underlying the functioning of these three processes is the supposition that affects are not directly and primitively expressed, except by an infant (Haan, 1977).

Hierarchy of Function

The main function of all of the ego processes is to help the individual maintain a consistent sense of self (Haan, 1977). Coping responses allow an individual to do this in an optimal manner, with little distortion of interpersonal reality. Defensive functions, on the other hand, result in "... self-compartmentalization rather than fragmentation" (Haan, 1977, p. 62), and consequently distortion of interpersonal reality. Fragmentation, a feebler attempt at the maintenance of self-consistency, engenders a total rejection of interpersonal objectivity.

The three general modes of ego processing form a functional hierarchy: "The person will cope if he can, defend if he must and fragment if he is forced, but whichever mode he uses, it is still in the service of his attempt to maintain organization" (Haan, 1977, p. 42). Implicit in this hierarchy is Haan's valuation of coping as normative, and defense and fragmentation as pathological. However, despite this judgment, success or failure in a given situation is not inherent to any one process. In other words, coping does not ensure success, while defense and fragmentation are not necessarily indicative of failure (Haan, 1993).

The Role of Accommodation and Assimilation

According to Haan (1977), the ego processes organize information and help maintain self-consistency through assimilation and accommodation. She defines these terms similar to how Piaget (1962) defines them. *Assimilation* involves integrating new information into already existing schemas or constructs.

Accommodation, on the other hand, involves creating new constructs to help integrate new experiences (Haan, 1977). Different ego processes will be employed depending on the balance of the use of assimilation and accommodation in maintaining self-consistency. For instance, defensive strategies are often invoked if there is a marked imbalance in assimilation and accommodation. Alternatively, fragmentation may occur when necessary accommodations are beyond the person's capacity and thus, a retreat to private assimilatory modes is more practical. Ultimately, whether a person copes, defends, or fragments is going to be dependent on the nature of the stressor, the individual's internal resources, and most significantly, the nature of the situation.

Discontinuity and Pathology

Discontinuity is another notion central to Haan's (1977) theory. At times, an individual who defends or fragments becomes "not himself" (p. 62) or is in a discontinuous state. At these times, the integrity of the cognitive, moral, and social structures remain intact. However, they may not be readily apparent in that the individual is in a temporary state of a new and "false equilibrium" (p. 56). Discontinuity seems to serve as the basis for the explanation of pathology in the Haan (1977) model.

The Relationship between Ego Processes and Cognitive, Moral, and Social Structures

Haan (1977) examined the relationship between the ego processes and the cognitive, moral, and social structures that govern thinking processes. An individual's level of cognitive development will dictate the extent to which the individual can potentially use reason and other formal thought-processes to solve problems or cope effectively. Ego processes develop in concert with ego structures. As children are less cognitively developed than adults, they are more likely to engage in defensive or fragmentary processes. Adults have more cognitive resources at hand and therefore have more choices over adaptive behavior. Likewise, the level of social and moral development is also dependent, but not solely, on the level of cognitive functioning. For instance, empathy and altruism are abstract concepts, which can only be understood once formal cognitive structures are developed.

Despite its importance, the final demonstration of behavior is not solely dependent on cognitive achievement. In fact, disparity is frequently seen between the ability to reason and subsequent behavioral responses. One of the reasons for this disparity is that the ego processes interact with the cognitive and moral structures to shape behavior. For instance, a nurse with a chronic illness may "know" that she must report her worsening symptoms to a doctor. However, she may tell the doctor that she is in fine health or not even consult a physician, because revealing her current symptoms might increase anxiety. This defense of denial may help restore equilibrium, but is not an optimal response in line with her level of cognitive development.

The Ego Processes and Their Relation to Affects

According to Haan (1977), affects are also mediated by cognitive structures. Affects dominate cognitive structures only in the youngest infants. In addition to cognition, however, the ego processes also mediate experience of emotion. For instance, during times of crisis, such as the initial diagnosis of a chronic illness, an individual may demonstrate significant strength and cope with the situation in an active and purposeful manner. Joining support groups and searching the internet for information may transform feelings of anxiety into feelings of purpose and mission. In this case, the level of perceived resilience may be surprising; the individual may be doing much better with the initial information than otherwise could have been imagined.

The behavior and affects of the same individual engaged in defensive processes may appear quite different than those noted above. For example, the individual may deny the emotional significance of the diagnosis, choosing instead to gather medical information without acknowledging the need for support from others. This form of isolation results in distortion in intrapersonal situations. Rather than feelings of anxiety, there is an absence of feeling, with the end outcome being a failure to seek appropriate care.

In conclusion, with regard to the relationship between ego processes, moral and social structures, and affect, the following may be stated. In normal circumstances, cognitive functioning is served by coping responses (Haan, 1977). The cognitive structures are then informed by moral and social structures, as well as affective responses. In aberrant situations, defenses and fragmentation distort cognitive processes or allow affective reactions to predominate cognitive experience.

Ego Processes and Stress

Rather than focusing on specific situations that are equated with a certain level of anxiety or arousal, Haan's (1993) model focuses on understanding stress by examining "how," or the *processes* by which the individual arrives at the determination that the event was stressful. Haan (1993) emphasizes that stressful experiences are idiosyncratically constructed by the individual. However, she does acknowledge that there are some experiences that would be universally considered stressful (e.g., being a prisoner of war).

The processes of assimilation and accommodation are continuously employed by the ego processes to help the individual adapt to stressful conditions. Certain environmental circumstances, however, hinder efforts at assimilation and accommodation (McGrath, 1970). Specifically, Haan (1993) argues that the *assimilation* of adverse circumstances is made more difficult under the following conditions: (a) when the aversive event had not been planned, or when hopes of a good

outcome do not come to fruition; (b) when there is no control over the occurrence of an event; (c) when situations are ambiguous; (d) when a situation is
assumed to be stressful; (e) when the situation is analogous to other aversive
and unresolved events; (f) when the individual is already stressed; or (g) when
important information cannot be secured. If one of these conditions exists, any
event, "good" or "bad," might be experienced as stressful.

According to Haan (1993), *accommodation* to stress is more difficult in the
following three situations: (a) when only limited control over diminishing the
amount of stress may be exercised, (b) when the stress is highly noxious, or
(c) when there is no prior experience with a certain type of stress.

Haan's focus on the cognitive processes, which result in the valuation of
stress, is consistent with her overall focus on the function of ego processes.
In both cases, the individual is actively constructing his or her experience and
is not a victim of a situation. Furthermore, stress does not automatically lead
to deterioration (Haan, 1993). Stressful experiences can enhance functioning,
resulting in greater insight or empathy. As in any situation, even in times of
stress, the ego processes come into play and lead the individual to cope, defend,
or fragment, in order to adapt to the situation.

Evaluation of Haan's Model

Numerous studies have been completed to examine the utility and construct
validity of Haan's model (1969). Morrisey (1977) provides a comprehensive
review of the early studies. Overall, the basic conclusion from this research is
that, methodological limitations aside, the model does show some promise as
a method for conceptualizing adaptive behavior. However, subsequent research
(Harder, 1992) failed to find support for six of Haan's defensive subtypes
(projection, repression, displacement, intellectualization, denial, and primitive
defense). Only primitive regression was found to be associated with symptom
variables in a manner that suggested it was a valid scale. Although the aggregate
analyses did not substantiate its validity, denial was associated with variables
indicative of psychological health. Future research should examine the generalizability of Harder's (1992) findings.

According to Haan (1977), denial is not conducive to health. Other forms of
negation, such as isolation, are also not believed to benefit the individual in the
long-term, even in the case of chronic illness. In addition to contradicting the
above research, her arguments differ from those of Lazarus (1983), who notes
that in some circumstances, there may be some benefit to using denial when
attempting to adapt to a chronically stressful situation. Clearly, the beneficial or
detrimental role of denial in adaptation to chronic illness remains a subject of
examination.

Some research has been completed using Haan's (1977) model to understand
the effects of chronic stress, such as long-term illness, on the development of
ego processes. Although the findings are somewhat limited because of methodological constraints, there is an indication that men and women adapt to chronic

illness differently. It appears that men's health difficulties are more closely associated with ego processes than are women's. Haan suggests that this is evidence that illness is a greater "social-psychological concern for men than women" (p. 190). Thus, gender differences in the use of specific ego processes should be a topic for future investigations.

In regard to the stress imposed by chronic illness, Haan (1977) also notes that individuals use a mixed pattern of coping and defense to adapt to the environment. Future research could address whether specific illnesses are associated with specific patterns of ego processing. A procedure for rating ego-functioning, which may be useful in these studies, can be found in Haan (1977, p. 299).

Lazarus and Folkman's Theory of Coping

When Lazarus and Folkman (Folkman & Lazarus, 1991; Lazarus, 1966, 1995; Lazarus & Folkman, 1984) proposed their theory of coping, it was distinguished from other coping theories by its focus on how coping interacts *transactionally* with cognition and emotion. In their view, the relationship between cognition, coping, and emotion was not static, but rather dynamic and variable, with a prominent role for cognition. Previously, coping had been viewed as a reaction to emotion (e.g., Menninger, 1963; Miller, 1980; Ursin, 1980; Vaillant, 1977). Such a view ignored that there is often a reciprocal and ongoing relationship between the two (Folkman & Lazarus, 1988; Lazarus, 1995).

Lazarus and Folkman's theory was also distinguished from other cognitive theories of emotion, in that coping was considered an inherent part of the *interaction* between cognition and emotion. Other prominent theories of cognition and emotion had emphasized either the primacy of cognition (e.g., Beck, Rush, Shaw, & Emery, 1979; Ellis, 1962), or emotion (e.g., Zajonc, 1980, 1984), giving relatively little attention to the intricate interplay between the two, and ignoring the important role that coping plays in the exchange. By putting forward a theory that placed coping squarely in a transactional relationship with cognition and emotion, Lazarus and Folkman (Folkman & Lazarus, 1988, 1991; Lazarus, 1966; Lazarus & Folkman, 1984) made a significant and innovative contribution to both theories of coping and theories of emotion and cognition.

Coping, Emotion, and Appraisal

To describe Lazarus and Folkman's theory of coping, it is first necessary to explain their definitions of emotion, coping, and appraisal. *Emotions* are "complex organized psychophysiological reactions, consisting of cognitive appraisals, action impulses, and patterned somatic reactions" (Folkman & Lazarus, 1991, p. 209). These elements are not construed as distinct responses, but instead are considered highly interrelated. It could be argued that they correspond to the cognitive, behavioral, and physiological modes of response, proposed by behavioral theorists (Cone, 1977, 1978, 1979) to delineate how humans respond to external stimuli. Folkman and Lazarus (1991) propose a central role for cognition, both in terms of their emphasis on the role of appraisal, and their use of the term "action impulses," which implies that *considered behavior* (as well as actual behavior) is part of the emotional experience.

Folkman and Lazarus (1991) define *coping* as "cognitive and behavioral efforts to manage specific external and/or internal demands that are appraised as taxing or exceeding the resources of the person" (p. 210). Construing coping as a dynamic process allows for a constant flux between appraisal and both emotional and behavioral responses. Moreover, as these emotional and behavioral responses are emitted, there is often an effect on the person-environment relationship, which in turn, can result in a reappraisal of the situation and possible changes in emotions and behavior. The encounter can remain fluid until the situation is resolved.

An *appraisal* is an evaluative judgment about the personal significance of an event (Lazarus, 1995). It is based on knowledge of that event and represents an attempt to determine the personal meaning of it, in order that a decision about whether, when, and how to respond can be made. In Lazarus's (1966) initial description of his coping model, he distinguished between primary and secondary appraisal. *Primary appraisal* is an estimation of the stress potential of an encounter, and affects both the type of emotion experienced (e.g., anger, sadness, or anxiety) and its strength. In response to the primary appraisal, a *secondary appraisal* is made whereby the individual takes stock of his or her resources, the coping options available, and the environment's probable reaction to these options if exercised. Based on these appraisals, especially in relation to each other, and their emotional consequences, a coping response is chosen which may engender a new emotional response, and which again interacts with appraisal and coping response, in an often rapid and dynamic interplay.

Coping Styles

Considering the broad and often diverse nature of coping responses, Folkman and Lazarus (1980) and others (e.g., Pearlin & Schooler, 1978) have proposed taxonomies for understanding the styles of coping that people use (Folkman & Moskowitz, 2004). One of the earliest and best-known conceptualizations of coping processes distinguished two coping styles: Problem-focused and emotion-focused coping (Folkman & Lazarus 1980). *Problem-focused coping* involves the utilization of active efforts to address the stressor. An example of problem-focused coping is active problem-solving that involves such behaviors as attempting to get more information about the problem and the resources and options that are available to deal with it. On the other hand, *emotion-focused coping* refers to coping efforts that do not seek to directly solve the problem, but instead center on managing the emotional reactions that result from the primary and secondary appraisals. An example of emotion-focused coping is escape/avoidance, which can involve the use of alcohol or other drugs, indicating an emotional avoidance of the real problem.

Subsequent efforts to delineate coping styles have supported the distinction between problem- and emotion-focused coping (e.g., Amirkhan, 1990; Billings and Moos, 1981; Carver, Scheier, & Weintraub, 1989; Pearlin & Schooler, 1978), but have also identified other coping styles (Folkman & Moskowitz, 2004). A three-factor model consisting of Active Behavioral (a form of problem-focused coping), Avoidance (a form of emotion-focused coping), and Active Cognitive styles of coping was proposed by Billings and Moos (1981) and is consistent with the Folkman and Lazarus (1980) model.

Based on a factor analysis of coping responses that resulted in a 17-factor solution, Pearlin and Schooler (1978) divided these factors according to their function. These functions (changing the situation, changing the meaning of the situation, and "controlling the stress itself") correspond almost exactly to the scheme proposed by Billings and Moos (1981). The factor of the "meaning-making" function (Folkman & Moskowitz, 2004) refers to a cognitive stratagem that is geared toward dealing with the meaning of a situation. Other factor analytic studies of coping inventories, such as the Coping Strategy Indicator (Amirkhan, 1990) and the COPE (Carver et al., 1989), identified an additional factor that involved seeking social support and interpersonal coping, in addition to the aforementioned coping styles.

Transaction and Variability

Folkman and Lazarus (1991; Lazarus, 1995; Lazarus & Folkman, 1987) emphasize the fluidity of the coping/emotion process within the context of the person-environment relationship, in contrast to viewpoints which place importance on specific structural patterns that occur. These structural models tend to be simpler and more static. Examples include both psychodynamic (e.g., the repression-sensitization scale developed from Minnesota Multiphasic Personality Inventory items; Byrne, 1961) and cognitive (e.g., Beck's cognitive distortions or Ellis's irrational beliefs) theories. Moreover, Folkman and Lazarus (1991; Lazarus & Folkman, 1987) contend that the high degree of variability, which is inherent in the temporal coping process, extends to the kinds of coping that individuals use in a given circumstance. In several studies (Folkman & Lazarus, 1985; Folkman, Lazarus, Dunkel-Schetter, DeLongis, & Gruen, 1986a; Folkman, Lazarus, Pimley, & Novacek, 1987) of the revised 67-item Ways of Coping Questionnaire (Folkman & Lazarus, 1980), eight types of coping were identified, specifically: Planful problem-solving, confrontative coping, escape-avoidance, emotional distancing, seeking social support, accepting responsibility or blame, positive reappraisal, and self-control of emotional expression. Problem-solving and confrontative coping can be considered problem-focused coping, while the remaining six are more typically emotion-focused types of coping (Folkman & Lazarus, 1991). However, there is a caveat to this classification, in that the function of a given type of coping will ultimately depend on the circumstance in which it occurs (Folkman & Lazarus, 1980; Lazarus & Folkman, 1984).

The Person-Environment Fit

Coping is hypothesized to serve a mediating function between situational appraisal, the person-environment relationship, and emotional response (Folkman & Lazarus, 1988; 1991). Initially, the individual will appraise an environmental transaction as personally important in some way – favorable, intimidating, damaging, or demanding. Based on this appraisal, coping strategies will be considered and one or more will be chosen and implemented. In doing so, the implementation of a coping response will affect the environment's response (hence, the person-environment fit), and consequently, the resultant emotions that the person will experience.

In attempting to ascertain how coping affects the person-environment fit, Folkman and Lazarus (1991) have proposed three putative pathways: (a) Degree of attentional focus, (b) alteration of meaning or importance of an event, and (c) changing the circumstances of the person-environment relationship. In the first pathway, coping can affect the person-environment fit, depending upon the degree to which the individual focuses attention on the stressor. This degree of attention can range from deliberate avoidance to hypervigilance. Depending on the circumstance, these responses may be adaptive or non-adaptive. For example, deliberate avoidance may be adaptive if the situation is beyond the individual's control, and non-adaptive if it prevents the individual from taking appropriate action. Similarly, hypervigilance may be adaptive in situations where there is excessive danger (e.g., combat), and non-adaptive when excessive attention on a specific transaction prevents the focus of attention on other important life events.

In the second pathway, coping efforts can affect the person-environment fit through changing the meaning or importance of an event (Folkman & Lazarus, 1991). These include the three strategies of *denial*, *distancing*, and *using positive cognitions*. In the former case, the individual may *deny* that a situation exists or is problematic to such an extent that his or her reality-testing is questionable. Denial may be adaptive in situations of crisis, such as learning of the diagnosis of a dangerous or chronic illness (Hackett & Cassem, 1973; Kortte & Wegener, 2004; Lazarus, 1983). At these times, the full comprehension of the implications of such news may be too much to take in all at once. However, if denial is used to an extent that it prevents the individual from engaging in strategic coping behaviors which would significantly improve his or her situation, then it is non-adaptive.

Distancing refers to coping through detachment where a problematic situation is acknowledged, but the individual makes conscious efforts to minimize or avoid thinking about it. Distancing can be very adaptive in highly stressful situations (e.g., health-care workers who deal with severely ill patients may need to distance themselves from the fates of those they care for to avoid being emotionally devastated when they die). On the other hand, distancing is an inappropriate strategy when serious problems that demand action are minimized or ignored. Finally, strategies that involve utilizing *positive cognition* include positive reappraisal (Folkman et al., 1986a) and cognitive restructuring (Pearlin & Schooler, 1978). These types of techniques typically involve reframing situations in a more positive light and are adaptive, in most cases.

The third pathway involves altering the nature of the person-environment fit, primarily through the use of the problem-focused coping strategies, confrontative coping, and problem-solving (Folkman & Lazarus, 1991). Confrontative coping strategies include aggressive efforts to alter the situation. These can be adaptive in some circumstances, such as when other milder coping efforts are unsuccessful. However, often confrontative coping involves the use of bullying tactics, which may be successful in the short-term but counterproductive in the long-term. Utilization of problem-solving strategies means that a great deal of thought is given to the implications of various courses of action, and that a balanced decision about a plan of action is carefully made. Although the outcome may not always be advantageous, these are generally considered adaptive forms of coping, except when so much thought is given (or the thinking occurs over too long of a period of time) that it either interferes with quality of life or effective functioning.

As is clear from the previous discussion, an important consideration in determining successful coping is the "fit" between the particular situation and the coping response (Folkman & Moskowitz, 2004). Every form of coping described may be adaptive in some circumstances and counterproductive in others, depending on the nature of the situation and how the coping response is executed. Hence, there are neither "good" coping responses nor "bad" ones; rather, all forms of coping must be evaluated within the context in which they occur.

Toward a Better Understanding of Cognition in Coping

In their initial work, Folkman and Lazarus (1980, 1991) did not propose a detailed conceptualization of appraisal, as other theorists had depicted for cognition in terms of beliefs (Ellis, 1962) or distortions (Beck et al., 1979). Later, Park and Folkman (1997) conceptualized how cognition played a role in the process of stress and coping by describing the role of beliefs, goals, and meaning in the coping process. In doing so, they have proposed an information-processing model of coping, which is a further development of Folkman and Lazarus's earlier work.

Park and Folkman's (1997) model distinguishes two types of meaning: *Global meaning* describes "people's basic goals and fundamental assumptions, beliefs, and expectations about the world" (p. 116), while *situational meaning* is derived from the interpretation of global meaning within the particular person-environment interaction. Hence, because global meaning is so fundamental to an individual's outlook, it is pervasive and will likely affect any and all situations that are considered important. Global meaning can be construed along two dimensions: namely, beliefs about *order* and decisions about defining *purpose* and life goals.

Beliefs about *order* refer to beliefs about the self, the world, and how the self relates to the world (Lazarus, 1991; Park & Folkman, 1997; Tunis, 1991). Examples of beliefs about the self include considerations of self-worth and the controllability of outcomes; examples of beliefs about the world include considerations of justice and fairness and how benevolent the world and other people are; and examples of beliefs about the self in the world include considerations of how beliefs about the self, such as self-worth, interact with beliefs about the world, such as the benevolence of others. In the latter case, for example, an individual with a positive sense of self-worth who believes that others are benevolent may believe that he or she is capable of having good social relationships and that these relationships are desirable and important.

Beliefs about *purpose* refer to decisions that validate and organize the course along which a person directs his or her efforts (Antonovsky, 1987; Csikszentmihalyi, 1990; Park & Folkman, 1997). Although these are often referred to as goals (e.g., Bandura, 1986; Carver & Scheier, 1991), recent work has focused more on the trajectory along which individuals strive for a sense of purpose without there necessarily being an endpoint (Hayes, Strosahl, & Wilson, 1999). This conception of purpose is similar to the categorization of distal, superordinate goals (e.g., health, environmentalism, career achievement; Powers, 1973), which guide proximal subordinate goals that are undertaken in everyday life. In this respect, it is just as important *how* a life is lived, regardless of whether any particular goal is achieved.

Park and Folkman's (1997) model of how meaning plays a role in stress and coping proposes that events occur that activate elements of global meaning. In this context, primary and secondary appraisals are made, resulting in appraised, situational meaning. The result of this appraised, situational meaning is then compared with the overriding global meaning to determine the extent of the congruence. If there is congruence, then the event is not considered stressful, and no further coping efforts are required. For example, if a person who values health and believes that the maintenance of good health is important (global meaning) bangs his or her elbow (event), he or she would likely see this occurrence as non-stressful (primary appraisal), and one that does not require any coping responses (secondary appraisal). Hence, the situational meaning that he or she would derive (i.e., the banged elbow is only temporarily painful and therefore inconsequential) would be largely congruent with the overall global value of good health and there would be no substantive stress. In this case, no significant coping efforts would be needed.

In contrast to the aforementioned example, if the situational meaning is *not* congruent with the global meaning, then the appraised, situational meaning is that the event is stressful and further coping is required. In this case, the individual may utilize various problem- and emotion-focused coping strategies in order to reduce the degree of incongruence between global and appraised situational meaning. For example, if the precipitating event is the diagnosis of a chronic, disabling illness, rather than a banged elbow, the appraised situational meaning would be that the person is not in good health, which obviously is not congruent with the global value of good health. In this circumstance, the person would likely utilize both problem-focused (e.g., pursuing good medical care) and emotion-focused (e.g., seeking social support) coping strategies to alter the appraised situational meaning of the event (toward better health status). However, if these problem-solving efforts are not successful and the incongruence between appraised situational meaning and global meaning persists, then the person may engage in a reappraisal process.

Typically, initial reappraisal efforts will focus on changing situational meaning, because doing so is usually preferable to changing a global belief system (Pargament, 1996; Park & Folkman, 1997; Tait & Silver, 1989; Thompson & Janigian, 1988). This initial reappraisal may involve a reattribution process, in which attributions about causality (why the event happened), selective incidence (why the event happened "to me" and not to someone else), and responsibility (who is responsible for the event's occurrence) are examined and possibly altered. In the event of a diagnosis of a chronic illness (e.g., diabetes), consideration of why it developed (e.g., weight gain), why it happened "to me" (e.g., family history), and who is responsible (e.g., a spouse who stocks the house with too many high calorie foods) may lead to situational reappraisal. In addition, attributions about controllability may be altered by making indirect attributions of control ("God's will" or post-hoc explanations), in lieu of primary control ("I can control the course of my disease"). Other strategies include delineating that there are perceived benefits (e.g., discovering heretofore unrecognized coping abilities) to a seemingly dire situation such as a chronic illness diagnosis; compensatory self-enhancement through recognition of other talents in a different domain (occupational success, as opposed to good health); downward comparison, whereby the individual recognizes how fortunate he or she is compared to others, despite the recent diagnosis; and perspective-taking, involving the adoption of a long-term perspective ("In five years, I'll adjust to having this condition").

Changing the global meaning of an event is considered a secondary option, available when the aforementioned cognitive strategies are not successful in accomplishing a reappraisal of situational meaning (Park & Folkman, 1997). Yet, it is doubtful that individuals systematically attempt all of these strategies. In our chronic illness diagnosis example, this may mean a revision of beliefs (good health may become less important) and/or goals (living well, as opposed to living a long time).

Efforts to change situational and/or global meaning may or may not be successful in realigning the two. In the event that they are successful, then an acceptable resolution is achieved. However, if these two forms of meaning remain divergent, then the individual may continue to experience distress, and may opt to attempt additional coping strategies.

Evaluation's of Lazarus and Folkman's Model

Folkman and Lazarus (e.g., Folkman & Lazarus, 1980, 1985, 1988) have conducted a substantial body of research that evaluates their model. Many of their findings have been replicated by other authors (e.g., Krantz, 1983; Pearlin & Schooler, 1978). Taken together, this body of research has largely corroborated the validity of the model. A detailed review of this literature is beyond the scope of this chapter, but studies have supported the mediating role of coping on emotion (Folkman, 1997; Folkman & Lazarus, 1988; Moskowitz, Folkman, Collette, & Vittinghoff, 1996), the influence of appraisal on coping (Baum, Fleming, & Singer, 1983; Folkman et al., 1986a) the distinction between problem- and emotion-focused coping (Amirkhan, 1990; Gottlieb and Gignac, 1996; Pearlin & Schooler, 1978; Zautra, Sheets, and Sandler, 1996), the variability of appraisal and coping as a function of intra-situational contextual change (Folkman & Lazarus, 1985), and the variability of some forms of coping, typically problem-focused, across situations (Folkman, Lazarus, Gruen, & DeLongis, 1986b). Although some inadequacies of this research have been noted, such as the narrow demographic profile of the samples (Lazarus & Folkman, 1987), the limitations of retrospective self-report measures (Folkman & Moskowitz, 2004), and the paucity of longitudinal research (Lazarus & Folkman, 1987), the overall conclusion that can be drawn from this work is that the model offers a valid framework for understanding cognition, appraisal, and emotion.

Conclusions

Although there are fundamental differences between Haan's psychodynamic and Lazarus and Folkman's cognitive theories, there are other areas of commonality. First, each model focuses on the processes by which an individual adapts to the environment. Haan (1977) and Folkman and Lazarus (1991) are primarily concerned with how the individual responds to the environment during periods of stress, and how he or she then evaluates the outcome. Both see the person-environment fit as central. Second, each theory emphasizes the importance of evaluating the efficacy of adaptive behavior, based on final outcome. An adaptive behavior is only considered a success or a failure when the full consequences of the outcome are examined. Finally, both theories emphasize the central role of cognition in adaptation. Haan (1977) notes that optimal coping responses can occur when the individual is able to rationally examine a situation, while Folkman and Lazarus (1991) place a great deal of emphasis on the role of appraisal in the coping process.

Both the psychodynamic and cognitive-behavioral models presented in this chapter provide useful heuristics for understanding adaptive behavior in chronic illness and disability (CID). First, a person actively responds to the environment and helps construct the outcome. Recognizing this can help empower the individual with CID, who may have relinquished a sense of control over his or her illness. Second, a myriad of cognitive factors intervene to help an individual cope with stress. Encouraging individuals to discuss their concerns and be aware of the cognitions surrounding their illness may improve adaptation (Sharoff, 2004).

Finally, adaptation or response to stress is idiosyncratic. The usefulness of any adaptive response can only be determined within a specific context. Therefore, as clinicians, we should not judge, a priori, a response to stress and assume that it is pathological. A full understanding of the individual, his or her illness or disability, and his or her environment, is needed before any evaluation can be made.[1]

References

Aldwin, C. (1994). *Stress, coping, and development: An integrative approach.* New York: Guilford.

Amirkhan, J. H. (1990). A factor analytically derived measure of coping: the coping strategy indicator. *Journal of Personality and Social Psychology, 59,* 1066–1074.

Antonovsky, A. (1987). *Unraveling the mystery of health: How people manage stress and stay well.* San Francisco: Jossey-Bass.

Bandura, A. (1986). *Social foundations of thought and action: A social cognitive theory.* Englewood Cliffs, NJ: Prentice Hall.

Baum, A., Fleming, I., & Singer, J. E. (1983). Coping with technological disaster. *Journal of Social Issues, 39,* 117–138.

Beck, A. T., Rush, A. J., Shaw, B. F., & Emery, G. (1979). *Cognitive therapy of depression.* New York: Guilford.

Billings, A. G., & Moos, R. H. (1981). The role of coping responses and social resources in attenuating the stress of life events. *Journal of Behavioral Medicine, 4*(2), 139–157.

Brenner, C. (1982). *The mind in conflict.* Guilford, CT: International Universities Press.

Byrne, D. (1961). The repression-sensitization scale: Rationale, reliability, and validity. *Journal of Personality, 29,* 334–349.

Carver, C. S., & Scheier, M. F. (1991). Self-regulation and the self. In J. Strauss & G. R. Goethals (Eds.), *The self: Interdisciplinary approaches* (pp. 239–254). New York: Springer-Verlag.

Carver, C. S., Scheier, M. F., & Weintraub, J. K. (1989). Assessing coping strategies: A theoretically based approach. *Journal of Personality and Social Psychology, 56,* 267–283.

Cone, J. D. (1977). The relevance of reliability and validity for behavioral assessment. *Behavior Therapy, 8,* 411–426.

Cone, J. D. (1978). The Behavioral Assessment Grid (BAG): A conceptual framework and a taxonomy. *Behavior Therapy, 9,* 882–888.

Cone, J. D. (1979). Confounded comparisons in triple response mode assessment research. *Behavioral Assessment, 1,* 85–95.

Csikszentmihalyi, M. (1990). *Flow: The psychology of optimal experience.* New York: Harper & Row.

Ellis, A. (1962). *Reason and emotion in psychotherapy.* Secaucus, NJ: Lyle Stuart.

[1] *Acknowledgments:* We would like to express our gratitude to Jennifer Schneider, Rachel Shechter, and Martha Sparks for their valuable assistance in preparing this manuscript.

Folkman, S. (1997). Positive psychological states and coping with severe stress. *Social Science and Medicine, 45,* 1207–1221.

Folkman, S., & Lazarus, R. S. (1980). An analysis of coping in a middle-aged community sample. *Journal of Health and Social Behavior, 21*(3), 219–239.

Folkman, S., & Lazarus, R. S. (1985). If it changes it must be a process: Study of emotion and coping during three stages of a college examination. *Journal of Personality and Social Psychology, 48,* 150–170.

Folkman, S., & Lazarus, R. S. (1988). *Manual for the ways of coping questionnaire.* Palo Alto, CA: Consulting Psychologists Press.

Folkman, S., & Lazarus, R. S. (1991). Coping and emotion. In A. Monat & R. S. Lazarus (Eds.), *Stress and coping: An anthology* (3rd ed., pp. 208–227). New York: Columbia University Press.

Folkman, S., Lazarus, R. S., Dunkel-Schetter, C., DeLongis, A., & Gruen, R. (1986a). The dynamics of a stressful encounter: Cognitive appraisal, coping and encounter outcomes. *Journal of Personality and Social Psychology, 50,* 992–1003.

Folkman, S., Lazarus, R. S., Gruen, R. J., & DeLongis, A. (1986b). Appraisal, coping, health status, and psychological symptoms. *Journal of Personality and Social Psychology, 50*(3), 571–579.

Folkman, S., Lazarus, R. S., Pimley, S., & Novacek, J. (1987). Age differences in stress and coping processes. *Psychology and Aging, 2,* 171–184.

Folkman, S., & Moskowitz, J. T. (2004). Coping: Pitfalls and promise. *Annual Review of Psychology, 55,* 745–774.

Freud, A. (1936). *The ego and the mechanisms of defense.* London: Hogarth Press.

Freud, S. (1923). Consciousness and what is unconscious, *Standard Edition* (Vol. 19, pp. 13–18). New York: W. W. Norton & Co.

Freud, S. (1936). *Inhibitions, symptoms, and anxiety.* London: Hogath Press.

Gottlieb, B. H., & Gignac, M. A. M. (1996). Content and domain specificity of coping among family caregivers of persons with dementia. *Journal of Aging Studies, 10*(2), 137–155.

Haan, N. (1963). Proposed model of ego functioning: Coping and defense mechanisms in relationship to IQ change. *Psychological Monographs, 77*(8), 1–23.

Haan, N. (1965). Coping and defense mechanisms related to personality inventories. *Journal of Consulting Psychology, 29*(4), 373–378.

Haan, N. (1969). A tripartite model of ego functioning values and clinical and research applications. *Journal of Nervous & Mental Disease, 148*(1), 14–30.

Haan, N. (1977). *Coping and defending: Processes of self-environment organization.* New York: Academic Press.

Haan, N. (1993). The assessment of coping, defense, and stress. In L. Goldberger & S. Breznitz (Eds.), *Handbook of stress: Theoretical and clinical aspects* (2nd ed., pp. 258–273). New York: Free Press.

Hackett, T. P., & Cassem, N. H. (1973). Psychological adaptation to convalescence in myocardial infarction patients. In J. P. Naughton, H. K. Hellerstein, & I. C. Mohler (Eds.), *Exercise testing and exercise training in coronary heart disease.* New York: Academic Press.

Harder, D. W. (1992). A construct validation study of the Haan defense scales. *Journal of Clinical Psychology, 48*(5), 606–616.

Hayes, S. C., Strosahl, K., & Wilson, K. G. (1999). *Acceptance and commitment therapy: An experiential approach to behavior change.* New York: Guilford Press.

Kortte, K. B. & Wegener, S. T. (2004). Denial of illness in medical rehabilitation populations: Theory, research, and definition. *Rehabilitation Psychology, 49*(3), 187–199.

Krantz, S. E. (1983). Cognitive appraisals and problem-directed coping: A prospective
study of stress. *Journal of Personality & Social Psychology, 44*(3), 638–643.

Lazarus, R. S. (1966). *Psychological stress and the coping process.* New York:
McGraw-Hill.

Lazarus, R. S. (1983). The costs and benefits of denial. In S. Breznitz (Ed.), *The denial
of stress* (pp. 1–30). New York: International Universities Press.

Lazarus, R. S. (1991). *Emotion and adaptation.* New York: Oxford University Press.

Lazarus, R. S. (1995). Cognition and emotion from the RET viewpoint. *Journal of
Rational-Emotive & Cognitive-Behavior Therapy, 13*(1), 29–54.

Lazarus, R. S., & Folkman, S. (1984). *Stress, appraisal, and coping.* New York: Springer.

Lazarus, R. S., & Folkman, S. (1987). Transactional theory and research on emotions and
coping. *European Journal of Personality, 1*, 141–169.

McGrath, J. E. (1970). *Social and psychological factors in stress.* New York: Houghton-
Mifflin.

Menninger, K. (1954). Regulatory devices of the ego under major stress. *International
Journal of Psychoanalysis, 35*(4), 412–420.

Menninger, K. A. (1963). *The vital balance: The life process in mental health and illness.*
New York: Viking.

Miller, S. (1980). When is a little information a dangerous thing? Coping with stressful
events by monitoring vs. blunting. In S. Levine & H. Ursin (Eds.), *Coping and health*
(pp. 145–170). New York: Plenum.

Morrisey, R. F. (1977). The Haan model of ego functioning: An assessment of empirical
research. In N. Haan (Ed.), *Coping and defending: Processes of self-environment
organization* (pp. 250–279). New York: Academic Press.

Moskowitz, J. T., Folkman, S., Collette, L., & Vittinghoff, E. (1996). Coping and mood
during AIDS-related caregiving and bereavement. *Annals of Behavioral Medicine, 18*,
49–57.

Nersessian, E., & Kopff, R. G. (1996). *Textbook of psychoanalysis.* Washington, DC:
American Psychiatric Press.

Pargament, K. I. (1996). Religious methods of coping: Resources for the conservation
and transformation of significance. In E. P. Shafranske (Ed.), *Religion and the clinical
practice of psychology* (pp. 215–240). Washington, DC: American Psychological
Association.

Park, C. L., & Folkman, S. (1997). Meaning in the context of stress and coping. *Review
of General Psychology, 1*(2), 115–144.

Pearlin, L. I., & Schooler, C. (1978). The structure of coping. *Journal of Health and
Social Behavior, 9*, 3–21.

Piaget, J. (1962). *Play, dreams, and imitation in childhood.* New York: Norton.

Powers, W. T. (1973). *Behavior: The control of perception.* Chicago: Aldine.

Pretzer, J. L., Beck, A. T., & Newman, C. F. (2002). Stress and stress management:
A cognitive view. In R. L. Leahy & E. T. Dowd (Eds.), *Clinical advances in cognitive
psychotherapy: Theory and application* (pp. 345–360). New York: Springer Publishing
Company.

Selye, H. (1976). *Stress in health and disease.* Reading, MA: Butterworths.

Shapiro, K. J. (1998). *Animal models of human psychology.* Seattle: Hogrefe & Huber.

Sharoff, K. (2004). *Coping skills therapy for managing chronic and terminal illness.* New
York: Springer Publishing Co.

Stroebe, M., & Schut, H. (1999). The dual process model of coping with bereavement: rationale and description. *Death Studies, 23*(3), 197–224.

Stroebe, M. S., & Schut, H. (2001). Meaning making in the dual process model of coping with bereavement. In R. Neimeyer (Ed.), *Meaning reconstruction and the experience of loss*. Washington, DC: American Psychological Association.

Tait, R., & Silver, R. C. (1989). Coming to terms with major negative life events. In J. S. Uleman & J. A. Bargh (Ed.), *Unintended thought* (pp. 351–382). New York: Guilford.

Thompson, S. C., & Janigian, A. S. (1988). Life schemes: A framework for understanding the search for meaning. *Journal of Social and Clinical Psychology, 7*, 260–280.

Tunis, S. L. (1991). Casual explanations in psychotherapy: Evidence for target- and domain-specific schematic patterns. In M. Horowitz (Ed.), *Person schemas and maladaptive interpersonal patterns* (pp. 261–276). Chicago: University of Chicago Press.

Ursin, H. (1980). Personality, activation, and somatic health: a new psychosomatic theory. In S. Levine & H. Ursin (Eds.), *Coping and health* (pp. 259–279). New York: Plenum Press.

Vaillant, G. E. (1977). *Adaptation to life*. Boston, MA: Little, Brown.

Vaillant, G. E. (1992). *Ego mechanisms of defense: A guide for clinicians and researchers.* Washington: American Psychiatric Association.

Zajonc, R. B. (1980). Feeling and thinking: Preferences need no inferences. *American Psychologist, 35*, 151–175.

Zajonc, R. B. (1984). On the primacy of affect. *American Psychologist, 39*, 117–123.

Zautra, A. J., Sheets, V. L., & Sandler, I. N. (1996). An examination of the construct validity of coping dispositions for a sample of recently divorced mothers. *Psychological Assessment, 8*, 256–264.

3
Hierarchical Coping: A Conceptual Framework for Understanding Coping Within the Context of Chronic Illness and Disability

Julie Chronister and Fong Chan

A considerable amount of interest in the construct *coping* has occurred over the past several decades (Billings & Moos, 1981; Byrne, 1964; Carver, Scheier, & Weintraub, 1989; Krohne, 1996; Lazarus & Folkman, 1984; Mullen & Suls, 1982; Pearlin & Schooler, 1978; Roth & Cohen, 1986). Emerging from the literature is a broad and complex conceptualization of coping, which generally refers to an array of dispositions, strategies, or efforts that people draw on or utilize, when faced with life stressors, in order to increase a sense of well-being and to avoid being harmed by stressful demands. Definitions of the construct encompass a range of personal dispositions, including stable and enduring traits, habitual styles or behavioral patterns, as well as situation-specific cognitive and behavioral efforts that are applied in a given circumstance. The most frequently-cited hypothesis is that coping – in any form – albeit a disposition, style, or effort, is a mediator or moderator of stress and well-being, which explains, in part, the persistent and theoretically-troubling, weak association between stress and well-being.

The taxonomic structure of coping is complex and multi-leveled. Krohne (1996) organized coping formulations into a hierarchical manner with broad, trans-situational coping dispositions comprising a higher level or *macroanalytic* category, and situation-specific, variable coping efforts comprising lower level or *microanalytic* categories. This hierarchical framework allows for the grouping of specific microanalytic coping efforts into broad macroanalytic coping categories. According to Krohne (1996), the macroanalytic approach "operates at a higher level of aggregation, or abstraction, thus concentrating on more fundamental constructs in coping research" (p. 384). In contrast, the microanalytic approach entails a large number of specific coping strategies (Krohne, 1996; Laux & Weber, 1990; Lazarus & Folkman, 1987). See Figure 3.1 for Krohne's (1993) hierarchical model of coping.

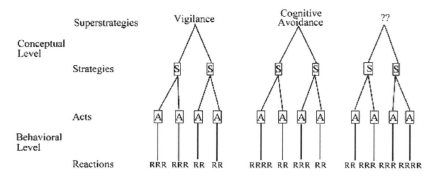

FIGURE 3.1. Krohne's Hierarchical coping model. (Adapted from Krohne, 1993)

There is some debate regarding how these coping levels should be investigated. Although Krohne's hierarchical model illustrates that different conceptual approaches lead to different behavioral strategies, rarely do coping formulations encompass all levels of the hierarchy. Most often, scholars define and investigate one level of coping. Some argue the emphasis should be on lower-level coping mechanisms, because higher-level coping is not situation-specific, and therefore does not adequately explain or predict the variability in coping behavior (Folkman, Lazarus, Dunkel-Schetter, DeLongis, & Gruen, 1986a; Lazarus & Folkman, 1987). Indeed, coping at the microanalytic level involves a more complex analysis of the transactional and temporal sequence of the stress–coping process. Nonetheless, others argue that microanalytic coping conceptions lack a theoretical basis, and that to understand and change a person's specific coping strategy, "a mere description of actual coping behavior with its antecedents and consequences is not satisfactory... Instead, it is crucial to identify the rules that the system follows in regulating itself, and this is only possible when the crucial effect mechanisms [macroanalytic concept] that this process is based on have been previously identified" (Krohne, 1996, pp. 382–383).

Krohne's framework of hierarchical coping offers a comprehensive yet parsimonious way to organize this multifaceted construct. Therefore, the present chapter will review the history and theoretical background of various coping models that comprise components of this framework, including various macroanalytic and microanalytic coping models. In addition, this chapter will provide a review of the empirical findings regarding these models and conclude with a discussion of the application of these models within the context of CID.

Theoretical and Historical Background

Macroanalytic Orientation

The explication of coping from the macroanalytic perspective has a long theoretical and empirical history with roots in psychoanalytic and phenomenological theories (Freud, 1957; Lewin, 1951). Generally, macroanalytic approaches depict coping as a personality trait or disposition that consistently emerge in antic- ipation of or in recovery from stressful events. For example, coping may include habitual preferences, such as withdrawing or moving closer to a person, denying or dwelling on difficulties, taking an active or reactive stance, or blaming others rather than oneself. Such coping typologies, by definition, assume some cross-situational, relatively stable problem-solving tendencies in individuals, and are typically described as "partial area" theories, whereby the models do not cover the full range of possible coping strategies, but concentrate on two specific, albeit fundamental, dimensions of coping (Krohne, 1996).

To date, numerous macroanalytic models exist (i.e., Byrne, 1964; Krohne, 1996; McGlashan, Levy, & Carpenter, 1975; Miller, 1987; Mullen & Suls, 1982; Roth & Cohen, 1986; Shontz, 1975). These models are generally dimensional conceptualizations and include such formulations as perceptual defense – perceptual vigilance (Bruner & Postman, 1947), repression – sensitization (Byrne, 1961), denial – intrusion (Horowitz, 1976), avoidance – vigilance (Cohen & Lazarus, 1973; Janis, 1977), monitoring – blunting (Miller, 1980), attention – rejection (Mullen & Suls, 1982), and vigilance – cognitive avoidance (Krohne, 1993). Macroanalytic models that are specific to recovery from trauma include Shontz' (1975) coping with disability models of retreat – encounter and fragmentation – containment, Horowitz's (1976, 1979) denial – intrusion mode, and McGlashan and colleagues' (1975) coping with schizophrenia model of integration – sealing. Theoretically, most of these models posit a curvilinear relationship between the bi-polar dimensions and emotional adjustment, with higher adjustment for those in the middle area of the distribution (Krohne, 1996).

Although there are a number of different macroanalytic coping formulations, central to all of these models are the concepts of *approach* and *avoidance* (Roth & Cohen, 1986). According to Roth and Cohen (1986), "one is struck by the extent to which the concepts of approach and avoidance underlie the personality or individual difference variables studied in the anticipatory threat literature, and also the dimensions of coping studied in traumatic stress reaction research" (p. 813). The approach – avoidance conceptualization refers to two basic modes of coping with stress, which involve a psychological orientation either towards or away from threat (Roth & Cohen, 1986). This model can be said to assume the highest conceptual level of the coping hierarchy. Subsumed under this prototypic category are numerous coping formulations, which correspond to this core conceptualization, yet differ in terms of theoretical orientation, motivating principles, measurement, and whether they are framed within the context of coping with anticipatory threat or in reaction to stress.

In the anticipatory threat literature for example, the repression – sensitization (Byrne, 1961) formulation reflects the approach – avoidance paradigm. This bi-polar concept is theoretically grounded in research on perceptual defenses (Bruner & Postman, 1947). Repression is defined as avoidance of anxiety- arousing stimuli and a general orientation away from threat; sensitization is an approach toward anxiety-arousing stimuli and an orientation toward threat monitoring—blunting

(Roth & Cohen, 1986). People who are located more towards the repression pole of this dimension are likely to deny or minimize the stressor or threat, fail to verbalize feelings of anxiety, and avoid thinking about the consequences of this encounter. People falling at the sensitization end of the pole are likely to react to threat or stressors by way of enhanced information search and obsessive and ruminative worrying (Krohne, 1996). Similarly, the monitoring – blunting hypothesis (Miller, 1987) posits that when faced with a threatening situation, individuals tend to moderate their anxiety by either directing their attention away from the stressor, either by employing blunting strategies, such as distraction, denial, or reinterpretation, or monitoring strategies, such as seeking information about the stressor.

In the literature on stress reactions, Horowitz's (1976, 1979) formulated a model of denial – intrusion, which corresponds with the approach – avoidance paradigm. In this model, denial (characterized by numbness, removal of material from consciousness, and avoidance of reminders of the stressor) is driven by the need to protect the ego from the impact of the stressful event, whereas intrusions (e.g., nightmares, negative feelings, and being reminded of the stressor from numerous external stimulus) involve an "intrinsic tendency towards repetition of representations of contents" (Roth & Cohen, 1986, p. 93). In this model, there can be vacillating periods of denial and intrusion, which ultimately become less powerful. Adaptation involves 'working through' the stressful event, which allows for a complete integration of the stressor (Roth & Cohen, 1986).

Without question, macroanalytic coping models have been central to the development and explication of coping. Nonetheless, scholars (Folkman & Lazarus, 1985; Krohne, 1996; Roth & Cohen, 1986) have criticized these approaches for weak discriminant validity, lack of explanatory power, and situational variability. For example, studies have shown that the repression – sensitization conception cannot be discriminated from other trait-based constructs, such as anxiety and defensiveness. In addition, many of the bi-polar anticipatory-threat models allow only for an explanation of those individuals who fall on either pole, but not for those that may utilize both approaches. Indeed, the accumulated knowledge about macroanalytic coping models suggests that approach- and avoidant-oriented coping tendencies are not mutually exclusive; people can not simply be placed in one category or the other, because most individuals use strategies from both (Roth & Cohen, 1986).

Finally, although these models posit situational invariability, research in this area is mixed (Averill & Rosenn, 1972; Cohen & Roth, 1984; Spence, 1957; Stein, 1953). Critics (Folkman et al., 1986a; Lazarus & Folkman, 1984) argue that these higher-order coping constructs cannot adequately explain the situational variability in coping behaviors, acts, and reactions, and are therefore considered unsuitable for adequately explaining or predicting the variability in coping behavior.

In response to these limitations, Krohne developed the personality model of coping modes (Krohne, 1993). This model considers the multiple levels of coping and addresses the necessity of providing an explanatory, theoretically based model. The core concepts of this model, *vigilance* (the intensified intake and processing of threatening information) and *cognitive avoidance* (the turning away from threat-related cues) correspond to the approach – avoidance prototype, yet differ from other personality-oriented coping models in several ways.

First, this model attempts to provide a more in-depth definition and explanation of the central constructs of vigilance and cognitive avoidance. Specifically, Krohne (1993, 1996) defines threatening situations as those which involve the presence of aversive stimuli and a high degree of ambiguity. These components correspond to specific reactions that are elicited in people, who are confronted with threatening situations; namely, the perception of emotional arousal (caused by the presence of aversive stimuli) and the experience of uncertainty (related to ambiguity). Krohne explained dispositional preferences for vigilance and cognitive avoidance by the constructs *intolerance of uncertainty* and *intolerance of emotional arousal*. Krohne proposed that individuals habitually vary in the extent to which they can tolerate uncertainty or emotional arousal, with individuals high in intolerance of uncertainty tending to employ vigilant coping, and those high in intolerance of emotional arousal using more cognitive avoidant strategies.

Similar to Byrne's "sensitizing" term and Miller's "monitoring" term, Krohne's model suggests that people, who use vigilant coping strategies, are especially sensitive to ambiguity. As a response, their primary concern is to construct a cognitive schema of the impending threat to avoid a "negative surprise." Consequently, people, who are dispositionally vigilant, tend to manifest a relatively consistent vigilant behavior and direct their attention continuously to threat–relevant information. Conversely, similar to Byrne's (1961) "repression" term and Miller's (1980) "blunting" term, those who employ cognitive avoidance utilize a class of coping strategies aimed at shielding the person from situations that induce emotional arousal. For these individuals, the emotional arousal produced by threatening situations is the central problem. They manage these situations by ignoring threatening cues and enduring the subsequent increase of uncertainty, because it is not particularly stressful for them.

A second aspect of this model that differs from other macroanalytic approaches is that Krohne (1993) delineated vigilance and cognitive avoidance to be conceptually separate personality dimensions, wherein the employment of one coping strategy does not preclude employment of the other. In Krohne's model, the specific configuration of a person's standing on both personality dimensions (e.g., high vigilance and low cognitive avoidance) is called "coping mode." See Figure 3.2 for schematic depiction. This model allows for making the distinction between vigilant coping and truly low anxious individuals, as well as avoidant coping and highly anxious individuals. Further, it gives those, who fall in the middle, a more defined status, wherein a person in the middle range may use an increased amount of both vigilance and cognitive avoidance; whereas an individual, who does not fall in the middle range, may tend toward using either form of coping (Krohne, 1996).

Cognitive Avoidance/Vigilance

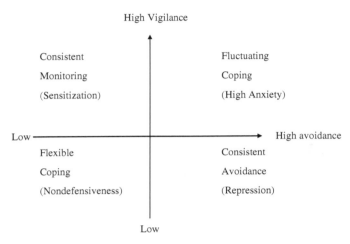

FIGURE 3.2. Krohne's Model of coping modes. (Adapted from Krohne, 1996.)

Third, although Krohne concentrated primarily on the explication of two specific higher-order concepts, he delineated a hierarchical model that includes both the macroanalytic, conceptual levels of coping, as well as the microanalytic, behavioral levels of coping. Specifically, Krohne outlined several behavioral coping groups, which included coping strategies, acts, and reactions, each of which is postulated to include various behaviors (Krohne, 1989). For example, the coping strategy "distraction from threatening cues" can manifest itself in different acts (e.g., listening to music with closed eyes or participating in an animated discussion), which may not only be directed at different partial goals, but also can be distinguished with regard to individual reaction components and their respective arrangements. Strategies, in turn, can also be categorized into behavioral classes of a higher order, or *superstrategies*. Examples of super-strategies include vigilance, approach, avoidance, monitoring or blunting.

Krohne cautions that the hierarchy described (i.e., reaction, act, strategy, superstrategy) is not meant to be a functional model that conceptualizes qualitatively different processes and their functional relationships. Instead, he describes this model as a "philosophy of science" approach, in that it gives an idea how to organize and differentiate the concepts that must be taken into account when analyzing coping. This model emphasizes the importance of distinguishing between observable behaviors (reactions and acts) and theoretical concepts (strategies and superstrategies). Further, it stresses that behaviors do not necessarily correspond neatly with theoretical classes.

Finally, Krohne (1989, 1996) acknowledged the transactional nature of the stress – coping process in his model. Specifically, he posited that the process of dealing with stress involves the selection of strategies, the employment of coping

Process of dealing w/ Stress

reactions or acts, and processing the potential consequences of these coping behaviors – the latter of which provides feedback to the individual that governs both the future process of coping and the emotional experience accompanying the stress process (Krohne, 1989).

The fundamental principles guiding macroanalytic coping models are that stable coping styles exist and these preferred ways of coping derive from traditional personality dimensions, such as approach – avoidance (Carver et al., 1989). With the advent of the "cognitive revolution," coupled with Lazarus and Folkman's (1984) transactional model of coping and mixed empirical support for personality-oriented models, a new direction in coping formulation and measurement emerged (Cohen & Lazarus, 1973; Folkman & Moskowitz, 2004). These approaches moved away from the psychodynamic models of defense to include a wider range of microanalytic level cognitive and behavioral responses that individuals use to manage stress (Folkman & Moskowitz, 2004). Today, these models maintain central stage in the literature and will be described below.

Microanalytic Orientation

The microanalytic level of coping entails more specific types of emotional, behavioral, and cognitive efforts that are used in anticipation of, response to, and recovery from stress. In Krohne's hierarchical framework, these include the lower level behavioral acts and reactions. Major contributors in this area include Lazarus and colleagues (Lazarus & Folkman, 1984), Carver and colleagues (Carver et al., 1989), Pearlin and colleagues (Pearlin, Menaghan, Lieberman, & Mullan, 1981; Pearlin & Schooler, 1978), Billings and Moos (1981, 1982), Stone and Neale (1984), McCrae (1984), and Endler and Parker (1990). These models are generally considered state- versus trait-oriented, and emphasize situational variability and processing. Microanalytic coping investigators typically analyze types of coping strategies that are used in specified contexts and their effectiveness.

A number of researchers have attempted to identify the basic dimensions of coping behavior at the microanalytic level. The most commonly cited dimensions include *emotion-focused* and *problem-focused* coping. Indeed, most of the current coping scales tap these two coping dimensions in some way (e.g., Billings & Moos, 1981, 1984; Carver et al., 1989; Folkman & Lazarus, 1980, 1985; Pearlin & Schooler, 1978). Pivotal to the development of these dimensions is the work of Lazarus and colleagues (Folkman & Lazarus, 1980, 1985), who used a rational approach to distinguish these two major, theory-based functions of coping. They posited that problem-focused coping involves addressing the problem that is causing distress, and includes such strategies as making a plan of action or concentrating on the next step. Emotion-focused coping involves ameliorating the negative emotions that are associated with the problem, and may include such strategies as engaging in distracting activities, acceptance, using alcohol or drugs, or seeking emotional support (Folkman & Moskowitz, 2004). According to Endler and Parker (1990), problem-focused coping is considered more task-oriented, whereas emotion-focused coping is more person-orientated. Lazarus and colleagues believe that people use *both* functions in stressful situations, which underscores the inadequacy of macroanalytic bipolar conceptualizations.

Although these two coping dimensions have been used extensively in the coping literature (Folkman & Moskowitz, 2004), there is disagreement about which specific coping responses constitute these domains. Critics argue that these two domains are limiting and not empirically stable (Carver et al., 1989). For example, studies have shown that Lazarus and Folkman's coping scale measures several factors, rather than just two (Aldwin, Folkman, Schaefer, Coyne, & Lazarus, 1980; Folkman & Lazarus, 1985; Scheier, Weintraub, & Carver, 1986). Scheier et al. (1986) found that factors other than problem-focused coping, which are typically considered variations of emotion-focused coping, often diverge significantly and are inversely correlated. For example, some emotion-focused responses involve denial, while others involve positive reinterpretation of events, and still others involve seeking out social support. Similarly, problem-focused coping can potentially involve several distinct activities, such as planning, taking direct action, seeking assistance, screening out other activities, and sometimes even forcing oneself to wait before acting. Carver et al. (1989) suggested that these responses are distinctly different from each other, and may have very different implications for a person's success in coping.

Consequently, additional dimensions have emerged in the literature such as avoidance coping and meaning-focused coping. Avoidance coping has a long research history, which dates back to the traditional macroanalytic paradigms that were discussed earlier. This construct developed as a result of the finding that avoidance coping can include either problem-focused or emotion-focused coping strategies (Endler & Parker, 1990). Particularly, individuals may avoid a stressful situation by getting support from other people (emotion-focused) or by engaging in another task rather than the task at hand (problem-focused). In regards to appraisal or meaning-making coping, Park and Folkman (1997) proposed that people draw on values, beliefs, and goals to modify the meaning of a stressful transaction. This may be true, especially in cases of chronic stress, which may not be amenable to problem-focused efforts (Folkman & Moskowitz, 2004). Gottlieb and Gignac (1996) found that meaning-making coping, which can include making causal attributions and searching for meaning in adversity, were coping strategies that caregivers most frequently reported as a way of coping with the behavior of care-recipients who had dementia.

There are a number of conceptualizations that coincide with the dimensions discussed above. For example, Pearlin and Schooler (1978) categorized coping behaviors into three major domains: (a) Responses that change the situation (problem-focused coping), (b) responses that change the meaning or the appraisal of the stress (meaning-making coping), and (c) responses aimed at controlling distressful feelings (emotion-focused coping). Billings and Moos (1981) conceptualized coping to include two components of problem-focused coping (active-behavioral and active cognitive coping) and one form of emotion-focused coping (avoidance coping). Later, Billings and Moos (1984) extended their work and developed a new classification scheme which had three domains of coping responses: (a) appraisal-focused coping, (b) problem-focused coping, and (c) emotion-focused coping. Endler and Parker (1990) conceptualized coping to include three dimensions: (a) task-oriented coping, (b) emotion-oriented coping, and (c) avoidant-oriented coping.

Finally, Carver et al. (1989) formulated a model of coping that included numerous distinct coping acts and behaviors, which could not necessarily be subsumed under two or three dimensions. Their model includes 13 theoretically derived scales that are differentiated primarily by their functional properties and include the following coping strategies: Active coping, planning, suppression of competing activities, restraint coping, seeking social support for instrumental reasons, seeking social support for emotional reasons, focusing on and venting emotions, behavioral disengagement, mental disengagement, acceptance, turning to religion, denial and alcohol-drug disengagement. While Carver et al. (1989) suggested that these dimension not be organized into broader emotion or problem-focused coping, these scales are often conceptualized in this manner in coping studies.

A more comprehensive formulation of coping was conceptualized by Moos and Schaefer (1993). They combined coping efforts and orientations into an integrated conceptualization by separating coping into macroanalytic-type approach and avoidance domains, and then dividing these domains into lower level cognitive and behavioral coping efforts. Accordingly, they proposed four basic types of coping processes: (a) *Cognitive approach coping*, which includes logical analysis and positive reappraisal; (b) *behavioral approach coping*, which includes seeking guidance and support and taking concrete action to deal directly with a situation or its aftermath; (c) *cognitive avoidance coping*, which comprises responses aimed at denying or minimizing the seriousness of a crisis or its consequences, as well as accepting a situation as it is and deciding that the basic circumstances cannot be altered; and (d) *behavioral avoidance coping*, which covers seeking alternate sources of satisfaction, wherein the person attempts to replace the loss involved in a crisis by becoming involved in new activities (Moos & Schaefer, 1993). This formulation incorporates a higher level, conceptual framework, as well as lower level coping actions and reactions – a model that supports a hierarchical formulation of coping.

Empirical Findings

Macroanalytic Models

Numerous studies have been conducted to determine the efficacy of approach versus avoidant coping styles. Although conclusions are difficult to draw due to the diversity in coping conceptualizations, measurement approaches,

avoidant Coping better for short-term stress
approach strategies are better in the long run.

all research studies were the same

outcomes, and types of stressors (Roth & Cohen, 1986), several findings consistently emerge, which are important in evaluating and understanding the effectiveness of macroanalytic coping models. First, researchers, who examined the efficacy of approach versus avoidance-oriented coping, have found no evidence that one strategy is better than the other (Suls & Fletcher, 1985; Thompson, 1981; Zeidner & Saklofske, 1996). Results from a meta-analytic review, which examined the efficacy of these coping orientations, show no strong evidence favoring either approach or avoidant coping (Suls & Fletcher, 1985). Additionally, in a lengthy review of reactions to stressful life events, Silver and Wortman (1980) concluded that there were no coping strategies that were uniformly effective.

Differences occur, however, when contextual and temporal factors are taken into consideration. Researchers have concluded that the point in time in which effectiveness is evaluated, the controllability of aspects of the stressful situation, and the fit between coping style and certain demands of the situations contribute to determining the efficacy of approach versus avoidant-coping styles.

In regards to time, a commonly held view in the literature is that avoidant strategies are considered more efficacious in the short-term or at an early stage of coping, whereas approach strategies are more effective in the long term at a later stage of recovery (Lazarus, 1983; Mullen & Suls, 1982; Shontz, 1975). The most compelling evidence comes from the work of Mullen & Suls (1982), who found a consistent pattern in two meta-analytic studies that avoidant coping was found to be effective when outcome measures were immediate or short-term, whereas approach strategies were found to be more effective when the outcome measures were long-term. Similarly, Wolff, Friedman, Hofer, and Mason (1964) found support for this concept in a study looking at parents of children with leukemia. In this study, parents who used avoidant strategies exhibited lower levels of corticosteroid secretion during the child's illness, than parents who did not use avoidant strategies. In contrast, nine months later, parents who had high secretion levels before the child's death, now had lower secretion levels. The implication is that avoidant strategies may have short-term benefits, but approach strategies are more beneficial in the long run (Hofer, Wolff, Friedman, & Mason, 1972).

These results are consistent with several theoretical perspectives. For example, Lazarus (1983) proposed that people may need to use avoidant strategies when initially faced with stressful events, because approach strategies may be too overwhelming. As time passes, the individual may be more capable of success-fully confronting the situation using approach strategies. In a similar vein, Horowitz's (1983) concept of "working through" a life stressor implies that at the outset the initial stressful information may be avoided because it does not fit with the individual's internal schema, but as the stressful experience continues, information will gradually be accepted. Horowitz's main point is that initial avoidant strategies are typically followed by a phase-like incorporation of new information until the stressor has been assimilated.

coping oriented

These perspectives about the temporal aspects of coping also provide some indirect support for models of stress adaptation (Crohn, 1962; Kubler-Ross, 1969; Livneh, 1986; Wright, 1983), whereby avoidant strategies are employed first, because they provide more benefits than approach strategies in the initial interval, but over time are replaced with approach strategies, which become more beneficial in the long-term. It has been suggested that long-term, enduring stressors require approach strategies, because continued use of avoidant tactics will prevent change and consume substantial effort, which over time, can deplete the individual's psychological and physical resources (Glass & Singer, 1972).

One exception to the proposition – that avoidant coping is more efficacious in the short-term than approach coping – is the perspective that an individual's interpretation set (i.e., whether the person uses emotional or sensory appraisals) should be considered. According to Leventhal and Everhart's (1980) parallel-processing model of emotion, a threatening event can be processed in terms of its emotional significance or in terms of its sensory elements.

Leventhal, Brown, Shacham, and Engquist (1979) found that individuals, who are instructed to focus on sensory elements during a stressful event, report less distress than individuals told to emote about the experience. Other empirical studies support this notion. For example, in Suls and Fletcher's meta-analytical study (1985), they found that in the short-term, individuals who used approach strategies that involved sensory interpretation rather than avoidant strategies, reflected better short-term health-related outcomes. Thus, approach tactics can be useful in the short-term, when they involve attending to sensory information instead of emotional processing. Often, however, sensory aspects are not easily identified and thus result in an emotional response, suggesting the need for intervention in this area (Suls & Fletcher, 1985). These results are consistent with models that emphasize the importance of the interpretation or appraisal when faced with stress (Lazarus, 1966).

In regards to the controllability of a situation, studies suggest that avoidant strategies are considered most useful in uncontrollable situations, whereas approach strategies are most effective in a controllable situation (Roth & Cohen, 1986). It is presumed that approach strategies allow an individual to take advantage of opportunities for control, if present. Katz, Weiner, Gallagher and Hellman (1970) found that people, who used avoidant strategies, delayed seeking diagnostic evaluations for breast cancer, and thus reduced their chances of effective intervention if they did have cancer. Similarly, Staudenmeyer, Kinsman, Dirks, Spector, and Wangaard (1979) found that people, who had asthma and who approached the onset of an attack, had fewer serious attacks than those who avoided. Lazarus (1983) concluded from these and related studies that coping effectiveness depends on controllability of the situation. Specifically, some illnesses, such as asthma, diabetes, and cancer, require approach strategies for appropriate treatment, whereas with uncontrollable illnesses, such as paralysis or traumatic brain injury, using avoidant strategies may provide advantages, such as a possible reduction of anxiety (Roth & Cohen, 1986).

Another area that has received empirical investigation is the trans-situational consistency of macroanalytic coping, or the salience of the fit between coping strategies used and the specific demands of the situation. Results in this area are generally mixed (Averill & Rosenn, 1972; Roth & Cohen, 1986; Stein, 1957). Averill and Rosenn (1972) found support for trans-situational consistency of coping strategies in a study in which participants under duress were given either approach or avoidant coping options. The results indicated that in the situations, which demanded a certain coping style, the majority of the participants continued to use another strategy. Similarly, researchers have found a high degree of consistency in coping responses over time among participants coping with abortion (Roth & Cohen, 1986) and cancer (Roth & Robinson, 1992). Importantly, studies in this area have found that, while people have utilized approach and avoidance coping in a highly consistent manner, utilization was not mutually exclusive; specifically, people could not simply be characterized as either using approach or avoidance, because most participants used strategies from both categories. It has been suggested that a vacillation between these coping approaches occurs throughout the stress process, with certain aspects of threatening material being avoided, while other aspects are approached. Indeed, research is sorely needed to shed light on the question of individual consistency in coping styles across time and situations (Byrne & Holcomb, 1962).

Microanalytic Models

Microanalytic models of coping have benefited from numerous empirical studies. Nonetheless, determining coping effectiveness at the microanalytic level is one of the most perplexing issues in coping research, due to its inter-action with contextual and dynamic factors (Somerfield & McCrae, 2000). Historically, studies have suggested that problem-focused coping is "adaptive," whereas emotion-focused and avoidant-focused coping are considered more "non-adaptive" (Billings & Moos, 1981; Dusenburg & Albee, 1988; Folkman, Lazarus, Gruen, & Delongis, 1986b; Sarason, 1973; Sarason & Sarason, 1981). Today, however, there is general consensus that these coping dimensions are not inherently good or bad (Lazarus & Folkman, 1984). Instead, the efficacy of a specific coping strategy is dependent, in large part, on its contextual and temporal nature. Thus, a coping strategy may be effective in one situation or at one point in time during the stress process, but not in another.

Contextual factors that have been studied include the type of stressor (work, death, illness, divorce, and caregiving), the psychological appraisal of the stressor (threat, loss, challenge), as well as the appraised controllability of the situation. Researchers have examined what strategies are used most often in these situations and their efficacy. For example, Folkman and Lazarus (1980) found that work-related stressors were associated with increased problem-focused coping, while illness-related stressors were associated with increased emotion-focused coping. They also have found that fewer problem-focused coping responses were used when coping with death, as compared to coping with an illness.

Conversely, Billings and Moos (1981) found that illness-related stressors elicited more problem-focused coping than did other categories, and death-related stress elicited the least amount of all coping strategies. Studies have also suggested that problem-focused coping tends to be highly variable across situations, whereas emotion-focused coping is more stable, suggesting that problem-focused coping is particularly responsive to contextual factors, whereas emotion-focused coping is more heavily influenced by personal factors (Folkman & Moskowitz, 2004).

An important contextual factor that has received considerable attention is the person's appraisal of the situation as a loss, threat, or challenge (Folkman & Lazarus, 1980). According to Lazarus and Launier (1978), a loss is a negative stressor that has occurred in the past; a threat is a negative stressor that is anticipated in the future; and a challenge, although similar to a threat, is generally more positive, but still requires effort from the individual. According to McCrae (1984), losses tend to be acute in nature, whereas threats and challenges are more likely to be chronic. Studies have shown that these appraisals affect the individual's choice of coping strategies. McCrae (1984) found that individuals experiencing a loss used faith, fatalism, and expression of feelings most frequently; whereas, when facing a threat, individuals most frequently used wishful thinking, faith, and fatalism. When faced with a challenge, individuals have been found to adopt a diverse number of coping strategies, including rational action, perseverance, positive thinking, intellectual denial, restraint, drawing strength from adversity, and humor.

Another contextual factor commonly studied is the controllability of the situation. The fit between the appraisal of controllability and coping is sometimes referred to as the goodness of fit (Conway & Terry, 1992; Folkman & Lazarus, 1980; Zeidner & Saklofske, 1996). Theoretically, appraisals of control demand more active, instrumental, problem-focused forms of coping, while appraisals of lack of control demand more emotion-focused coping (Folkman & Moskowitz, 2004). Therefore, it is presumed that people, who choose coping strategies that fit the appraised controllability of a stressor, will experience better outcomes than those who do not. Nonetheless, there is mixed support for this hypothesis (Folkman & Moskowitz, 2004).

Pearlin and Schooler (1978) found that stressful circumstances, over which one had little control, were less amenable to problem-focused coping. In a study of hemodialysis patients and adherence, Christensen, Benotch, Wiebe and Lawton (1995) found that coping involving planful problem-solving was linked to better adherence, when the stressor involved a controllable aspect of hemodialysis. For stressors that were less controllable, emotional self-control, a form of emotion-focused coping, was linked to better adherence. In a study of women coping with in-vitro fertilization, which was considered uncontrollable, Terry and Hynes (1998) found that direct attempts to manage the problem (a form of problem-focused coping) was related to poorer adjustment, and emotion-focused coping was related to better adjustment. Park, Folkman and Bostrom (2001) found support for the fit between problem-focused coping and controllability in a sample of HIV+ men, but the evidence for a fit between the emotion-focused coping and lack of control was less strong. Conversely, Macrodimitris and Endler (2001) found a link between lower perceived control and high emotion-oriented coping for the psychological adjustment of people with type 2 diabetes, but did not find evidence for the fit between higher perceived control and instrumental coping in this group.

The dynamic nature of the stress process also plays a role in how coping effectiveness is determined. Specifically, what might be considered effective coping at the beginning of a stressful situation may be less effective as time passes. Further, studies have found that the coping process typically includes both problem-focused and emotion-focused functions, suggesting that people use different strategies at different stages of the coping process (Folkman & Lazarus, 1980, 1985). Researchers propose, for example, that in preparing for an exam, it is adaptive to engage in problem-focused coping prior to the exam and to distance oneself while waiting for the results (Folkman & Lazarus, 1985). Conversely, when dealing with a major loss, such as the death of a spouse, it may be adaptive initially to engage in some emotional coping to deal with the loss and then later, after emotional equilibrium has been restored, to engage in more instrumental coping, in order to deal with future plans (Stroebe & Schut, 2001).

Numerous studies have also looked at the role of personal factors in coping. This area has assumed less importance over the years as context and temporality have assumed greater roles. Nonetheless, studies have suggested that factors, such as age, gender, education, income, personality, and psychological functioning, affect the types of strategies used and moderate their level of effectiveness.

In regards to gender, it has been posited that women are more emotionally responsive and sensitive, while men tend to be more analytic and task-oriented. Thus, women are presumed to use emotion-oriented coping more often, and are less likely to use problem-oriented coping than men (Billings & Moos, 1981). Findings in gender-related differences have been mixed and often confounded by type of stressor experienced. For example, Billings and Moos (1981) found that woman used problem-, avoidance-, and emotion-focused coping more frequently than did men, and that these strategies were less effective in attenuating the depressive effects of stress.

In a study investigating how men and woman coped with stressful events of daily living over the course of a year, Folkman and Lazarus (1980) found that women used less effective coping methods than men; yet, the gender differences in coping were relatively small after controlling for the source of stressors. Endler and Parker (1990) found that women used more emotion- and avoidant-coping than men. However, when examining within-group differences, men used more problem-focused than emotion-focused or avoidant coping, and women used more problem- than emotion-focused coping, more problem than avoidant coping, and more emotion than avoidant coping. Stone and Neale (1984) found that men used significantly more direct action, whereas women used more distraction, catharsis, seeking social support, relaxation, religion, and other types of coping. Studies have also suggested that people with more education and higher income are more likely to use problem-focused coping and are less likely to use avoidance coping. For example, Cronkite and Moos (1984) found that problem-focused forms of coping were more prevalent among better educated men.

A number of studies suggest that psychological functioning and personality traits play a role in the effectiveness of coping. For example, studies show that people with depression use more emotion-focused coping than do non-depressed individuals (Billings, Cronkite, & Moos, 1983; Billings & Moos, 1984, 1985; Mitchell, Cronkite, & Moos, 1983; Rosenberg, Peterson, & Hayes, 1987). Specifically, Rosenberg et al. found that people with higher levels of depression reported more use of confrontive coping, self-control, escape avoidance, self-blame, and emotionally reacting with more disgust/anger and worry/fear, than those who reported fewer symptoms.

Billings and Moos (1981) found that the use of avoidant strategies were associated with greater depression, whereas the use of active or approach strategies attenuated the effects of depression on stressful events. Endler and Parker (1990) also found a positive link between depression and anxiety and emotion-focused coping for both men and women, and a negative link between problem-focused coping and depression and anxiety. Similarly, Mitchell and Hodson (1983) found a negative relationship between problem-focused behaviors and depression, and a positive relationship between avoidant coping and depression. Finally, studies have also suggested that Type A behavior is associated with avoidant-coping behaviors (Greenglass, 1988). Specifically, it has been show that Type A individuals have a tendency to use more denial and cognitive avoidance strategies than Type B individuals (Pittner, Housten, & Spiridigliozzi, 1983; Weidner & Mathews, 1978). Endler (1990) found a positive link between Type A and emotion-focused coping in men and women, and a positive association between Type A behavior and avoidant coping in men.

Coping within the Context of Chronic Illness and Disability

Coping with chronic illness and disability (CID) has been an important research and clinical area in rehabilitation. Most of the research in this area can be considered microanalytic in nature, with a focus on the effect of various cognitive and behavioral strategies on psychosocial adjustment to CID (e.g., Livneh & Wilson, 2003). One exception is Shontz's (1975) model of coping within the context of CID, which can be classified as a macroanalytic model.

Shontz's model is quite similar to Horowitz's (1976, 1979) denial-intrusion model, which was previously mentioned in the macroanalytic model section. In Shontz's model, there are cycles of encounter and retreat, wherein encounter signifies both cognitive and emotional approaches to the stressor, while retreat indicates avoidance of thinking about the trauma and its consequences. Shontz describes the coping process to include intense periods of encounter and retreat, which are gradually replaced by a more stable equilibrium. In this model, adaptation to CID occurs when the threat is safely incorporated into an "integrated self structure" (Shontz, 1975, p. 115). When adaptation does not occur, the person remains either overwhelmed by the threat or may become fragmented, splitting the illness off from the self (Roth & Cohen, 1986).

At the microanalytic level, Wright (1983) advocated that psychosocial adjustment to disability could be considered from a positive coping framework, based on her disability acceptance model. She viewed acceptance of disability as paramount to the psychosocial adjustment of people with traumatic disabilities. In Wright's model, positive coping is related to making the following value shifts toward self-acceptance by: (a) Enlarging the scope of values, (b) subordinating physique relative to other values, (c) containing the effects of disability, and (d) transforming comparative-status values to asset values. Conversely, succumbing (negative coping) is characterized by: (a) Denial, (b) idolizing normal standards, (c) eclipsing behavioral possibilities, and (d) overcompensation.

There is some empirical support for the notion that disability acceptance is related to psychosocial adjustment. Specifically, Linkowski and Dunn (1974) surveyed a sample of undergraduate and graduate students with disabilities and found a significant, moderate, positive correlation between disability acceptance and self-esteem, social relationships, and vocational satisfaction. Heinemann and Shontz (1982) also found a significant and positive correlation between disability acceptance and self-esteem, masculinity, femininity, and achievement among a group of high-school seniors with hearing impairments.

In a sample of individuals with physical disabilities from a VA hospital, Grand (1972) found that participants in the high disability-acceptance group were less anxious, than participants in the low self-acceptance group, in responding to negative reactions from people without disabilities. Osuji (1985, 1987) also found that acceptance of loss was related to completion of an industrial rehabilitation program and counselors' ratings of employability of the participants. More recently, Ferrin (2002) examined the relationships among disability acceptance, self-esteem, and quality of life with people among paraplegia and found that disability acceptance was significantly related to self-esteem, as well as to quality of life.

In a review and synthesis of the phase theories, Livneh (1986) and Livneh and Antonak (2005) suggested that coping and psychosocial adaptation to disability can be conceptualized as progressing through three distinct phases: Earlier (proximal) reactions (shock, anxiety, and denial), intermediate reactions (depression, internalized anger, and externalized hostility), and later (distal) reactions (acknowledgment and adjustment). According to Livneh and Wilson (2003), defense and coping strategies are mobilized during this time, in order to lessen the threat of stressful situations that is related to traumatic injury and chronic illness. Both problem-focused coping and avoidance-coping strategies are deemed appropriate along this psychosocial adaptation continuum. Livneh and Antonak (2005) also viewed self-acceptance as important to psychosocial adjustment to CID, because it signals that the person has cognitively reconciled with or accepted the inescapable existence of the condition, along with its future ramifications.

Livneh and his colleague (e.g., Livneh, 1986, 2000; Livneh & Wilson, 2003) have conducted research on the types of coping that can foster psychosocial adaptation to CID. They found that coping strategies contributed above and beyond disability-related variables (e.g., functionality and visibility) to psychosocial adjustment to CID. They also consistently found problem-focused coping to be the most powerful predictor of psychosocial outcomes, whereas avoidance- focused coping tended to predict poor psychosocial adjustment.

There is a large volume of research investigating the relationship between various microanalytic coping strategies, psychosocial adjustment, and health outcomes among people with CID. For example, Fitchett, Rybarczyk, DeMarco and Nicholas (1999) found a positive relationship between negative religious coping and activities of daily living. Pakenham (1999) showed that coping style predicted adjustment in people with multiple sclerosis. Kosciulek (1994) reported that individuals, who had a family member with a traumatic brain injury, utilized positive reappraisal, and successfully managed family tension, also reported better family adaptation. Finally, Chronister and Chan (2006) found that individuals, who had a family member with a traumatic brain injury and who used problem-focused and avoidant-focused coping, more frequently experienced higher levels of perceived burden.

Within the area of psychiatric rehabilitation, coping has been conceptualized as a skill, as well as a strategy. From this perspective, coping skills help people with severe mental illness address unexpected barriers that block attainment of social goals. Frequently-identified, successful coping skills among people with psychiatric disabilities include medication management, symptom management, sleep management, relaxation, and basic hygiene. Studies have found a positive relationship between these coping skills and quality of life (Corrigan, Rao, & Lam, 2005). A more in-depth review of coping among people with specific disabilities is beyond the scope of this chapter and is provided in other chapters of this book.

successful coping skills.

Conclusion

Considerable research, regarding macroanalytic and microanalytic coping approaches, has occurred over the past several decades. In fact, coping is considered one of the most active research areas in psychology and behavioral medicine (Ptacek & Pierce, 2003). Within the areas of rehabilitation and disability studies, researchers have repeatedly demonstrated a link between coping and adjustment (e.g., Chronister & Chan, 2006; Fitchett et al., 1999; Kosciulek, 1994; Pakenham, 1999). Nonetheless, conclusions are muddled by poor conceptual frameworks, psychometrically-weak coping measures, and reliance on retrospective reports.

Moreover, measuring the effectiveness of these strategies, as well as the contextual, temporal, and dynamic nature of the stress process, adds to the difficulties inherent in coping research. Despite these challenges, the salience of investigating coping with CID cannot be underscored. Chronic illnesses and disabilities can create major life stressors and, therefore, understanding which coping dispositions and strategies are most effective, in regards to acceptance and adjustment to CID and to positive quality of life, remains central to research and practice.

Thus, rehabilitation researchers need to consider a broader and more comprehensive framework, such as Krohne's model of coping modes, which takes into account both the dispositional and the situational aspects of coping, and to test this model with populations of people with CID. Specifically, dispositional or macroanalytic coping styles are personal resources, which should relate to situational or microanalytic coping styles through secondary appraisals. Researchers, then, should focus on assessing both areas of coping, as each may contribute substantially to understanding psychosocial adjustment to CID.

References

Aldwin, C., Folkman, S., Schaefer, C., Coyne J., & Lazarus, R. (1980, September). *Ways of coping: A process measure*. Presented at the 88th annual meeting of the American Psychological Association, Montreal, Quebec, Canada.

Averill, J. R., & Rosenn, M. (1972). Vigilent and nonvigilent coping strategies and psychophysiological stress reactions during anticipation of electric shock. *Journal of Personality and Social Psychology, 23*, 128–141.

Billings, A. G., Cronkite, R. C., & Moos, R. H., (1983). Social-environmental factors in unipolar depression: Comparisons of depressed patients and nondepressed controls. *Journal of Abnormal Psychology, 92*, 119–133.

Billings, A., & Moos, R. H. (1981). The role of coping responses and social resources in attenuating the stress of life events. *Journal of Behavioral Medicine, 4*, 139–157.

Billings, A. G., & Moos, R. H. (1982). Psychological theory and research on depression: An integrative framework and review. *Clinical Psychology Review, 2*, 213–237.

Billings, A. G., & Moos, R. H. (1984). Coping, stress, and social resources among adults with unipolar depression. *Journal of Personality and Social Psychology, 46*, 877–891.

Billing, A. G., & Moos, R. H. (1985). Psychosocial stressors, coping, and depression. In E. E. Beckham & W. R. Leber (Eds.), *Handbook of depression: Treatment, assessment and research* (pp. 940–974). Homewood, IL: Dorsey Press.

Bruner, J. S., & Postman, L. (1947). Tension and tension-release as organizing factors in perception. *Journal of Personality, 15*, 300–308.

Byrne, D. (1961). The repression-sensitization scale: Rationale, reliability, and validity. *Journal of Personality, 29*, 334–349.

Byrne, D. (1964). Repression-sensitization as a dimension of personality. In B. A. Maher (Ed.), *Progress in experimental personality research* (Vol. 1, pp. 169–220). New York: Academic Press.

Byrne, D., & Holcomb, J. (1962). The reliability of response measure differential recognition- threshold scores. *Psychological Bulletin, 59*, 70–73.

Carver, C. S., Scheier, M. F., & Weintraub, J. K. (1989). Assessing coping strategies: A theoretically based approach. *Journal of Personality and Social Psychology, 56,* 267–283.

Christensen, A. J., Benotch, E. G., Wiebe, J. S., & Lawton, W. J. (1995). Coping with treatment-related stress. Effects on patient adherence in hemodialysis. *Journal of Consulting and Clinical Psychology, 63,* 454–459.

Chronister, J., & Chan, F. (2006). A stress process model of caregiving for individuals with traumatic brain injury. *Rehabilitation Psychology, 51,* 190–201.

Cohen, F., & Lazarus, R. S. (1973). Active coping processes, coping dispositions, and recovery from surgery. *Psychosomatic Medicine, 35,* 375–389.

Cohen, L., & Roth, S. (1984). Coping with abortion. *Journal of Human Stress, 10,* 140–145.

Conway, V. J., & Terry, D. J. (1992). Appraised controllability as a moderator of the effectiveness of different coping strategies: A test of the goodness of fit hypothesis. *Australian Journal of Psychology, 44,* 107.

Corrigan, P., Rao, D., & Lam, C. S. (2005). Psychiatric rehabilitation. In F. Chan, M. J. Leahy, & Saunder, J. L. (Eds.), *Case management for rehabilitation health professionals* (Vol. 2, pp. 132–163). Osage Beach, MO: Aspen Professional Services.

Crohn, B. B. (1962). An historic note on ulcerative colitis. *Gastroenterology, 42,* 366–370.

Cronkite, R. C., & Moos, R. H. (1984). The role of predisposing and moderating factors in the stress-illness relationship. *Journal of Health and Social Behavior, 25,* 372–393.

Dusenburg, L., & Albee, G. W. (1988). Primary prevention of anxiety disorders. In C. G. Last & M. Hersen (Eds.), *Handbook of anxiety disorders* (pp. 571–583). New York: Pergamon Press.

Endler, N. S., & Parker, J. D. A. (1990). Multidimensional assessment of coping: A critical evaluation. *Journal of Personality and Social Psychology, 58,* 844–854.

Ferrin, J. M. (2002). *Acceptance of loss after an adult-onset disability : Development and psychometric validation of the Multidimensional Acceptance of Loss Scale.* Unpublished doctoral dissertation, University of Wisconsin-Madison.

Fitchett, G., Rybarczyk, B. D., DeMarco, G. A., & Nicholas, J. J. (1999). The role of religion in medical rehabilitation outcomes: A longitudinal study. *Rehabilitation Psychology, 44,* 333–353.

Folkman, S., & Lazarus, R. S. (1980). An analysis of coping in a middle aged community sample. *Journal of Health and Social Behavior, 21,* 219–239.

Folkman, S., & Lazarus, R. S. (1985). If it changes it must be a process: Study of emotion and coping during three stages of a college examination. *Journal of Personality and Social Psychology, 48,* 150–170.

Folkman, S., Lazarus, R. S., Dunkel-Schetter, C., DeLongis, A., & Gruen, R. J. (1986a). Dynamics of a stressful encounter: Cognitive appraisal, coping, and encounter outcomes. *Journal of Personality and Social Psychology, 50,* 992–1003.

Folkman, S., Lazarus, R. S., Gruen, R., & Delongis, A. (1986b). Appraisal, coping health status, and psychological symptoms. *Journal of Personality and Social Psychology, 50,* 571–579.

Folkman, S., & Moskowitz, J. T. (2004). Coping: Pitfalls and promise. *Annual Review of Psychology, 55,* 745–774.

Freud, S. (1957). Instincts and their vicissitudes. In J. Strachey (Ed.), *Standard edition of the complete psychological works of Sigmund Freud* (pp. 111–142). London: Hogarth.

Glass, D. C., & Singer, J. E. (1972). *Urban stress: Experiments on noise and social stressors.* New York: Academic.

Gottlieb, B. H., & Gignac, M. A. M. (1996). Content and domain specificity of coping among family caregivers of persons with dementia. *Journal of Aging Studies, 10,* 137–155.

Grand, S. A. (1972). Reactions to unfavorable evaluations of the self as a function of acceptance of disability: A test of Dembo, Leviton, and Wright's misfortune hypothesis. *Journal of Counseling Psychology, 19,* 87–93.

Greenglass, E. R., (1988). Type A behavior and coping strategies. *Applied Psychology: An International Review, 37,* 271–288.

Heinemann, A. W., & Shontz, F. C. (1982). Acceptance of disability, self-esteem, sex role identity, and reading aptitude in deaf adolescents. *Rehabilitation Counseling Bulletin, 25,* 197–203.

Hofer, M. A., Wolff, C. T., Friedman S. B., & Mason, J. W. (1972). A psychoendocrine study of bereavement. Parts I & II. *Psychosomatic Medicine, 34,* 481–504.

Holahan, C. J., & Moos, R. (1990). Life stressors, resistance factors, and improved psychological functioning: An extension of the stress-resistance paradigm. *Journal of Personality and Social Psychology, 58,* 909–917.

Horowitz, M. (1976). *Stress response syndromes.* New York: Jason Aronson.

Horowitz, M. (1979). Psychological response to serious life events. In V. Hamilton & D. M. Warburton (Eds.), *Human stress and cognition: An information processing approach* (pp. 237–265). Chichester, England: Wiley.

Horowitz, M. (1983). Psychological responses to serious life events. In S. Breznitz (Ed.), *The denial of stress* (pp. 129–161). New York: International Universities Press.

Janis, I. L. (1977). *Decision making.* New York: Free Press.

Katz, J., Weiner, H., Gallagher, T., & Hellman, L. (1970). Stress, distress, and ego defenses. *Archives of General Psychiatry, 23,* 131–142.

Kosciulek, J. F. (1994). Relationship of family coping with head injury to family adaptation. *Rehabilitation Psychology, 39,* 215–230.

Krohne, H. W. (1989). The concept of coping modes: Relating cognitive person variables to actual coping behaviors. *Advances in Behavioral Research and Therapy, 11,* 235–248.

Krohne, H. W. (1993). Vigilance and cognitive avoidance as concepts in coping research. In H. W. Krohne (Ed.), *Attention and avoidance: Strategies in coping with aversiveness* (pp. 19–50). Seattle, WA: Hogrefe & Huber.

Krohne, H. W. (1996). Individual differences in coping. In M. Zeidner & N. S. Endler (Eds.), *Handbook of Coping: Theory, research, applications* (pp. 381–409). New York: Wiley.

Kubler-Ross, E. (1969). *On death and dying.* New York: Macmillan.

Laux, L., & Weber, H. (1990). Coping with emotions. In K. R. Scherer (Ed.), *Enzyklopadie der Psychologie: Serie Motivation une Emotion: Band 3. Psychologie der Emotion* (pp. 560–629). Gottingen: Hogrefe.

Lazarus, R. S. (1966). *Psychological stress and the coping process.* New York: McGraw-Hill.

Lazarus, R. S. (1983). The costs and benefits of denial. In S. Breznitz (Ed.), *The denial of stress* (pp. 1–30). New York: International Universities Press.

Lazarus, R. S., & Folkman, S. (1984). *Stress, appraisal, and coping.* New York: Springer.

Lazarus, R. S., & Folkman, S. (1987). Transactional theory and research on emotions and coping. *European Journal of Personality, 1,* 141–169.

Lazarus, R. S., & Launier, R. (1978). Stress-related transactions between person and environment. In L. A. Pervin & M. Lewis (Eds.), *Perspectives in interactional psychology* (pp. 287–327). New York: Plenum.

Leventhal, H., Brown, D., Shacham, S., & Engquist, G. (1979). Effect of preparatory information about sensations, threat of pain and attention on cold pressor distress. *Journal of Personality and Social Psychology, 37*, 688–714.

Leventhal, H., & Everhart, D. (1980). Emotion, pain, and physical illness. In C. E. Izard (Ed.), *Emotions and psychopathology* (pp. 263–299). New York: Plenum.

Lewin, K. (1951). *Field theory in social science*. New York: Harper & Row.

Linkowski, D. C., & Dunn, M. A. (1974). Self-concept and acceptance of disability. *Rehabilitation Counseling Bulletin, 18*, 28–32.

Livneh, H. (1986). A unified approach to existing models of adaptation to disability. Part I: A model of adaptation. *Journal of Applied Rehabilitation Counseling, 17*(1), 5–17, 56.

Livneh, H. (2000). Psychosocial adaptation to cancer: The role of coping strategies. *Journal of Rehabilitation, 66*, 40–49.

Livneh, H., & Antonak, R. F. (2005). Psychosocial aspects of chronic illness and disability. In F. Chan, M. J. Leahy, & J. L. Saunder (Eds.), *Case management for rehabilitation health professionals* (Vol. 2, pp. 3–43). Osage Beach, MO: Aspen Professional Services.

Livneh, H., & Wilson, L. M. (2003). Coping strategies as predictors and mediators of disability-related variables and psychosocial adaptation: An exploratory investigation. *Rehabilitation Counseling Bulletin, 46*, 194–208.

Macrodimitris, S. D., & Endler, N. S. (2001). Coping control and adjustment in Type 2 diabetes. *Health Psychology, 20*, 208–216.

McCrae, R. R. (1984). Situational determinants of coping: Loss, threat, and challenge. *Journal of Personality and Social Psychology, 46*, 919–928.

McGlashan, T. H., Levy S. T., & Carpenter, W. T. (1975). Integration and sealing over. *Archives of General Psychiatry, 32*, 1269–1272.

Miller, S. M. (1987). Monitoring and blunting: Validation of a questionnaire to assess styles of information seeking under threat. *Journal of Personality and Social Psychology, 52*, 345–353.

Miller, S. M. (1989). Cognitive informational styles in the process of coping with threat and frustration. *Advances in Behavioral Research and Therapy, 11*, 223–234.

Mitchell, R. E., Cronkite, R. C., & Moos, R. H. (1983). Stress, coping and depression among married couples. *Journal of Abnormal Psychology, 92*, 433–448.

Mitchell, R. E., & Hodson, C. A. (1983). Coping with domestic violence: Social support and psychological health among battered women. *American Journal of Community Psychology, 11*, 629–654.

Moos, R. H., & Schaefer, J. A. (1993). Coping resources and processes: Current concepts and measures. In L. Goldberger & S. Breznitz (Eds.), *Handbook of stress: Theoretical and clinical aspects* (2nd ed., pp. 234–257). New York: Free Press.

Mullen, B., & Suls, J. (1982). The effectiveness of attention and rejection coping styles: A meta-analysis of temporal differences. *Journal of Psychosomatic Research, 26*, 43–49.

Osuji, O. N. (1985). Personality factors in acceptance of loss among the physically disabled. *The Psychological Record, 35*, 23–28.

Osuji, O. N. (1987). "Acceptance of loss" and industrial rehabilitation: An empirical study. *International Journal of Rehabilitation Research, 10*, 21–27.

Pakenham, K. I. (1999). Adjustment to multiple sclerosis: Application of a stress and coping model. *Health Psychology, 18*, 383–392.

Park, C. L., & Folkman, S. (1997). Meaning in the context of stress and coping. *Review of General Psychology, 1*, 115–144.

Park, C. L., Folkman, S., & Bostrom, A. (2001). Appraisals of controllability and coping in caregivers and HIV+ men: Testing the goodness of fit hypothesis. *Journal of Consulting and Clinical Psychology, 69,* 481–488.

Pearlin, L. I., Menaghan, E. G., Lieberman, M. A., & Mullan, J. T. (1981). The stress process. *Journal of Health and Social Behavior, 22,* 337–356.

Pearlin, L. I., & Schooler, C. (1978). The structure of coping. *Journal of Health and Social Behavior, 19,* 2–21.

Pittner, M. S., Housten, B. K., & Spiridigliozzi, G. (1983). Control over stress. Type A behavior pattern, and response to stress. *Journal of Personality and Social Psychology, 44,* 627–637.

Ptacek, J. T., & Pierce, G. R. (2003). Issues in the study of stress and coping in rehabilitation settings. *Rehabilitation Psychology, 48,* 113–124.

Rosenberg, S. J., Peterson, R. A., & Hayes, J. A. (1987). Coping behaviors among depressed and non-depressed medical inpatients. *Journal of Psychosomatic Research, 31,* 653–658.

Roth, S., & Cohen, L. J. (1986). Approach, avoidance, and coping with stress. *American Psychologist, 41,* 813–819.

Roth, S. L., & Robinson, S. E. (1992). Chronic disease in women: The role of the mental health counselor. *Journal of Mental Health Counseling, 14,* 59–72.

Sarason, I. G. (1973). Test anxiety and cognitive modeling. *Journal of Personality and Social Psychology, 28,* 58–61.

Sarason, I. G., & Sarason, B. R. (1981). Teaching cognitive and social skills to high school students. *Journal of Consulting and Clinical Psychology, 49,* 908–918.

Scheier, M. F., Weintraub, J. K., & Carver, C. S. (1986). Coping with stress: Divergent strategies of optimists and pessimists: *Journal of Personality and Social Psychology, 46,* 892–906.

Shontz, F. C. (1975). *The psychological aspects of physical illness and disability.* New York: Macmillan.

Silver, R. & Wortman, C. B. (1980). Coping with undesirable life events. In J. Garber & M. E. P. Seligman (Eds.), *Human helplessness* (pp. 279–340). New York: Academic Press.

Somerfield, M. R., & McCrae, R. R. (2000). Stress and coping research. Methodological challenges, theoretical advances, and clinical applications. *American Psychologist, 55,* 620–625.

Spence, D. P. (1957). A new look at vigilance and defense. *Journal of Abnormal Social Psychology, 54,* 103–108.

Staudenmeyer, H., Kinsman, R. A., Dirks, J. F., Spector S. L., & Wangaard, C. (1979). Medical outcome on asthmatic patients: Effects of airways hyperactivity and symptom-focused anxiety. *Psychosomatic Medicine, 41,* 109–118.

Stein, K. B. (1953). Perceptual defense and perceptual sensitization under neutral and involved conditions. *Journal of Personality, 21,* 467–478.

Stone, A., & Neale, J. (1984). New measure of daily coping: Development and preliminary results. *Journal of Personality and Social Psychology, 46,* 892–906.

Stroebe, M. S., & Schut, H. (2001). Meaning making in the dual process model of coping with bereavement. In R. A. Neimeyer (Ed.), *Meaning reconstruction and the experience of loss* (pp. 55–73). Washington, DC: American Psychological Association.

Suls, J., & Fletcher, B. (1985). The relative efficacy of avoidant and non-avoidant coping strategies: A meta-analysis. *Health Psychology, 4,* 249–288.

Terry, D. J., & Hynes, G. J. (1998). Adjustment to a low control situation: Re-examining the role of coping responses. *Journal of Personality and Social Psychology, 74,* 1078–1092.

Thompson, S. C. (1981). Will it hurt less if I can control it? A complex answer to a simple question. *Psychological Bulletin, 90,* 89–101.

Weidner, G., & Mathews, K. A. (1978). Reported physical symptoms elicited by unpredictable events and the Type A coronary-prone behavior pattern. *Journal of Personality and Social Psychology, 36,* 1213–1220.

Wolff, C. T., Friedman, S. B., Hofer, M. A., & Mason, J. W. (1964). Relationship between psychological defenses and men urinary 170HCS excretion rates. Parts I & II. *Psychosomatic Medicine, 26,* 576–609.

Wright, B. (1983). *Physical disability – a psychosocial approach.* (2nd ed.) New York: Harper Collins.

Zeidner M., & Saklofske, D. (1996). Adaptive and maladaptive coping. In M. Zeidner & N. S. Endler (Eds.), *Handbook of coping: Theory, research, application* (pp. 505–531). New York: Wiley.

4
The Social Context of Coping

John F. Kosciulek

No man is an island,
entire of itself every man is a piece of the continent,
a part of the main if a clod be washed away by the sea,
Europe is the less, as well as if a promontory were,
as well as if a manor of thy friends or of thine own were,
any man's death diminishes me, because I am involved in mankind,
and therefore never send to know for whom the bell tolls – it tolls for thee.

John Donne, 1624

The above poem by the seventeenth-century English author John Donne (Shawcross, 1967) provides insight to the significance of the social context of coping with a chronic illness or disability (CID). Donne suggests that no one is completely self-sufficient, that everyone relies on others, and that human beings do not thrive when isolated from others. From this perspective, the process of coping with CID does not occur in isolation. On the contrary, coping with CID occurs in broader social contexts, which include family, friends, neighbors, the community, employers, schools, and rehabilitation and health-care service providers. This chapter is intended to extend and expand the reader's understanding and knowledge regarding the social context of coping with CID.

Developmental research on coping with CID has relied heavily on models of the appraisal and coping process, such as proposed by Lazarus and Folkman (1984). According to Lazarus and Folkman's (1984) approach, individuals cognitively appraise a potential stressor through a transaction between environmental demands and individuals' perceptions of the resources that they have to cope with demands. In models of stress and coping across the lifespan (e.g., Billings & Moos, 1981), researchers, who perceive coping from a cognitive orientation, view a person who copes as one who "individually" appraises and copes with stressors. From this perspective, each individual has a unique way of coping, a view which precludes the ability to examine coping trends across individuals. For instance, an individual might appraise memory deficits associated with a traumatic brain injury as stressful and might be asked by researchers to describe his or her coping strategies for dealing with the stress.

Such an "individual" approach to stress and coping, however, neglects the fact that individuals experience stressors within a social context and may cope with stressors related to CID in a collaborative fashion with other individuals (Berg, Meegan, & DeViney, 1998).

Using the example of memory deficits related to a brain injury, this stress may influence not only the individual who sustained the injury, but also may influence a spouse, child, other family members, friends, and co-workers (Kosciulek, 1995). In fact, the stress may not be something that the individual alone deals with, but other individuals are required to assist and to become intimately involved in the coping process. Family members may provide overt cognitive, emotional, and physical support in the home environment, friends may structure social engagements around familiar people and environments, and co-workers may adjust their roles and responsibilities to compensate for their colleague's CID-related difficulties. The stressor soon becomes the province of a social unit, rather than solely the individual.

The stress of one person is not necessarily confined to the person alone, but can be experienced indirectly by another person. In addition, other individuals may not only act as sources of stress, but may also be involved in the coping process – either as sources of information, advice, or support, models for functional or dysfunctional coping, or as collaborators engaged in mutual or compensatory coping efforts (Berg et al., 1998; Hobfoll, 1998). The coping literature currently does not illuminate how CID-related stressors may be experienced by social units and thus may be solved through *interdependent* coping efforts of individuals within a social unit.

The purpose of the present chapter, therefore, is to illustrate the importance of examining coping within a social context across the lifespan and to examine the ways that others are not only supportive of a person's "individual" coping efforts, but are involved in collaborative coping efforts with CID-related stressors, which can be viewed as the property of a social unit rather than of an individual. A primary tenet in this chapter is that efforts to cope with CID are embedded in a rich social context, are appraised within that context, and frequently involve the receiving the help of others in ways that extend beyond social support. From this perspective, the current chapter attempts to include a more dynamic view of coping with CID than has been presented in the literature to date. To this end, the chapter initially addresses the social coping tasks associated with CID. In the next section, readers are provided content related to the theoretical and historical background of the social context of coping. General social models of coping are then discussed. In the final section of the chapter, two areas of the social context of coping of particular relevance to CID – work and family – are presented.

Social Coping with Chronic Illness and Disability

Given the potential enormity of the tasks of coping with CID and the significant social aspects of the CID coping process, it is instructive to provide the reader with information on the social coping tasks associated with CID. Social coping tasks are those particular challenges that must be faced and overcome so that the individual preserves integrity, restores or maintains a positive self-concept, and functions effectively in relationships and life-roles. Individuals with CID may be challenged to cope with multiple, complex, social tasks. According to Miller (2000), the major social coping tasks for individuals with CID include maintaining a sense of normalcy, adjusting to altered social relationships, dealing with role change, dealing with the social stigma of illness or disability, and maintaining a feeling of being in control. Each of these CID-related social coping tasks is discussed below.

Maintaining a Sense of Normalcy

Normalization is a process by which individuals and families cope with CID (Riding, 1997). That is, individuals view and describe their lives as normal, despite significant illness or impairment and disruption of family routines. Normalization depends on a cognitive reframing of a difficult life challenge into one that is manageable and "normal."

Maintaining a sense of normalcy involves keeping the signs and symptoms of CID under control. It includes a mental review of existing abilities, functions, and relationships with significant others. The ideal of being and feeling normal is fostered, if individuals with CID engage in a personal reaffirmation of being as capable as others in their personal social network.

Adjusting to Altered Social Relationships

CID may result in social isolation and loneliness. The person with CID may withdraw because of a depleted energy-reserve or poor self-concept, feeling unworthy of social contacts, or simply being physically unable to participate in social events (Miller, 2000). If CID encapsulates more and more of an individual's time, both thought and behavior processes may be dominated by the existence of a CID, its symptoms, and obtaining relief from emotional or physical discomfort. Only the most loyal family and friends may persist in being supportive during this phase of adaptation to CID. As such, the person with CID may need to cope with having fewer social interactions with people and with receiving a decreased level of confirmation of being a capable individual.

Dealing with Role Change

Role changes for persons with CID may be conceptualized in terms of loss and replacement. Role losses can include the loss of social roles (e.g., church participant, member of a sports team, and officer in a community group). Lost social roles may be replaced by the roles of having a CID, and/or being a client of a complex health-care or rehabilitation system. Thus, one task of social coping with CID may involve giving up pre-CID life roles and choosing new, non-medically related roles.

Managing Social Stigma

One of the most challenging tasks of coping with the social aspects of CID involves dealing with social stigma. Managing the social stigma of CID may involve dealing with second looks, stares from children, physical avoidance by others, and the inconvenience and embarrassment of being unable to enter buildings or restrooms. Wright (1983) described three types of responses of individuals to stigmatizing behavior: (a) Ignore it, bury one's head in the sand; (b) overreact with rage, retaliation, and overt hostility; and (c) use humor, which may result in further self-depreciation. Mature self-acceptance and self-confidence by the individual will help facilitate positive adaptation to CID.

Maintaining a Feeling of Being in Control

Controlling a deteriorating or unstable physical or emotional state may not always be possible. Individuals with CID may find it difficult to maintain feelings of control over certain aspects of their lives, because of intrusions into their privacy by rehabilitation and health-care providers. Social coping in relation to being in control includes the ability to control environmental intrusion, while maintaining a sense of privacy. If such a balance is struck, personal dignity can be maintained (Lemaistre, 1995).

Theoretical and Historical Background of the Social Context of Coping

Coping, defined as the thoughts and behaviors used to manage the internal and external demands of situations that are appraised as stressful, has been a focus of research in the social sciences for more than three decades (Folkman & Moskowitz, 2004). The dramatic proliferation of coping research has spawned healthy debate and criticism and offered insight into the question of why some individuals fare better than others do, when encountering stress in their lives.

The past 35 years have seen a dramatic proliferation of coping research across the social and behavioral sciences, medicine, public health, and nursing. Studies on coping have ranged from small-sample qualitative studies to large-scale population-based studies, with content ranging from the exploration of abstract theoretical relationships to applied studies in clinical settings. Some disability and rehabilitation investigators undertook such research with the hope that the concept of coping might help explain why some individuals fare better than others do when encountering CID-related stress in their lives (e.g., Iwasaki & Mactavish, 2005; Ptacek & Pierce, 2003). While other concepts, such as culture, developmental history, or personality, can also help explain these individual differences, coping is unlike these other concepts in that it lends itself to cognitive-behavioral intervention. As such, the allure of coping is not only as an explanatory concept regarding variability in response to stress, but also as a portal for interventions (Folkman & Moskowitz, 2004).

It is clear that the concept of coping, like that of stress, is not a unified construct with readily agreed-upon meaning. Rather, coping more accurately represents a general rubric or meta-construct, under which a number of phenomena are embedded (Eckenrode, 1991). What distinguishes coping from other aspects of human behavior is its relevance to adaptation in the face of stressful life experiences or conditions. As such, a prerequisite for coping is the presence of an event or condition that is appraised as harmful or threatening to the individual, such as a CID.

During the past two decades, substantial gains have been made in understanding coping (Parker & Endler, 1996). Yet, more clinical and research work is needed to further enhance our grasp of the ways in which coping affects psychological, physiological, and behavioral outcomes, both in the short- and long-term. The discovery task is not simple. Coping is not a stand-alone phenomenon: it is embedded in complex, dynamic stress processes that involve the person, the environment, and the relationship between them. Further, individuals with whom one is emotionally close can play a role in the etiology, maintenance and resolution of stress. Nevertheless, the role of close relationships in affecting individual coping is only beginning to be explored (Wethington & Kessler, 1991). A full account of coping, then, must consider characteristics of the social context and the fit between those characteristics and various types of coping.

General Social Models of Coping

While some models of coping view the individual as embedded in a social context, the literature on coping is dominated by individualistic approaches that generally give short shrift to social aspects. Themes of personal control, personal agency, and direct action are central to most theories of coping (e.g., Aspinwall & Taylor, 1997; Pearlin & Schooler, 1978), all of which reflect the emphasis on the individual. The coping literature has developed largely within the tradition of psychology and psychiatry. As a result, much of the literature emphasizes the individual and his or her cognitive and emotional processes. Dunahoo, Hobfoll, Monnier, Hulsizer, and Johnson (1998) described these individualistic approaches as a "Lone Ranger, 'man against the elements' perspective," but as they point out, "even the Lone Ranger had Tonto" (p. 137).

Coping rarely takes place in a social vacuum; many stressful events of daily living involve other persons. Further, interpersonally created traumas (e.g., acts of terrorism) have higher levels of stress reactions than other types of trauma (e.g., natural disasters) (Stout, 2004). As such, coping must be viewed within a social context and as part of a dynamic social process. In addition, despite many admirable and theoretically provocative attempts to understand the role of coping in the stress process, issues about the social and situational aspects of coping remain relatively unexplored. To address this gap in the coping literature, several authors have attempted to advance our understanding of coping, beyond an emphasis solely on individual appraisals and responses, by delineating the complex social, situational, and environmental aspects and determinants of coping. Noteworthy theoretical discussions on the social aspects of coping include communal coping (Wells, Hobfoll, & Lavin, 1997), situational determinants of coping (Wethington and Kessler, 1991), social support as coping assistance (Thoits, 1986), conservation of resources theory (Hobfoll, 1989), and a model of social coping with everyday problems (Berg et al., 1998). Each theory will be described below.

Communal Coping

As a counterpoise to the emphasis on individualistic coping, Hobfoll and his colleagues developed a multiaxial coping model that takes both individualistic and communal perspectives into account. It includes a prosocial-antisocial dimension and a passive-active dimension (Wells et al., 1997). The communal perspective is contained in the prosocial-antisocial dimension and refers to coping responses that are influenced by and in reaction to the social context. Thus, a person may delay or not engage in a direct action to solve a problem if that action is perceived as causing distress to another member of the social environment.

Communal coping can be prosocial (e.g., "Join together with others to deal with the situation together," "Think carefully about how others feel before deciding what to do"), or antisocial (e.g., "Assert your dominance quickly," "Be firm, hold your ground") (Monnier, Hobfoll, Dunahoo, Hulsizer, & Johnson, 1998). In a series of studies, Hobfoll and his colleagues found that active, prosocial coping was associated with better emotional outcomes (Wells et al., 1997), and that women use more prosocial and men use more antisocial coping (Dunahoo et al., 1998).

Situational Determinants of Coping

Wethington and Kessler (1991) described the social context of coping in relation to the situational determinants of coping. These authors hypothesized that situational determinants were a critical factor in coping strategies and coping effectiveness. Wethington and Kessler divided situational determinants into two types: the situational context surrounding the individual who is coping, and the type of event that occurs. In this model, the situational context of coping includes the social resources that are available to the individual, as well as the characteristics of an individual, such as age, gender, and personality traits.

Event types are characterized by: (a) The type of situation (e.g., a financial problem or marital difficulty), which specifies the tasks presented for coping; and (b) severity of the situation, defined in terms of the degree to which the situation involves the loss of valued persons or objects, or a threat of future harm. These factors influence an individual's cognitive and affective responses such as emotion management, constructive problem-solving, and vigilance for the future. The type and severity of situational demands are particularly relevant for evaluating the efficacy of different coping strategies. Wethington and Kessler (1991) suggest that, in order to promote good emotional adjustment, coping should not only fit the demands of the situation, but also alleviate the emotional and practical difficulties facing the individual.

Social Support as Coping Assistance

Perhaps the most commonly discussed aspect of the social context of coping is that of social support (Eckenrode, 1991; Hobfoll, 2002). The belief in the potential of social support to decrease stress and enhance coping has been widely supported in both the professional and lay literature during the past three decades. No other coping resource has received such widespread attention. The existence of numerous lay and professional support groups, for all manner of health and social challenges, attests to an inherent belief in the positive difference that this factor can make when an individual or family is dealing with CID (Underwood, 2000).

Considerable research indicates that social support reduces, or buffers, the adverse psychological impacts of exposure to stressful life events and ongoing life-strains (e.g., Folkman & Moskowitz, 2004, Ptacek & Pierce, 2003). Relationships with others, especially with intimates or confidants, can significantly lower the risk of psychological disturbance in response to stress exposure. Social support is an important factor in the prevention of and susceptibility to illness, disease, and disability (Pierce, Sarason, & Sarason, 1996). There is widespread consensus that social support is positively related to health and well-being. Researchers have found positive relationships between social support and a variety of outcomes associated with health, well-being, and coping (Chronister, 2005; Vash & Crewe, 2004).

In a seminal paper that links coping and social support, Thoits (1986) urged clinicians, theoreticians, and researchers to view social support as coping assistance. Thoits indicated that coping and social support have a number of functions in common. These include: (a) Instrumental functions, which in terms of social support include tangible assistance and aid, and in terms of coping include problem-focused coping; (b) emotional functions, which in terms of social support include emotional support, and in terms of coping include emotion-focused coping; and (c) perceived support, which in terms of social support includes informational support that alters perceptions of meaningful aspects of stressful situations, and in terms of coping includes cognitive reappraisal or restructuring. Thoits hypothesized that the same coping methods used by individuals in response to their own stressors are also the methods that they apply to others as assistance.

Thoits' (1986) purpose in linking coping and social support was to explicate how and when attempts at support work. Most research which investigated the effects of social support has focused primarily on establishing that there is a buffering effect (Folkman, 1992). By describing social support as coping assistance, Thoits provided a model for testing hypotheses about the conditions under which various types of support are used, and the conditions under which they may or may not be effective in reducing distress and solving problems.

Conservation of Resources Theory

Hobfoll (1989) developed a theory, called the conservation of resources (COR), which is instructive as a framework for describing the social aspects of coping. This model depicts resources as a product of widely-shared values and of meanings about what is valuable to people. The role of resources is the pivotal construct in COR theory; the central tenet is that individuals (alone and in systems) strive to maximize resource gain and minimize resource loss.

Resources are defined as those things that people value or that act as a means of protecting what they value. COR theory posits four principal resource categories: (a) Object resources (e.g., transportation); (b) condition resources (e.g., good marriage); (c) personal resources (e.g., self-esteem); and (d) energy resources (e.g., money). The theory further proposes that what an individual or social system, such as a family or work group, has to offset resource loss is other resources (Hobfoll & Spielberger, 1992).

The COR theory posits that loss and gain cycles do not have equal intensity or velocity, because losses are more highly weighted by both individuals and social groups than are gains (Hobfoll, Lilly, & Jackson, 1992). In the COR model, it is predicted that loss cycles will have greater intensity and momentum than gain cycles, and that loss cycles will be harder to interrupt and reverse than gain cycles. Such thinking is helpful to guide social coping research, as more emphasis is placed on resource models.

Social-Contextual Model of Coping with Everyday Problems

Berg, Meegan, DeViney (1998) presented a comprehensive model of the social context of coping. These authors described a process whereby individuals, in connection with others, anticipate and cope with everyday life problems. In Berg, Meegan, and Deviney's model, appraisal and stress are conceptualized at a variety of levels, ranging from solely individual appraisals of everyday problems to integrated and shared relational appraisals by a social unit. Coping efforts likewise are hypothesized to range from solely individual efforts to highly collaborative efforts.

Within Berg, Meegan, and Deviney's model, appraisal and coping with everyday stressors span from being highly individual in focus, to being coordinated and/or shared with other individuals through mutual reciprocal influence. The extent of influence ranges from a lack of relation and influence, when individuals use distinctive modes of coping, to a shared and coordinated relation and mutual influence, such as when individuals share similar appraisals and approaches to coping with stress. In this manner, the social aspects of coping facilitate the development and expansion of individual coping repertoires.

Berg, Meegan, and Deviney suggest that coping efforts are embedded in a social context, are appraised within that context, and frequently involve the use of others, in ways that extend beyond using individuals for support. One of the important implications of Berg, Meegan, and Deviney's model is that it illustrates the importance of studying coping within a social context across the lifespan.

It also examines the ways that others not only support a person's "individual" coping efforts, but are involved in a collaborative coping effort, with the stressor often better described as the property of a social unit rather than of an individual. Berg, Meegan, and Deviney recommend that coping research is reoriented away from documenting general developmental differences in coping strategies, and instead, is focused on understanding the process whereby individuals and others in their social context cope with everyday stressors.

Coping with CID in the Context of Work and Family

As previously stated, coping rarely takes place in a social vacuum. Most stressful events of daily living involve other persons. Thus far, this chapter has emphasized the importance of understanding the social nature of coping with general life stressors. Similarly, the specific case of coping with CID must be viewed within a social context. Unfortunately, the social and situational aspects of coping with CID have been minimally explored in the literature. To address this void, this section focuses on two areas of the social context of coping of particular relevance to CID: work and family. To enhance reader understanding of the dynamic social process of coping with CID, both the employment and family context of coping with CID are presented.

Employment Context of Coping with CID

One of the most significant challenges relative to social coping with CID is in the context of work. Work is a complex social activity that is deeply connected to psychological well-being. Further, work is social, cultural, psychological, and economic in nature. It is a social endeavor; its meaning and value determined by social values and beliefs (Rothman, 1987).

The world of work is changing at a rapid pace, and the changes are likely to accelerate during the twenty-first century. Employment arrangements, such as temporary employment, short-term hires, contractual positions, leased workers, and on-call and part-time workers, have and will continue to influence the career development of all workers (Institute on Rehabilitation Issues, 1999). These changes are having a substantial impact on the life roles of people with CID, the settings in which they live and work, and the events that occur in their lives.

The ever-changing nature of work presents new problems for people with CID in finding and maintaining suitable employment. Major trends, such as globalization of the American economy, technology, and population shifts, are changing the nature of work and worker skill-requirements (Friedman, 2005). Despite rehabilitation efforts, a majority of Americans with disabilities between the ages of 16 and 64 are not employed; that disparity has not changed since 1986, despite the fact that a majority of non-employed people with disabilities in the working-age population want to work (National Organization on Disability, 2000). In general, the vocational adjustment of individuals with CID has been characterized by limited, marketable work-skills, low income, under-employment, and unemployment (Stapleton & Burkhauser, 2003).

Given that work is a central force in people's lives, dramatically high rates of unemployment and underemployment can adversely affect not only the economic and social status of individuals with CID, but also their self-image. A distinct employment and career challenge encountered by many people with disabilities, which can be used as a reference point for conceptualizing the social context of coping with CID, is a negative worker self-concept that originates from numerous sources.

Szymanski and Trueba (1994) maintained that at least some of the difficulties faced by people with disabilities are not the result of functional impairments related to the disability, but rather are the result of "castification" processes embedded in societal institutions for rehabilitation and education, which are enforced by well-meaning professionals. Castification processes have their roots in a determinist view, in which people who are different are viewed as somehow less "human" or less capable. Problems of castification, stigma, and stereo-typing plague services to people with disabilities, because, in general, the same categories of impairment and functional limitation are used to determine eligi-bility for services, to prescribe interventions and, on occasion, to explain failure. The constructs about disability and those who use them become agents of casti-fication, or limit to individuals with CID in ways that are harmful to them, especially in the employment sphere.

Thus, complexities in the work-context of coping with CID are not solely the result of CID, but are also an outcome of social attitudes and stereotypes. Social attitudes toward CID may be as important as the CID itself, because the negative attitude of others plays a part in shaping the life-roles of the individual with CID. The outcome of long-term exposure to prejudicial attitudes may result in a negative self-appraisal and a negative worker self-concept.

Coping with CID in the Family Context

In addition to the demands of coping with CID in work contexts, a significant social aspect of coping with CID involves the family. As emphasized at the beginning of this chapter, individual approaches to stress and coping neglect the fact that individuals experience stressors within the social context of family, and may cope with stressors related to CID with the support of family members. Further, demands and stress resulting from CID influence not only the individual, but also a spouse, child, parent, or other family members. Rather than dealing with the CID alone, an individual may experience the assistance of family members. Through such assistance, family members become intimately involved in the coping process. As a result, CID-related stressors soon become the province of family units, rather than solely a domain of the individual.

Unfortunately, the stress and coping literature is quite limited in its attention to the family/social context of coping, particularly in the milieu of CID. Thus, in order to add to this area of the coping literature, this chapter further explicates how CID-related stressors are experienced by family units and how the stress may be resolved through family coping efforts.

A model useful for conceptualizing how families deal with the CID-related demands and stressors (i.e., the family social context of coping with CID) is the Resiliency Model of Family Stress, Adjustment, and Adaptation (Kosciulek, 2004). This model, which is a stress and coping framework that is based on a family-systems approach, is a clinical and conceptual framework that is particularly useful for describing a family's response to CID. The Resiliency Model has as its origin the seminal family stress and coping work of Reuben Hill (1958) and the Double ABCX Model of Family Adjustment (McCubbin & Patterson, 1983). Further, the model focuses on the following primary factors: (a) CID as potential family stressor, leading to family crisis; (b) family resistance resources (e.g., economic, psychological); (c) the family's appraisal of the CID situation; and (d) family coping patterns that are designed to protect the family from breakdown and facilitate effective family adaptation to CID. Each of these factors will be discussed briefly in the following sections.

Family Demands and Crisis

In the Resiliency Model, CID is considered a family crisis (McCubbin & McCubbin, 1991). Family crisis is a continuous condition, denoting the amount of disruptiveness, disorganization, or incapacitation in the family system. Families in crisis after CID-onset have a situational inability to restore stability, and are often trapped in a cyclical trial-and-error struggle to reduce tensions, which tends to make matters worse rather than better. Family crisis denotes family disorganization and a demand for basic changes in the family patterns of functioning, in order to restore stability, order, and a sense of coherence.

Because family crises after the onset of CID evolve and are resolved over a period of time, families are seldom dealing with CID in isolation. A pile-up of demands following CID-onset is commonplace and thus is a critical factor that should be taken into account when examining the family context of coping with CID. Stresses and strains resulting from CID, which contribute to a pile-up of demands on the family system, include the following six broad categories:

1. CID-related hardships over time (e.g., ambiguity surrounding the CID, marital or sibling relationship-strains, increased financial hardship);
2. Normative transitions (e.g., normal development of young family members, career development of adult members);
3. Prior strains accumulated over time (e.g., pre-CID family psychological and physical health);
4. Situational demands and difficulties (e.g., interfacing with medical and rehabilitation systems, over-protectiveness of children with CID);
5. Consequences of family efforts to cope (e.g., increased family rigidity, suppression of anger, acting-out behavior, co-dependency); and
6. Intra-family and social ambiguity (e.g., role changes, responsibility for long-term care needs) (Kosciulek, McCubbin, & McCubbin, 1993; Walsh, 2002).

Family Resources

Family resources are defined as the potentiality of the family for meeting its demands (Kosciulek, 1995). Three types of resources available to the family after CID-onset include the personal resources of individual family members, the family system itself, and community resources and supports. The personal resources of individual family members include innate intelligence, personality traits (e.g., sense of humor), physical health, and self-esteem. Primary family-system resources, which are necessary for successful adaptation to CID, include cohesion and flexibility. Cohesion is the unity running through the family, while flexibility is the family's capacity to meet obstacles and shift course. Finally, community resources and supports include social, rehabilitation, and friendship activities outside the family, which the family unit faced with CID may call upon, access, and use to cope with the CID situation and to bring demands under control.

Family Appraisal

One of the primary components of the Resiliency Model is family appraisal. Families assess the degree of controllability of the CID situation, the amount of change expected in the family system, and whether or not the family is capable of responding effectively to the situation. Given the often ambiguous nature of CID, family appraisal is critical in shaping positive family adaptation. Viewing CID as a manageable family challenge, rather than a catastrophe, will affect how a family adapts over time.

Family Coping

The process of acquiring, allocating, and using resources for meeting demands is a critical aspect of family adaptation to CID. In this context, the family can be viewed as a resource-exchange network. Coping is viewed as the action for this exchange. In the Resiliency Model, a coping behavior is a specific effort, by which singular family members or the family unit attempts to reduce or manage a demand on the family (Kosciulek, 2004). Coping patterns may be generalized responses or stressor-specific reactions to different types of demanding situations. Four categories characterize the ways in which coping facilitates family adaptation to CID:

1. Coping can involve direct action to eliminate or reduce the number and/or intensity of CID-related demands.
2. Coping can involve direct action to acquire additional resources that are not already available to the family faced with a CID-related situation.
3. Coping can involve managing tension that is associated with ongoing strains, which result from CID.

4. Coping can also involve family-level appraisal to create, shape, and evaluate meanings, which families may give to a CID-related situation to make it more constructive, manageable, and acceptable.

These coping strategies, which operate simultaneously following a CID-induced family crisis, can serve as a useful guide for understanding the family aspect of the social context of coping.

Conclusion

The process of coping with CID does not occur in isolation. On the contrary, coping with CID occurs in broader social contexts, which include family, friends, neighbors, community, employers, schools, and rehabilitation and health-care service settings. This chapter opened with a discussion of the social coping tasks associated with CID, followed by the theoretical and historical background of the social context of coping and then a brief description of five social models of coping. In the final section of the chapter, two areas of the social context of coping of particular relevance to CID, work and family, were presented. One model for understanding coping in the family context was the Resiliency Model, which emphasized that efforts to cope with CID are embedded in a social context, are appraised within that context, and frequently involve the assistance of others in ways that extend beyond social support.

There are many aspects of the social context of coping that future research could investigate, including: (a) What kinds of coping are more effective for addressing the six categories of stresses that affect the family system (see p. 83 in this chapter); (b) empirically studying CID-related social support using a theoretical model that includes both personal and environmental factors and the interaction of the two (De Ridder & Schreurs, 1996; Kosciulek, 2004; Livneh, 2001; Maes, Leventhal, & de Ridder, 1996; Moos & Holahan, 2006; (c) a broad range of definitional, conceptual, and contextual issues related to social support, as well as therapeutic findings that focus on social support in the context of CID (De Ridder & Schreurs, 1996; Ell, 1996); (d) critical examination of instruments used to assess family systems (e.g., the Moos Family Environmental Scale, see Ell, 1996, p. 176 for more instruments) as applied to the context of coping with CID; (e) an investigation of specific CID-related characteristics (e.g., prognosis, functional limitations of the CID) on the family coping processes (De Ridder & Schreurs, 1996); (f) exploration of problematic social and family support, including unrealistic expectations, miscommunication, misguided support, or interpersonal conflict that affect interdependent and interactive coping strategies within family systems when a CID is present (Ell, 1996); and (g) transforming social support research into social relationship research that includes the perspective that there can be both distressing or positive social interactions (De Ridder & Schreurs, 1996).

References

Aspinwall, L. G., & Taylor, S. E. (1997). A stitch in time: Self-regulation and proactive coping. *Psychological Bulletin, 121*, 417–436.

Berg, C. A., Meegan, S. P., & Deviney, F. P. (1998). A social contextual model of coping with everyday problems across the lifespan. *International Journal of Behavioral Development, 22*(2), 239–261.

Billings, A. G., & Moos, R. H. (1981). The role of coping responses and social resources in attenuating the stress of life events. *Journal of Behavioral Medicine, 4*, 139–157.

Chronister, J. A. (2005). *Social support and rehabilitation counseling: Challenges and future directions.* Paper presented at the NRCA Professional Development Symposium, Memphis, TN.

De Ridder, D., & Schreurs, K. (1996). Coping, social support, and chronic disease: A research agenda. *Psychology, Health, and Medicine, 1*(1), 71–82.

Dunahoo, C. L., Hobfoll, S. E., Monnier, J., Hulsizer, M. R., & Johnson, R. (1998). There's more than rugged individualism in coping. Part 1: Even the Lone Ranger had Tonto. *Anxiety, Stress, & Coping: An International Journal, 11*(2), 137–165.

Eckenrode, J. (Ed.). (1991). *The social context of coping.* New York: Plenum Press.

Ell, K. (1996). Social networks, social support, and coping with serious illness: The family connection. *Social Science and Medicine, 42*(2), 173–183.

Folkman, S. (1992). Making the case for coping. In B. N. Carpenter (Ed.), *Personal coping: Theory, research, and application* (pp. 31–46). Westport, CT: Praeger.

Folkman, S., & Moskowitz, J. D. (2004). Coping: Pitfall and promises. *Annual Review of Psychology, 55*, 745–774.

Friedman, T. L. (2005). *The world is flat.* New York: Farrar, Straus, and Giroux.

Hill, R. (1958). Generic features of families under stress. *Social Casework, 49*, 139–150.

Hobfoll, S. E. (1989). Conservation of resources: A new attempt at conceptualizing stress. *American Psychologist, 44*, 513–524.

Hobfoll, S. E. (1998). *Stress, culture, and the community: The psychology and philosophy of stress.* New York: Plenum.

Hobfoll, S. E. (2002). Social and psychological resources and adaptation. *Review of General Psychology, 6*, 307–324.

Hobfoll, S. E., Lilly, R. S., & Jackson, A. P. (1992). Conservation of social resources and the self. In H. O. F. Veiel & U. Bauchmann (Eds.), *The meaning and measurement of social support* (pp. 125–141). Washington, DC: Hemisphere.

Hobfoll, S. E., & Spielberger, C. D. (1992). Family stress: Integrating theory and measurement. *Journal of Family Psychology, 6*, 99–112.

Institute on Rehabilitation Issues. (1999). *Meeting future workforce needs.* Menomonie, WI: Stout Vocational Rehabilitation Institute, University of Wisconsin-Stout.

Iwasaki, Y., & Mactavish, J. B. (2005). Ubitiquitous yet unique: Perspectives of people with disabilities on stress. *Rehabilitation Counseling Bulletin, 48*(4), 194–208.

Kosciulek, J. F. (1995). Impact of head injury on families: An introduction for family counselors. *The Family Journal: Counseling and Therapy for Couples and Families, 3*(2), 116–125.

Kosciulek, J. F. (2004). Family counseling. In F. Chan, N. L. Berven, & K. R. Thomas (Eds.), *Counseling theories and techniques for rehabilitation health professionals* (pp. 264–281). New York: Springer Publishing Company.

Kosciulek, J. F., McCubbin, M. A., & McCubbin, H. I. (1993). A theoretical framework for family adaptation to head injury. *Journal of Rehabilitation, 59*(3), 40–45.

Lazarus, R. S., & Folkman, S. (1984). *Stress, appraisal, and coping.* New York: Springer.

Lemaistre, J. (1995). *After the diagnosis: From crisis to personal renewal for patients with chronic illness.* Berkeley, CA: Ulysses Press.

Livneh, H. (2001). Psychosocial adaptation to chronic illness and disability. *Rehabilitation Counseling Bulletin, 44,* 151–160.

Maes, S., Leventhal, H., & de Ridder, D. T. (1996). Coping with chronic diseases. In M. Zeidner & N. S. Endler (Eds.), *Handbook of coping: Theory, research and applications* (pp. 221–251). New York: John Wiley & Sons.

McCubbin, M. A., & McCubbin, H. I. (1991). Family stress theory and assessment: The Resiliency Model of family stress, adjustment, and adaptation. In H. I. McCubbin & A. I. Thompson (Eds.), *Family assessment inventories for research and practice* (pp. 3–32). Madison, WI: University of Wisconsin-Madison.

McCubbin, H. I., & Patterson, J. M. (1983). The Double ABCX model of adjustment and adaptation. In H. I. McCubbin, M. B. Sussman, & J. M. Patterson (Eds.), *Social stress and the family: Advances and developments in family stress theory and research* (pp. 7–37). New York: Haworth Press.

Miller, J. F. (Ed.). (2000). *Coping with chronic illness: Overcoming powerlessness* (3rd ed.). Philadelphia: Davis.

Monnier, J., Hobfoll, S. E., Dunahoo, C.L., Hulsizer, M. R., & Johnson, R. (1998). There's more than rugged individualism in coping. Part 2: Construct validity and further model testing. *Anxiety, Stress, Coping: An International Journal, 11*(3), 247–272.

National Organization on Disability. (2000). *Survey of the status of people with disabilities in the United States: Employment.* Washington, DC: Author.

Parker, J. D., & Endler, N. S. (1996). Coping and defense: A historical overview. In M. Zeidner & N. S. Endler (Eds.), *Handbook of coping: Theory, research, applications* (pp. 3–23). New York: Wiley.

Pearlin, L. I., & Schooler, C. (1978). The structure of coping. *Journal of Health & Social Behavior, 9,* 3–21.

Pierce, G. R., Sarason, I. G., & Sarason, B. R. (1996). Coping and social support. In M. Zeidner & N. S. Endler (Eds.), *Handbook of coping: Theory, research, applications* (pp. 434–451). New York: Wiley.

Ptacek, J. T., & Pierce, G. (2003). Issues in the study of stress and coping in rehabilitation settings. *Rehabilitation Psychology, 48*(2), 113–124.

Riding, T. M. (1997). Normalization: Analysis and application within a specialty hospital. *Journal of Psychiatric and Mental Health Nursing, 4,* 23–28.

Rothman, R. A. (1987). *Working: Sociological perspectives.* Englewood Cliffs, NJ: Prentice Hall.

Shawcross, J. T. (1967). *The complete poetry of John Donne.* Garden City, NY: Anchor Books.

Stapleton, D. C., & Burkhauser, R. V. (Eds.). (2003). *The decline in employment of people with disabilities: A policy puzzle.* Kalamazoo, MI: W. E. Upjohn Institute.

Stout, C. E. (2004). *Psychology of terrorism: Coping with the continuing threat.* Westport, CT: Praeger.

Szymanski, E. M., & Trueba, H. T. (1994). Castification of people with disabilities: Potential disempowering aspects of classification in disability services. *Journal of Rehabilitation, 60*(3), 12–20.

Thoits, P. (1986). Social support as coping assistance. *Journal of Consulting & Clinical Psychology, 54,* 416–423.

Underwood, P. W. (2000). Social support: The promise and the reality. In V. H. Rice (Ed.), *Handbook of stress, coping, and health: Implications for nursing research, theory, and practice* (pp. 367–391). Thousand Oaks, CA: Sage.

Vash, C. L., & Crewe, N, M. (2004). *Psychology of disability* (2nd ed.). New York: Springer Publishing Company.

Walsh, F. (2002). A family resilience framework: Innovative practice applications. *Family Relations, 51*(2), 130–137.

Wells, J. D., Hobfoll, S. E., & Lavin, J. (1997). Resource loss, resource gain, and communal coping during pregnancy among women with multiple roles. *Psychology of Women Quarterly, 21*(4), 645–662.

Wethington, E., & Kessler, R. C. (1991). Situations and processes of coping. In J. Eckenrode (Ed.), *The social context of coping* (pp. 13–30). New York: Plenum Press.

Wright, B. A. (1983). *Physical disability: A psychosocial approach* (2nd ed.). New York: Harper & Row.

5
Reauthoring the Self: Chronic Sorrow and Posttraumatic Stress Following the Onset of CID

Susan Roos and Robert A. Neimeyer

Complications stemming from her delivery left Jackie traumatized from birth, having suffered a vaguely-diagnosed brain injury, resulting in a cerebral palsy-like disorder—walking with a halting gait and a "spastic condition" that was exacerbated when she was fatigued. Now in her mid-fifties, she sought counseling for pervasive feelings of grief, sadness, anxiety, and insufficiency, especially in social and work situations, and a deep sense of aloneness and isolation. As a lay minister in her church, Jackie's fears currently focused on her concern that, despite her apparent intelligence and sensitivity, she "might actually be harmful" to the people she attempted to serve.

Echoing the implicit, lifelong attitude of her highly protective mother and sister, she sensed that she was "always a problem for people," and that her "vulnerability and helplessness" were "encoded in her body" from her near-suffocation at the moment of birth. Her subsequent life, marked by a series of losses following the early death of her father and divorce from her husband, seemed to validate her core fear that others would always reject her in the end. As a consequence, Jackie's self-isolation was protective of both herself and others, a way of defending herself from abandonment, and of sparing others contact with a self she presumed to be deficient at best, and toxic at worst.

Jackie's self-criticism found dramatic expression in the second session of therapy when the second author invited her to enact her internal dialogue by taking an empty chair, lending her inner critic her own voice, before resuming her seat and responding, allowing the dialogue to unfold in whatever direction it did. Immediately the "critic" savaged Jackie for her brokenness and inadequacy, admonishing her with the statement, "You're a lost cause. You do everything late! You'll never get things done! Never! What makes you think that you have anything to say that people want to hear? You are a *wrong*! People are not supposed to look like you, to move like you. Nothing you do will ever be right! You can never be a *right*, because people know you're a *wrong*!" Taking her own seat, Jackie's initial responses were weak and ineffectual, because, as she noted, "Part of me believes this, part of me believes that it's not okay to be me." Unsurprisingly, Jackie was left with a "deep heaviness" and a tendency to retreat to a "wilderness" of self-isolation, the pain of which ultimately prompted her to seek psychotherapeutic help.

The study of acute and posttraumatic stress reactions to the onset of chronic illness and disability (CID) and its aftermath would not be complete without an understanding of attendant grief responses. When confronted by a significant loss that is ongoing, unrelenting, and has no foreseeable end, the affected person is frequently launched, by way of traumatic disruptions, into a never-imagined life. The unchosen life of coping with permanent disability or chronic, debilitating illness is characterized by profound challenges, related to the imposed demand resulting from loss of the expected, assumed, dreamed-of, or normative future, and its replacement by an unwanted, often initially terrifying, new reality. Our goal in the present chapter is to examine posttraumatic adaptation to the experience of disability, using the dual lenses of narrative theory (Neimeyer, 2006) and chronic sorrow (Roos, 2002), to suggest ways to facilitate coping with the distinctive problems and prospects faced by individuals, like Jackie, who are dealing with these life-altering conditions.

The Self-Narrative and its Disruption

Isak Dineson once said in an interview that "all sorrows can be borne if you put them into a story" (Mohn, 1957, p.49). The immense variety of story-telling devices and media, contemporary and historical, attest to the ubiquitous human penchant for meaning-making through narrative discourse. Life narratives are evident in songs, novels, biographies, fiction, fables, folklore, movies, TV programming, plays, and poetry, as well as in intimate and social interactions and family life. We use story lines in order to teach, we tell children bedtime stories, and we share stories about our lives and even "our day" with partners and friends (Neimeyer & Levitt, 2001). Storying, as an internal resource for achieving coherent accounts of self and experience, has been the basis for psychological theories, such as script theory (Berne, 1973), and for a number of therapeutic modalities, such as journaling, psychodrama, and family reconstruction.

Interdisciplinary interest in narrative therapy has been increasing. Cognitive science research suggests that the way in which we organize stories into sequences, with beginnings, middles, and endings, may constitute the basic schematic structure for much of human thought (Barsalou, 1988; Mandler, 1984). Social psychologists, who have studied autobiographical accounts, have emphasized the means by which we subtly position ourselves as characters of moral worth in our stories (Wortham, 2001). Developmental psychologists have noted the gradual emergence of narrative capacities in children. Further, the neuroanatomy of autobiographical memory and narrative reasoning—processes that are difficult to disrupt even in the presence of brain lesions—is being mapped and better understood (Damasio, 1994; Rubin & Greenberg, 2003).

The last 15 years have witnessed a burgeoning application of these narrative models and findings in the context of clinical psychology and bereavement research, resulting in greater emphasis on meaning reconstruction and the organizing role of narrative in human life (Neimeyer, 1995, 2000, 2001). From this perspective, people are viewed as attempting to construct, revise, and enact a *self-narrative*, defined as "an overarching cognitive-affective-behavioral structure that organizes the 'micro-narratives' of everyday life into a 'macro-narrative' that consolidates our self-understanding, establishes our characteristic range of emotions and goals, and guides our performance on the stage of the social world" (Neimeyer, 2004, pp. 53–54). Thus, identity can be considered a narrative achievement, because it is through stories—those we tell about ourselves, those that relevant others tell about us, and those we enact or participate in with others—that we establish and strengthen a sense of self.

This emphasis on the construction of self in the social world carries the further, and darker, implication that the processes by which identity is established can also be disrupted in any of a number of ways, three of which have special relevance to CID. The first of these, *narrative disorganization*, arises when the self-narrative is shaken or splintered by a seismic event, such as a traumatic loss, and the world and the self as they were previously experienced no longer exist (Neimeyer, 2000, 2006). For many people, catastrophic injury or the diagnosis of a debilitating life-condition in oneself or a loved one can devastate the thematic coherence of one's self-narrative, representing a traumatic event that is difficult to integrate into the plot structure of one's previous life-story (McAdams, 2006). As Currier, Holland, and Neimeyer (2006) have demonstrated empirically, the resulting inability to "make sense" of a traumatic loss mediates the impact of such loss on complicated grief, accounting for essentially all of the variance between the objective situation and the chronic and intense devastation experienced on a subjective level. Likewise, much of what can be so traumatic in CID is the inability to find coherence and meaning in a life circumstance that is seemingly beyond comprehension. Practices of the narrative review of catastrophic life-events can therefore be helpful in promoting sense-making and the reestablishment of a sense of continuity and direction in a life-story gone tragically awry (Neimeyer, Herrero, & Botella, 2006).

A second form of narrative disruption of particular relevance to acute onset conditions, such as physical trauma to oneself or a significant other, is *narrative dissociation*: silent stories of loss that are largely "unvoiced" to others, or even to the self (Neimeyer, 2006). In such cases, critical aspects of the experience can become dissociated in both the classic psychodynamic sense, unintegrated into one's conscious story of self, as well as being deprived of an audience in the social world. As Stiles and his colleagues (2004) have demonstrated, unassimilated life experiences can take many forms, ranging from a vague or emerging awareness of something psychologically painful, through "screen memories" and active avoidance of unwanted thoughts, to entirely warded-off, unconscious material that can take the form of somatic symptoms or abrupt switches in psychological states or personalities. In many forms of CID, the obvious physical limitations usually force the affected individual to acknowledge their reality, however reluctantly; yet, their subtler impacts and meanings are often integrated into the person's self-narrative and disclosed in public only gradually and with difficulty. Efforts to help the person give voice to these silent narratives in a setting in which they can be validated can therefore have a healing function (Rynearson, 2001).

Finally, a third form of disruption of high relevance to CID is *narrative dominance*, in which a particular story of self comes to "colonize" one's sense of identity and possibility, crowding out all others (Neimeyer, 2000, 2006; White & Epston, 1990). For many with CID conditions, the illness or disability can become the dominant story of their lives, the thematic structure in which all life experience is framed. Jackie, for example, apparently viewed herself as pervasively defective and isolated by her disability, viewing all significant life struggles through this lens. As her case further illustrates, this form of dominance often reflects the attributions of others in the family or broader social world, underscoring the pernicious role of social attitudes toward disability in configuring a self-concept (Wright, 1983). In such cases, resistance to dominant narratives of disability could take the form of seeking out an individual's choices and actions, which undermine the oppressive story that is often associated with "disability," and drawing on them to affirm a preferred story of hope and competence, even in the face of severe stress (White & Epston, 1990). Taken together, attempts to counter narrative disorganization, dissociation, and dominance in rehabilitation counseling and therapy are congruent with models of adaptation to CID, which focus on the individual's capacity for identity reconstruction and self-reorganization in the aftermath of a potentially traumatizing life-disruption (Livneh & Parker, 2005).

Chronic Sorrow

A second lens through which CID can be usefully viewed is that of chronic sorrow, a common and ongoing form of grief resulting from confrontation with the persistent, and often escalating losses that arise from significant, permanent injury, or the progressive deterioration of oneself or a loved one (Roos, 2002). As first introduced in the 1960s (Olshansky, 1962, 1966), the concept of chronic sorrow referred to understandable, non-pathological, profound, pervasive, and resurgent parental grief responses to having a child with permanent and severe developmental disabilities (e.g., neural tube defects, cerebral palsy, autism, mental retardation, congenital metabolic disorders, etc.). The concept was a compassionate paradigm shift away from previously-held professional views of ongoing and periodically exacerbated parental distress as pathological. Parents themselves had been recipients of such negative labels as "neurotic," "chronically depressed," "schizophrenogenic," "autistogenic," "never satisfied," and "unable to accept" their children's severe disabilities and mental deficiencies.

Olshansky, a rehabilitation counselor, administrator, and researcher, reasoned that because the child continues to live and to require constant care, permanent adaptations cannot occur, and grief cannot be resolved, as it might be in cases of loss due to finality (e.g., death, divorce, loss of a job). Despite the ongoing nature of chronic sorrow, Olshansky observed that most parents meet their challenges with tenacity, function effectively, and take pride and pleasure in their child. They learn to be more comfortable with the child's disabilities and develop ways to help the child. However, Olshansky expected that parents would understandably have periodic resurgence of grief intensity, probably as long as the child lives.

Since the early 1990s, when professional interest in chronic sorrow re-emerged, primarily from the field of nursing, the concept has been found to have much wider applicability. Chronic sorrow has now been documented in a variety of conditions involving CID, and is currently being usefully applied to many individuals, who are themselves the locus of the loss, as well as to those who love and care for them (Burke, 1998; Hainsworth, 1994; Lindgren, 1992, 1996; Lindgren et al., 1992). Understandably, there are differences in perspective and in how chronic sorrow is experienced by persons with CID, who are the locus of the loss, and by those who are emotionally close to them (e.g., parents, siblings, partners, devoted friends). Individual and situational variables are so extensive and complex that these differences have yet to be delineated.

Social support can be meager for those who are coping with chronic sorrow and its accompanying stress. Whether due to self-loss or other-loss, this type of grief is largely disenfranchised (Doka, 2002; Doka & Aber, 1989). Because the person has not died, there is usually no social recognition of the loss and, sadly, often little recognition of the *person* who is the source of the loss. There are no rituals, no customary social supports, and no acceptable ways to grieve the loss. Often, there is no time and space in which to grieve, because the loss demands drastic and immediate actions, related to diagnosis and treatment, and because often the person requires complicated, 24-hour care. Further, as the research of Braun and Berg (1994) illustrates, this disenfranchisement can create a kind of "double loss" in instances in which a chronic sorrow condition, such as the birth of a child with a severe disability, is followed years later by the loss of the child through death. In such cases, not only can the legitimacy of the family caregiver's grief be discounted during the child's life, but her or his loss can also be invalidated following the child's death, as others in the social world fail to recognize the real grief experienced, offering reassurances that the death is "a blessing," that the parents can devote more attention to their "normal" children, and other similarly hurtful attempts at comforting. Thus, chronic sorrow is not simply an internal psychic process, but is also a condition that can be exacerbated by observable practices and processes in the social world, such as the subtle attribution of blame and personal deficiency from which Jackie suffered.

The meaning attached to losing the life that was assumed, imagined, and expected in the natural course of events, is shaped by countless variables (e.g., age at onset and severity of condition; cultural, social, and family impacts; identity development; strength of the attachment to life dreams and expectations;

economic resources). Whether the loss is of crucial aspects of oneself (self-loss) or another living person (other-loss) to whom there is a deep attachment, the way in which the loss is perceived determines the existence of chronic sorrow, as well as its intensity and extent (Roos, 2002). Thus, although chronic sorrow is a common concomitant of CID, it is not inevitable, and even when present, need not be debilitating. It does, however, tend to color the lives of those whose losses have no clear endpoint, and in this sense, is an important, if often invisible, dimension of adaptation to CID.

The experiential core of chronic sorrow is a painful discrepancy between what is perceived as reality and what continues to be dreamed of (Roos, 2001, 2002). Although Jackie had never experienced herself as unfettered by disability, she obviously could—and did—see and comprehend the self, as was meant to be, and the self in reality. In the case of CID that develops in later childhood or adulthood, that moment of first realization of the loss is the trauma that launches chronic sorrow. As an initiation, it is the moment of one's expulsion from a metaphorical Eden. This realization can be of the birth of a child with severe congenital defects, the moment one learns of a diagnosis of HIV in oneself or a lover, the determination that a loved one's vegetative state is permanent, or the graduation from an uncertain prognosis to being an individual with quadriplegia, multiple sclerosis, or cancer. That moment—just before the realization of the loss—is one that will never be again. Eternity will not return it. Events conspire to produce a double plot: anxiety and grief.

Considering this largely "hidden" shadow of CID is important, because it is likely that the prevalence of chronic sorrow is escalating. As a result of technological improvements in medical care, the life-span of extremely low birth-weight infants and individuals with severe conditions is lengthening. Survival rates for stroke victims and individuals with major head injuries are increasing. Casualties of war and protracted, large group conflicts throughout the world add to the toll. Advancements in military medicine have permitted unusually high survival rates; consequently, military casualties involving permanent, extensive disabilities, such as limb amputations and major organ, skeletal, craniofacial, and brain damage, are accruing alarmingly. Due to its increasing prevalence, the need for an understanding of chronic sorrow by all helping professionals has never been greater.

Until recently, stress and chronic sorrow applicable to caregivers have received more attention than have their effects on individuals with CID. The psychological side to a new onset physical disability or debilitating chronic illness is extreme in its significance, yet frequently is minimized within the clinical domain. Nonetheless, its importance is paramount for physical rehabilitation, good professional care, and the ultimate reclaiming of a changed self. Although a person may have learned to adapt to and cope with circumstances, chronic sorrow is lodged in the matrix of meaning through which the person views the self and world. Thus, even when excluded from conscious awareness, chronic sorrow can affect perception, coloring—often darkly—every aspect of one's experience (Roos, 2001). As Jackie noted, it permeated her life to such an extent that it seemed "encoded in her body."

From a life-span perspective, individuals who are coping with chronic sorrow often have been sensitized to traumatic experiences. They, therefore, may experience complex posttraumatic stress disorder (PTSD) and other trauma-related disruptions of the self, including dissociation, relationship difficulties, revictimization, somatization, affect dysregulation, and disruptions in identity (Herman, 1992; Neimeyer et al., 2006). As a consequence, any distinction between the self and symptoms may become blurred; the person becomes at risk for taking on a defective, "disabled," or otherwise problematic identity, as a dominant narrative of whom he or she is in a more comprehensive or essential sense, a process that is often reinforced by social stereotypes. In the disability literature, a similar phenomenon has been recognized in the concept of "spread," which occurs when a single salient characteristic (e.g., a physical limitation) evokes similar inferences about a person's handicaps in other domains (Wright, 1983).

Adaptation to CID as a Trauma Response

The pain and stress of the onset of CID can often be seen as a psychological emergency. In the literature on disability, adaptation to this severe stressor is often depicted as a series of non-linear but hierarchical phases, including: (a) *Shock* and associated numbness and depersonalization, (b) *anxiety,* with attendant disorganization and fears of the future, (c) *denial* or minimization of the impact of the disability, (d) *depression* and hopelessness over loss of physical integrity or ability, (e) *internalized anger* and self-blame, (f) *externalized hostility* and blaming others, (g) gradual *acknowledgement* of the condition's implications and growing self-acceptance, and (h) eventual *adjustment* and the pursuit of new goals (Livneh and Antonak, 1997). In contemporary formulations of this model, these phases of adaptation are viewed as overlapping and continuous, with early reactions gradually being supplemented and ultimately supplanted by later ones, under favorable circumstances (Livneh and Antonak, 1997). Indeed, recent chaos theory applications to CID suggest that the process of adaptation may be even more complex, characterized by a non-linear, dynamic, and self-organizing course that defies clear prediction (Livneh & Parker, 2005).

A chronic sorrow conceptualization is broadly consonant with this model. From this perspective, the sudden onset of CID disorganizes a self-narrative that is constructed around assumptions of physical wellness. As Janoff-Bulman (1992) has noted, tragedy forces a reappraisal of the very beliefs in life's predictability and fairness that have defined our existence, as we are confronted by their naiveté. In the relatively extensive literature on adaptation to HIV or AIDS, for example, acute depression, fear, and specifically death anxiety have been associated with both the initial diagnosis and subsequent exacerbation of the disease (Neimeyer, Stewart, & Anderson, 2005), which are times that require substantial revisions of life assumptions. Unfortunately, in the unremitting or deteriorating courses that accompany many forms of CID, such revision and concomitant distress can be an ongoing challenge that requires ongoing coping efforts. Even with successful acknowledgement and behavioral adaptation to a life-limiting condition, the penumbra of chronic sorrow can darken daily life, yielding only gradually to the ironic "gifts" of the condition: opportunity for change, for growth, for deepening wisdom, and for reconstructing a more interesting and worthwhile life—one that includes a keen appreciation for the humor embedded in the absurdity of life that is lived in a permanently warped world (Roos, 2002).

Coping with and adapting to a CID can be especially challenging, however, in cases of a relapsing or episodic CID that involves periods of stabilization or improvement alternating with periods of exacerbation. Examples include multiple sclerosis, seizure disorders, hydrocephalic conditions (i.e., unpredictable and recurrent shunt blockages associated with increased intracranial pressure), chronic mental illness, autism, cystic fibrosis, and so on. The large discrepancy between crisis and non-crisis is psychologically taxing, as it is difficult to look forward to anything or to plan ahead. Even in periods of relative quiescence, affected individuals and their caregivers or families may adopt a stance of vigilance, anxiety, and wariness (Rolland, 1989; Roos, 2002). In narrative terms, a frequent additional aspect of the experience of chronic sorrow is the living of a life that is "marker bereft," devoid of the conventional milestones of a normally progressive life-course (Roos, 2002).

By facing a life that is fraught with both ambiguity and unpredictability, those who sustain a loss of ability, and their close family members, confront recurrent cycles of *primary* and *secondary* stress (Hewson, 1997). Primary episodes refer to extremely emotional and life-changing events, such as the time of first diagnosis (when recognition and adjustment are demanded), and when there are subsequent major crises (e.g., ventricular shunt failure, seizures). Secondary stress episodes refer to periods when the appraised stress is not so inherently challenging to daily routine or the future (e.g., cumulative stress, constancy of reality demands, fatigue, lack of support, etc.). The range of responses to these two conditions can fluctuate considerably on the continuum of responses described by Livneh and Antonak (1997), featuring prominent emotional states, such as shock, sadness, anger or guilt; physical responses, such as headaches, feeling hollow, and fatigue; cognitive responses, such as denial, confusion, rumination, and a sense of going crazy; and behavioral responses, such as social withdrawal, sleep disturbances, restless hyperactivity, and crying.

Particularly in periods of primary stress, when disabling illness or injury first occurs or is diagnosed, it is appropriate to speak of potential trauma, which carries the prospect of long-term consequences. As a relatively new diagnostic category, the term posttraumatic stress disorder (PTSD) first appeared in the *Diagnostic and Statistical Manual of Mental Disorders,* 3rd Edition (DSM-III: APA, 1980). The 1980 definition was problematic in its over-emphasis on the objective characteristics of the overt stressor. Thus, it was revised in *DSM-IV* (APA, 1994), and retained in *DSM-IV-TR* (APA, 2000). More diagnostic emphasis is now placed on the subjective experience of the traumatized individual, leading to recognition of the traumatogenic aspects of a wider variety of life events—including CID.

As an anxiety disorder, PTSD is defined by the existence of several major characteristics, including: (a) Exposure or witness to an event that is threatening and overwhelming in nature; (b) persistent reexperiencing of the event in varying sensory forms (e.g., flashbacks, nightmares, intrusive thoughts, physiological reactivity to associative cues); (c) marked avoidance of stimuli associated with or serving as reminders of the trauma experience, memory impairments, narrowing of affective range, and a sense of foreboding; and (d) increased arousal in the autonomic nervous system, such as sleep disturbances, inappropriate anger and irritability, problems with concentration, hypervigilance, and elevated startle response. Symptoms must impair functioning and persist for at least a month following the trauma, leading to impairment in social, occupational, or other important areas of functioning.

In keeping with the diagnostic shift in the DSM, Pearlman (2004) uses the term "trauma" as designating the response, not the stressor. Such a term aptly describes the experience of many individuals who suffer disabling injuries. For example, Martz and Cook (2001) found current rates of PTSD ranging from 8% to 13% in veterans suffering from major chest trauma, amputations, spinal cord injuries, and burns. Even more alarmingly, lifetime rates of the disorder have been reported for as many as 30–40% of survivors of life-threatening physical assault (Resnick, Kilpatrick, Dansky, Saunders, & Best, 1993), burns (Patterson, Carrigan, Questad, & Robinson, 1990), cardiac arrest (Ladwig, Schoefinius, Dammann, Danner, Gurtler, & Hermann, 1999), and spinal cord injury (Radnitz et al., 1995). Moreover, accumulating evidence indicates that PTSD is a persistent disorder, as survivors of violent attack, man-made disasters, and combat frequently meet criteria for PTSD even several years following the original trauma (Dirkzwager, Bramsen, & van der Ploeg, 2001; Green, Lindy, Grace, & Leonard, 1992; Kilpatrick, Saunders, Veronen, Best, & Von, 1987). Prospective studies of PTSD related to traffic accidents indicate that victims report approximately a 50% chance of continuing to suffer from PTSD symptoms after an interval of three years (Koren, Amon, & Klein, 2001; Mayou, Ehlers, & Bryant, 2002). Thus, it is clear that for a substantial subset of those with sudden-onset CID, the traumatic disruption of their self-narrative by serious injury or illness and its aftermath can prove disorganizing over a protracted period.

Although factors distinguishing those who develop PTSD remain unclear, Rothschild (2000) has identified several non-clinical factors that mediate traumatic stress. These include preparation for expected stress, successful fight or flight responses, developmental history, the person's belief system, prior experience, internal resources, and support (e.g., from family, community, and social networks). For those who do develop PTSD, however, it is clear that in some cases (e.g., complex PTSD), trauma can produce a profound discontinuity in one's identity and life narrative, affecting existential meaning and agency

(Neimeyer & Stewart, 1998; Watkins & Watkins, 1997). In the context of chronic sorrow, PTSD symptoms may be a factor in stress and grief responses during the life-span, especially during shifts in life-course developmental trajectories.

In the immediate aftermath of traumatic events, these symptoms are considered to be normal. When chronic, however, they can lead to a host of disturbances. Rothschild (2000) has argued that somatic disturbance is at the core of PTSD. Its symptoms can be incited by internal, as well as external, reminders of the traumatic event(s), and somatic symptoms alone can trigger a PTSD reaction; therefore, PTSD can become a vicious circle. For instance, the concept of "loss spirals,"* introduced by Roos (2002) as a complicating component of chronic sorrow, refers to intense, frequently disorienting responses to new or additional losses in the ordinary course of living. Often insignificant in and of itself, a current loss places the person at risk of rekindling affective flooding, in which one is launched into a review of virtually all past losses, the current loss, and anticipated losses well into the future. Just this sort of pattern was evident for Jackie, as minor reversals at work or in other domains reverberated with her deep and ongoing sense of insufficiency, disability, and vulnerability.

Based on cognitive therapy theory, Roos (2001, 2002) hypothesized that loss may be the central aspect of certain schemas. Current loss may tap into the brain's confirmatory function that crystallizes schemas about losses. Spirals may also lead to non-adaptive avoidance behaviors. Life decisions, large or small, may become associated with an overriding fear of potential losses and fears regarding one's ability to withstand or manage loss spirals in the event of their recurrence. Fears of positive expectations, emotional attachments, spontaneity, and feelings of want and desire can lead to avoidance and withdrawal. The vicious circle is perpetuated in many ways, including personal relationship patterns that, in fact, lead to further losses and, hence, the likelihood of increasing loss spirals, rather than preventing them. A life-long spiral of this sort seemed to be operating in the case of Jackie, for whom the concept of her disability and vulnerability to further loss came to occupy a central role in her sense of self, world, and future, engendering patterns of self-isolation that continued the spiral.

Suicide and Associated Problems

Individuals affected by PTSD are at greater risk of developing other Axis I disorders and usually have characteristics of at least one other psychiatric diagnosis. The most common of these co-occurring disorders are major depression, panic disorder, substance abuse or dependence, and dissociative

---

* Hobfall (1989) attaches a different meaning to the term "loss spiral" in his Conservation of Resources model of stress. He refers to the series of losses that occur in the context of trauma, in which internal and external resources become depleted, often in rapid succession

disorder (Kennedy & Duff, 2001). Professionals should be especially aware of the high incidence of suicidal thinking among individuals with CID. Based on a review of 73 studies of neurological disease, Arciniegas and Anderson (2002) found the risk of attempted or completed suicide is increased in patients with migraine with aura, epilepsy, stroke, multiple sclerosis, traumatic brain injury, and Huntington's disease. Several studies also suggest that the risk of suicide in patients with Alzheimer's, and other conditions involving dementia, increases relative to the general population. Individuals who are at risk for certain neurological disorders are also at increased risk for suicide; risk is especially high among individuals who have a genetic propensity for developing Huntington's disease, independent of the known presence or absence of the Huntington's gene mutation (Farrer, 1986; Kessler, 1987; Sorensen, 1992).

The risk of attempted or completed suicide in neurological illnesses (e.g., migraine with aura, epilepsy, stroke, multiple sclerosis, traumatic brain injury, and Huntington's disease) is strongly associated with depression and social isolation, as well as cognitive impairment, age under 60 years old, moderate physical disability, recent change in illness status, prior psychiatric illness or suicidal behaviors, and most importantly in our view, *a lack of future plans or perceived meaning in life* (Arciniegas and Anderson, 2002). Although the chaotic disruption of life patterns associated with the onset of CID can indeed set the stage for functional adaptation to chronic sorrow (Roos, 2002), posttraumatic growth (Calhoun & Tedeschi, 2006), or the creative evolution of the person's system at new levels of complexity (Livneh & Parker, 2005), the possibility of adverse outcomes, and the attendant need for intervention to bolster coping abilities, should not be minimized.

Case Illustration

Amir, age 49, was born in Sierra Leone, which is currently rated the world's poorest country by the World Health Organization. His family is Muslim. Amir's father took him to England at age 3 when Amir contracted polio. Ironically, Amir was born on the same day that world press headlines announced Jonas Salk's achievement of a successful immunization, but the vaccine was slow to reach West Africa. In England, "It was just the two of us—my father and me." His father studied law and became a barrister, while Amir attended a craft school for crippled children ("craft" and "crippled children" defined the perspective on disability at that time). Impressively, Amir obtained an economics degree before moving to the United States, where he obtained Bachelor's, Master's, and Ph.D. degrees through scholarships resulting from his involvement in wheelchair basketball, including the Paralympics. He is a professor and teaches physical education (pedagogy track). His loss history for the past decade is notable, including: a brief marriage and divorce; the deaths of a brother and both parents; and retirement from basketball, which was a source of belongingness and an identity characterized by coping, protest, and mastery. A woman, with whom he was intimately involved, had recently broken off their relationship. Indicating an understanding of collateral loss and limitations in CID, Amir remarked that enduring intimacy was more likely in relationships with other individuals with physical disabilities or with nurses and rehabilitation professionals "because they know the real deal."

Amir appeared to be a troubled, hurt, uncomfortable, yet determined, man in "new territory." He brought a feature story in a leading newspaper about himself and his involvement in wheelchair basketball, which was a tangible source of validation and a bridge for our first encounter. In narrative terms, two story motifs were represented: one from the old self-narrative (the article) and one from the new (his need for psychotherapy). Thus, at the very outset, he seemed to be underscoring the disruption in a previously coherent life-story that had been organized along hopeful and heroic lines.

Amir had recently been discharged from inpatient and outpatient psychiatric programs. He was on escitalopram oxalate (Lexapro) and temazepam (Restoril) for acute symptoms of depression and wary sleeplessness. He was attending AA and had 40 days of sobriety. He recounted recent events in a regressed, flat, dissociated manner, indicative of difficulty in assimilating the reality of what had happened. He had suffered a trauma. Selecting words carefully, he described a pattern of drinking during semester breaks and becoming increasingly solitary. Within these circumstances, he was denied tenure. He responded catastrophically. The denial signified failure. He said, "I was destroyed. Everything I've done and all I've accomplished will never be good enough." He felt dead. He had suffered a shattering of his previous consolidation of self and a massive narrative disorganization. He wondered what people would think and, ultimately, "What would my father say?"

He stayed alone in his house, not answering the phone and drinking "way too much." He re-read *Tuesdays with Morrie* (Albom, 1997), an account of one man's deepening maturity through conversations with a former professor, Morrie, who was in the end stages of amyotrophic lateral sclerosis (ALS) and philosophically confronting an imminent and inevitable death. In a distorted way, Amir's internal dialogue mirrored *Tuesdays* . . . . Due to his isolation, however, an external source of challenge or correction of distorted thinking was lacking. Cognitive function was impaired by alcohol, and reality-testing became increasingly tenuous. He became immobilized and "stuck in paradox," a solipsistic, repetitive, and circular consciousness that was fixated on polarities (e.g., "If I do this (go outside), then that will happen, but if I do another thing (stay indoors), then this other thing will happen, but if I don't do. . ., then. . . ."). He researched the term "mental collapse" on the internet. He had ideas of reference (i.e., an impression of meanings in internet-content as intended only for him). He became convinced he was dying. He stated, "I was going mad." Desperate, incapacitated, and unable to make any decisions for himself, he managed to call his ex-girlfriend. He asked her to keep him from dying. She took him to an emergency room, and he was transferred to a psychiatric hospital.

Amir realized that he had damaged himself physically with alcohol. His mind had suffered an insult; it had lost its quickness and resiliency. "My thinking doesn't flow well now, and my head hurts when I think too hard." The first author, as his therapist, sensed that he was asking for gentle, well-paced handling and that he was afraid to put his trust in me, a stranger with whom he would engage in the hard work of self-reconstruction and restoration. I saw this distrust as evidence of basic good sense. He identified one of his issues as "externality," referring to: "What do people think and say about me?" He said, "I don't know where the depression started." He described his role as an advocate, in which he "questioned the system," stressed the need for disability sports, and spoke on what it was like growing up with a disability. In this role, he was brought into opposition with the "medical model" (i.e., a perspective of disability as defined by pathology and deficit) and medical professionals, "so I have been living a life of opposites." He further pointed out that he was a "multiple minority" in a country in which he has no vote. He retains citizenship in Sierra Leone, is culturally British (though usually defined as African–American), black, has a disability, and is a United States resident, who is Muslim and living in the South. Contradictions in his self-narrative seemed palpable. Amir seemed to struggle to integrate opposing story lines of his life, with their contrasting images of his obvious abilities and equally obvious disability, and how each was received in the social world.

Lindy's (1985; Lindy & Wilson, 2004) therapeutic metaphor of the "trauma membrane" was applicable to this client. The trauma membrane, often initially a barrier constructed by supportive others to protect the traumatized individual, develops in time as an internal defense, a thin but vital boundary or "membrane" that covers the tear in the repression barrier that was created by the trauma experience. Its function is to decrease vulnerability to re-traumatization and to preserve the integrity of the survivor's life-experience. I would always respect this delicate semi-permeable membrane, yet I needed to find a way to interact with Amir that would both soothe his wounds and support moving to the next chapter of his life story, a not-so-unusual dialectic of therapy, especially when dealing with trauma and loss. Interestingly, in light of narrative theory, I had a vivid mental image of expensively bound books lying on their backs, open to the breeze, their pages rustling and rippling back and forth in dappled sunlight, as Amir struggled to reconstruct the events in his story. I had said very little, but had reflected his content well enough to convey understanding and the desire to better understand him and his situation. Conveying reasonable hope, I said, "We don't know yet exactly what paths we will take, but I do know that you have more options than we can possibly know about right now."

Amir has worked diligently in therapy, never missing an appointment and maintaining sobriety. He values his sessions as "the only place I can have conversations about the things we talk about." Regular attendance of AA meetings supports his individual progress. We began on a once-weekly schedule with gradual decreases in frequency. We currently meet every three weeks. Our initial focus was on: (a) Developing an intersubjective space of safety and mutual authenticity; (b) monitoring Amir's fragile state of consciousness; (c) restoring resiliency; and (d) getting to know Amir as a whole person, with a richly complex and unique past, a wounded present, and a reasonably hopeful future, yet he viewed it as highly conditional, due to his religious beliefs about fate. I have been comfortable with Amir's complexity and have found a sense of personal completion in the space that we have carefully created. Amir gained security by seeing his therapist pass the test of trustworthiness; e.g., I use the language of disability and loss, know the history of disability, make a distinction between normalization and access, and so on. As Amir regained resiliency, I inquired about how he had successfully coped with past disappointments. He began to revalue his "old" narrative, in which a sense of security was derived from the pride that was expressed by his idealized father (his "icon").

The idea of returning to the university was fraught with dread for Amir. An empowering step toward this goal occurred in mutual problem-solving to reorder boundaries with his AA sponsor. After he had successfully set limits with the sponsor, he returned to campus to retrieve his mail and felt intimations of the self-confidence that he needed to meet his next semester's classes. I asked, "What might your father be thinking?" He said, "He's proud, but he's also sad about how poorly I was taking care of myself, the drinking, and about what happened. He's worried it could happen again." Asked if his father blamed him, Amir replied, "I don't know. I can't answer that."

A few months ago, Amir was recruited as a consultant to a prestigious rehabilitation facility. He saw this opportunity as not being possible had he been granted tenure. "I'm doing what other faculty aren't doing, and I have time to do it well." The same week he signed the contract, he adopted a kitten, a sign of future projection and reconnection. His fragmented narrative had begun to cohere. He was making new meanings, revising out-of-date perceptions, and committing to a new attachment. I then reintroduced his pre-trauma motif of his life as an adventure.

Recently returning to Amir's trauma of relational and academic losses and, with careful titration of the retelling, he has expanded and elaborated a more detailed and meaningful account. I asked him to imagine his father sitting across the room or in his mind's eye. "Your father has heard and observed everything. Pay close attention to his facial expressions. Be open to what they tell you." I spoke of Amir's anguished devastation when tenure was denied and asked, "How does your father look to you?" "Distressed." "Is he angry with you?" "No, but he's agitated, upset." "Is he turning away from you?" "He would never do that!" After a period of silence, Amir stated: "My whole existence was dependent on making my father proud of me." "Yes," I said, "but I think you've been wrong about something, Amir. He not only saw to it that you lived and would have the best life possible, he also embraced his new life as a barrister. You both turned tragedy into triumph. You told me he took tough cases, those no one else would touch. His indomitable sense of justice included everyone. He would not have faulted you; he would see the injustice immediately, something he may have learned from you. He would ferret it out and expose it." After another silence, Amir said, "When I've thought that I've disappointed and failed him, I've misjudged him. Getting tenure would give me back the security I had with him. But I have to live my own life and face that it's up to me. It's me I must contend with. That's OK with my father. It's what a man does."

Amir chooses not to read the proceedings that led to denial of tenure. He does not do special projects, as he once did, and is more distant from some department faculty. Although scarred by trauma and many losses, he has nevertheless made good progress in therapy. He has achieved more differentiation from his father, values life more, and sees it as precious in light of its fragility. I can now imagine the expensively bound books of his life stacked in a chosen order. One book is open, and there is a bookmark on the open page. In fact, there are bookmarks in all the books, and Amir can now more easily refer to those markers and what they signify to him.

Conclusion

Whether having a disability or not, most people who seek psychotherapy do so when there has been a breakdown in the thematic motif of their life story. It no longer holds events together; it doesn't make sense any more. As co-authors, clients and therapists then collaborate in re-writing the story into what Hillman (1983) calls a "collaborative fiction" (i.e., a revisioning of the story into a more intelligent, more imaginative plot, one more open to possibility). Relationally, we search for a new story, but we also need to find a way to reconnect meaningfully to the old one. With work, luck, and fortitude, we attempt to make the story integrative, meaningful, and coherent. It is a process of growth, self-acceptance, maturing, and of finding a way to move beyond trauma and loss. Amir's story and that of many with chronic illnesses and disabilities symbolize this quest for triumph in the context of coping with tragedy.

References

Albom, M. (1997). *Tuesdays with Morrie*. New York: Doubleday.

American Psychiatric Association. (1980). *Diagnostic and statistical manual of mental disorders* (3rd ed.). Washington, DC: Author.

American Psychiatric Association. (1994). *Diagnostic and statistical manual of mental disorders* (4th ed.). Washington, DC: Author.

American Psychiatric Association (2000). *Diagnostic and statistical manual of mental disorders* (4th ed., TR). Washington, DC: Author.

Arciniegas, D. B., & Anderson, C. A. (2002). Suicide in neurologic illness. *Current Treatment Options in Neurology, 4*, 457–468.

Barsalou, L. W. (1988). The content and organization of autobiographical memories. In U. Neisser & E. Winograd (Eds.), *Remembering reconsidered* (pp. 193–243). Cambridge, UK: Cambridge University Press.

Berne, E. (1973). *What do you say after you say hello?* New York: Bantam Books.

Braun, M. J., & Berg, D. H. (1994). Meaning reconstruction in the experience of parental bereavement. *Death Studies, 18*, 105–129.

Burke, M. (1998). Chronic sorrow in mothers of school-age children with a myelomeningocele disability (Doctoral dissertation, Boston University, School of Nursing). (University Microfilms No. AAD89-20093.)

Calhoun, L., & Tedeschi, R. (Eds.). (2006). *Handbook of posttraumatic growth: Research and practice.* Mahwah, NJ: Lawrence Erlbaum.

Currier, J., Holland, J., & Neimeyer, R. A. (2006). Sense-making, grief, and the experience of violent loss: Toward a mediational model. *Death Studies*, 30, 403–428.

Damasio, A. R. (1994). *Descartes' error: Emotion, reason, and the human brain.* New York: Putnam.

Dirkzwager, A., Bramsen, I., & van der Ploeg, H. (2001). The longitudinal course of posttraumatic stress disorder among aging military veterans. *Journal of Nervous & Mental Disease, 189*, 846–853.

Doka, K. (Ed.). (2002). *Disenfranchised grief* (2nd ed.). Champaign, IL: Research Press.

Doka, K., & Aber, R. (1989). Psychosocial loss and grief. In K. Doka (Ed.), *Disenfranchised grief* (pp. 187–198). Lexington, MA: Lexington Books.

Farrer, L. A. (1986). Suicide and attempted suicide in Huntington's disease: Implications for preclinical testing of persons at risk. *American Journal of Medical Genetics, 24*, 305–311

Green, B. L., Lindy, J. D., Grace, M. C., & Leonard, A. C. (1992). Chronic posttraumatic stress disorder and diagnostic comorbidity in a disaster sample. *Journal of Nervous & Mental Disease, 180*, 760–766.

Hainsworth, M. (1994). Living with multiple sclerosis: The experience of chronic sorrow. *Journal of Neuroscience Nursing, 26*, 237–240.

Herman, J. L. (1992). Complex PTSD: A syndrome in survivors of prolonged and repeated trauma. *Journal of Traumatic Stress, 5*, 377–391.

Hewson, D. (1997). Coping with loss of ability: "Good grief" or episodic stress responses? *Social Science Medicine, 44*, 1129–1139.

Hillman, J. (1983). *Healing fiction.* Woodstock, CT: Spring Publications, Inc.

Hobfall, S. (1989). Conservation of resources: A new attempt at conceptualizing stress. *American Psychologist, 44*, 513–524.

Janoff-Bulman, R. (1992). *Shattered assumptions.* New York: Free Press.

Kennedy, P., & Duff, J. (2001). Post-traumatic stress disorder and spinal cord injuries. *Spinal Cord, 39*, 1–10.

Kessler, S. (1987). Psychiatric implications of presymptomatic testing for Huntington's disease. *American Journal of Orthopsychiatry, 57*, 212–219.

Kilpatrick, D. G., Saunders, B. E., Veronen, L. J., Best, C. L., & Von, J. M. (1987). Criminal victimization: Lifetime prevalence, reporting to police and psychological impact. *Crime & Delinquency, 33*, 479–489.

Koren, D., Amon, I., & Klein, E. (2001). Long-term course of chronic posttraumatic stress disorder in traffic accident victims: A three-year prospective, follow-up study. *American Journal of Psychiatry, 156*, 1449–1458.

Ladwig, K., Schoefinius, A., Dammann, G., Danner, R., Gurtler, R., & Hermann, R. (1999). Long-acting psychotraumatic properties of a cardiac arrest experience. *American Journal of Psychiatry, 156*(6), 912–919.

Lindgren, C. (1992). Current knowledge and research on chronic sorrow. *Death Studies, 16*, 231–245.

Lindgren, C. (1996). Chronic sorrow in persons with Parkinson's and their spouses. *Scholarly Inquiry for Nursing Practice, 10*, 351–366.

Lindgren, C., Burke, M., Hainsworth, M., & Eakes, G. (1992). Chronic sorrow: A lifespan concept. *Scholarly Inquiry for Nursing Practice, 6*, 27–40.

Lindy, J. D. (1985). The trauma membrane and other concepts derived from psychotherapeutic work with survivors of natural disaster. *Psychiatric Annals, 15*, 153–160.

Lindy, J. D., & Wilson, J. P. (2004). Respecting the trauma membrane: Above all, do no harm. In J. P. Wilson, M. J. Friedman, & J. D. Lindy (Eds.), *Treating psychological trauma and PTSD*. New York: Guilford Press.

Livneh, H., & Antonak, R. F. (1997). *Psychosocial adaptation to chronic illness and disability*. Gaithersburg, MD: Aspen.

Livneh, H., & Parker, R. M. (2005). Psychological adaptation to disability: Perspectives from chaos and complexity theory. *Rehabilitation Counseling Bulletin, 49*, 17–28.

Mandler, J. (1984). *Scripts, stories, and scenes*. Hillsdale, NJ: Erlbaum.

Martz, E., & Cook, D. (2001). Physical impairments as risk factors for the development of posttraumatic stress disorder. *Rehabilitation Counseling Bulletin, 44*, 217–221.

Mayou, R. A., Ehlers, A., & Bryant, B. (2002). Posttraumatic stress disorder after motor vehicle accidents: 3-Year follow up of a prospective longitudinal study. *Behavioral Research & Therapy, 40*, 665–675.

McAdams, D. P. (2006). The problem of narrative coherence. *Journal of Constructivist Psychology, 19*, 109–125.

Mohn, B. (1957, November 3). Talk with Isak Dinesen. *New York Times Book Review*, p. 49.

Neimeyer, R. A. (1995). Client-generated narratives in psychotherapy. In R. A. Neimeyer & M. J. Mahoney (Eds.), *Constructivism in psychotherapy* (pp. 231–246). Washington, DC: American Psychological Association.

Neimeyer, R. A. (2000). Narrative disruptions in the construction of self. In R. A. Neimeyer & J. D. Raskin (Eds.), *Constructions of disorder* (pp. 207–241). Washington, DC: American Psychological Association.

Neimeyer, R. A. (Ed.). (2001). *Meaning reconstruction and the experience of loss*. Washington, DC: American Psychological Association.

Neimeyer, R. A. (2004). Fostering posttraumatic growth: A narrative contribution. *Psychological Inquiry, 15*, 53–59.

Neimeyer, R. A. (2006). Re-storying loss: Fostering growth in the posttraumatic narrative. In L. Calhoun & R. Tedeschi (Eds.), *Handbook of posttraumatic growth: Research and practice*. Mahwah, NJ: Lawrence Erlbaum.

Neimeyer, R. A., Herrero, O., & Botella, L. (2006). Chaos to coherence: Psychotherapeutic integration of traumatic loss. *Journal of Constructivist Psychotherapy, 19*, 127–145.

Neimeyer, R. A., & Levitt, H. (2001). Coping and coherence: A narrative perspective on resilience. In D. Snyder (Ed.), *Stress and coping* (pp. 47–67). New York: Oxford University Press.

Neimeyer, R. A., & Stewart, A. E. (1998). Trauma, healing, and the narrative emplotment of loss. In C. Franklin & P. A. Nurius (Eds.), *Constructivism in practice* (pp. 165–183). Milwaukee, WI: Families International Press.

Neimeyer, R. A., Stewart, A. E., & Anderson, J. (2005). AIDS-related death anxiety: A research review and clinical recommendations. In H. E. Gendelman, S. Swindells, I. Grant, S. Lipton, & I. Everall (Eds.), *The neurology of AIDS* (2nd ed.) (pp. 787–799). New York: Chapman & Hall.

Olshansky, S. (1962). Chronic sorrow: A response to having a mentally defective child. *Social Casework, 43*, 190–193.

Olshansky, S. (1966). Parent responses to a mentally defective child. *Mental Retardation, 4*, 21–23.

Patterson, D. R., Carrigan, L., Questad, K. A., & Robinson, R. (1990). Posttraumatic stress disorder in hospitalized patients with burn injuries. *Journal of Burn Care Rehabilitation, 11*, 181–184.

Pearlman, L. A. (2004). Treatment of persons with complex PTSD and other trauma-related disruptions of the self. In J. P. Wilson, M. J. Friedman, & J. D. Lindy (Eds.), *Treating psychological trauma & PTSD*. New York: Guilford.

Radnitz, C. L., Schlein, I. S., Walczak, S., Broderick, P., Binks, M., Tirch, D. D. et al. (1995). The prevalence of posttraumatic stress disorder in veterans with spinal cord injury. *SCI Psychosocial Process, 8*, 145–149.

Resnick, H. S., Kilpatrick, D. G., Dansky, B. S., Saunders, B. E., & Best, C. L. (1993). Prevalence of civilian trauma and posttraumatic stress disorder in a representative national sample of women. *Journal of Consulting and Clinical Psychology, 61*, 984–991.

Rolland, J. (1989). Chronic illness and the family life cycle. In B. Carter & M. McGoldrick (Eds.), *The changing family life cycle* (2nd ed.). New York: Allyn & Bacon.

Roos, S. (2001). Theory development: Chronic sorrow and the Gestalt construct of closure. *Gestalt Review, 5*, 289–310.

Roos, S. (2002). *Chronic sorrow: A living loss*. New York: Brunner-Routledge.

Rothschild, B. (2000). *The body remembers: The psychophysiology of trauma and trauma treatment*. New York: Norton.

Rubin, D. C., & Greenberg, D. L. (2003). The role of narrative in recollection. In G. D. Fireman, T. E. McVay, & O. J. Flanagan (Eds.), *Narrative and consciousness* (pp. 53–85). New York: Oxford.

Rynearson, E. K. (2001). *Retelling Violent Death*. Philadelphia: Brunner-Routledge.

Sorensen, S. A. (1992). Causes of death in patients with Huntington disease and in unaffected first degree relatives. *Journal of Medical Genetics, 29*, 911–914.

Stiles, W., Osatuke, K., Glick, M., & MacKay, H. (2004). Encounters between internal voices generate emotion: An elaboration of the assimilation model. In H. Hermans & G. Dimaggio (Eds.), *The dialogical self in psychotherapy* (pp. 91–107). London: Routledge.

Watkins, J. G., & Watkins, H. H. (1997). *Ego states*. New York: Norton.

White, M., & Epston, D. (1990). *Narrative means to therapeutic ends*. New York: Norton.

Wortham, S. (2001). *Narratives in action*. New York: Teachers College.

Wright, B. A. (1983). *Physical disability—A psychosocial approach* (2nd ed.). New York: HarperCollins.

6
Adaptive Tasks and Methods of Coping with Illness and Disability

Rudolf H. Moos and Charles J. Holahan

An acute health crisis and its progression into a chronic illness or disability (CID) is a turning point in an individual's life. The vivid confrontation with a severe physical illness or injury, prolonged treatment and uncertainty, and intense personal distress has a profound and lasting impact. Most individuals cope reasonably well with such a crisis and are able to recover and achieve a new equilibrium. Some individuals emerge with a more mature outlook and a richer appreciation of life, but others are demoralized and suffer lasting psychological problems. What are the main determinants of individuals' psychosocial adaptation to CID? What adaptive tasks do individuals confront and what coping skills do they use to manage the initial crisis and its aftermath? What coping responses promote psychosocial recovery? To address these issues, we offer a conceptual framework that considers CID as an extended life crisis, describe relevant adaptive tasks and coping skills, and identify the primary determinants and outcomes of adaptive coping.

Historical and Theoretical Background

Current perspectives on coping with CID have been shaped by crisis theory, a biopsychosocial orientation, and diverse models of coping processes and resources.

Crisis Theory

Crisis theory focuses on how individuals confront and manage major life crises and disruptions to their established patterns of personal and social identity (Caplan, 1964; Lindemann & Lindemann, 1979; for recent overviews, see Roberts, 2000; Schaefer & Moos, 1998). A situation, which is so novel or all-encompassing that habitual responses are inadequate, engenders psychological turbulence, accompanied by heightened fear, distress, and/or anger. Because an individual cannot remain in a state of extreme disequilibrium, a crisis is self-limited. Even though it may be temporary, a resolution must be found and some equilibrium reestablished within a few days or weeks. The new balance may represent a healthy adaptation, which promotes personal growth and maturation, or a less adaptive response, which foreshadows psychological deterioration and decline.

Due to its typically sudden and unexpected appearance and its threat to an individual's life and well-being, the onset and development of a CID is an especially potent crisis. Moreover, even though individuals may achieve a tentative equilibrium, it may be shattered at any moment by unforeseen events. According to crisis theory, an individual is more receptive to outside influence at a time of disequilibrium. Such accessibility offers health professionals and other caregivers an unusual opportunity for constructive interventions for individuals with CID and their families.

A Biopsychosocial Perspective

The biopsychosocial orientation to health-care grew out of psychosomatic and behavioral medicine. The psychosomatic perspective focused primarily on personal and environmental factors and their connections to the onset and progression of chronic disorders, such as diabetes, hypertension, and rheumatoid arthritis. Evidence showed that these disorders were more likely to begin and to have a stormier course in the context of interpersonal conflicts and life crises (Backus & Dudley, 1974; Selye, 1956; for recent overviews, see Krantz & McCeney, 2002; Levenson, 2005). The psychosomatic orientation focused on the influence of personal and social factors in the onset and course of illness, but tended to neglect the role of adaptive coping skills in recovery.

These issues were addressed more directly by behavioral medicine, which emphasized problem-solving coping skills and the active role of the individual in managing and controlling some of the consequences of illness and disability. The biopsychosocial perspective integrated these ideas in a holistic systems approach to maximizing health and well-being. This view encompassed personal and environmental factors, coping processes, and the participation of the individual with CID and family members in all aspects of health-care (Leigh & Reiser, 1992).

Coping Resources and Processes

Theoretical formulations of coping processes began with psychoanalysis and the idea that ego defenses helped to resolve conflicts between an individual's impulses and external reality. Subsequently, theorists emphasized reality-oriented coping processes of the "conflict-free" ego sphere, such as attention, perception, and memory (Angyal, 1941; Haan, 1977; Hartman, 1950). In addition to highlighting defense and coping processes, these theorists formulated a developmental view of the accumulation of coping resources over an individual's life span (Erikson, 1963).

In a separate but parallel development, learning theory led to an emphasis on problem-solving behavior and behavior modification procedures. Initial applications of this tradition focused only on behavior, but quickly evolved to attend to cognitive components of coping. Cognitive behaviorism emphasizes the active role of the individual in self-regulation and highlights the sense of self-efficacy as a coping resource (Bandura, 1977). Individuals must believe they can succeed in an endeavor, in order to actively try to master the tasks involved. Successful coping promotes future expectations of self-efficacy, which inspire vigorous and persistent efforts at mastery.

The next step was the development of a transactional approach to the stress and coping process (Lazarus & Folkman, 1984). A stressful experience begins with primary appraisal, which involves awareness of an actual or threatened change and includes an initial evaluation of its potential significance. Secondary appraisal involves an evaluation of the options for coping and the extent to which the individual may be able to control or change the situation. The individual's belief that there is a strategy, which can achieve the desired outcome (outcome efficacy), and that he or she can effectively exercise that strategy (self-efficacy) are important determinants of coping.

An Integrative Conceptual Framework

Consistent with other conceptual models of adaptation to health problems (Livneh & Antonak, 1997; Livneh & Parker, 2005; Walker, Jackson, & Littlejohn, 2004), we constructed a framework to guide an understanding of the process of coping with CID. This framework offers a way of conceptualizing coping skills and integrates coping in a broader predictive model. According to the model (Figure 6.1), five sets of factors are associated with the selection and choice of coping skills: health-related factors, personal resources, the social and physical context, cognitive appraisal, and adaptive tasks.

Personal resources (Panel I), health-related factors (Panel II), and the social and physical context (Panel III) influence appraisal of a health condition (Panel IV) and the formulation of adaptive tasks (Panel V). These factors shape the choice of coping skills (Panel VI), which then mediate between the influences in Panels I through V and health-related outcomes (Panel VII). In a mutual feedback cycle, health-related outcomes may alter the preceding sets of factors and consequently, change longer-term health outcomes.

Personal Resources

Personal resources include intellectual ability, ego strength and self-confidence, religious beliefs, and prior health-related and coping experiences, as well as such

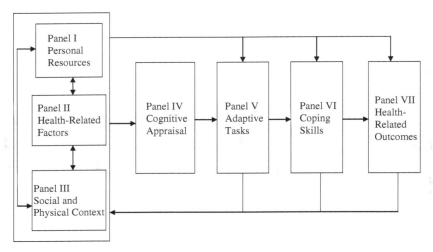

FIGURE 6.1. Conceptual model of the determinants of health-related outcomes of chronic illness and disability.

demographic characteristics as age, gender, and education. Personal resources also encompass relatively stable personality characteristics, such as extroversion, optimism, internal control, and sense of coherence, as well as broad cognitive and problem-solving styles, such as autonomy and dependency (Moos & Holahan, 2003). Individuals, who have a more internal locus of control, higher self-confidence and self-efficacy, and a stronger sense of coherence, are more likely to rely on problem-solving and other aspects of approach coping (De Ridder & Schreurs, 1996; Kemp, Morley, & Anderson, 1999; Lustig, 2005). Optimistic individuals tend to rely more on seeking social support and problem-solving coping, whereas pessimistic individuals tend to rely more on denial, resignation, and venting affect (Scheier & Carver, 1987).

 ## Health-Related Factors

Health-related factors include the rapidity of onset and progression of a condition, the location of symptoms, the stage and severity of illness, such as whether a cancer is localized or widespread, and the type of disability. They also encompass the health-care environment and treatment procedures, including unfamiliar technical equipment, such as scanners and lasers, examinations by seemingly aloof strangers, dependence on other people for basic needs, and mandatory consent forms that graphically outline the risks of complex surgical procedures, total body irradiation, and exposure to invasive tests, such as cardiac catheterization (Groves & Muskin, 2005).

Individuals facing a life-threatening illness, such as cancer and myocardial infarction, initially rely more on problem-focused coping than do individuals who face a non-life-threatening illness, such as arthritis and dermatitis (Feifel,

Strack, & Nagy, 1987). Overall, however, coping may vary more in relation to stage than type of illness. For example, women with newly diagnosed breast-cancer initially rely heavily on approach coping, but then decline in their use of these skills over time (McCaul et al., 1999).

Social and Physical Context

The social context encompasses relationships between individuals with CID and their family members and friends, and the support and expectations of other members of their social network, such as caregivers and coworkers. A supportive social context can enhance self-efficacy, appraisal of a health condition as more of a challenge than a threat, and reliance on approach coping (Rohrbaugh et al., 2004). Conversely, a lack of spouse support has been associated with lower self-efficacy and more reliance on avoidance coping among individuals with cancer (Manne & Glassman, 2000). When family members or friends convey criticism or a lack of interest, individuals with a serious health condition may avoid talking about their problems and may be less likely to cope with illness-related demands (Norton et al., 2005).

The physical features of a home and workplace, including ease of access, can markedly influence individuals' range of mobility and autonomy. The aesthetic quality of the surroundings, the type of personal space and privacy, and the amount of sensory stimulation, all affect the adaptive tasks individuals face and their choice of coping responses. In combination with the trauma of a health crisis, the cumulative burden of adversity that individuals with CID experience may heighten a reliance on avoidance coping and lead to non-adherence to health-care, including failure to return for follow-up visits, to adhere to therapeutic regimens, and to institute exercise and life-style changes (Alonzo, 2000).

Cognitive Appraisal and Adaptive Tasks

Cognitive Appraisal

The way in which individuals appraise a crisis is the first step in construing adaptive tasks and choosing potential coping strategies. The key aspects of appraisal include the context of the stressor, such as whether it was expected and there was adequate time to prepare for it. Appraisal also encompasses whether the problem is seen as a challenge or a threat, how much it seems changeable or controllable, and the extent to which it is seen as caused by one's self. Related aspects of illness perceptions include individuals' beliefs about the causes and probable consequences of the illness, expectations about its duration and course, and potential controllability or cure (Scharloo & Kaptein, 1997). To note, self-blame and catastrophic thinking have sometimes been conceptualized as coping responses; however, because they reflect the perception that a stressor was self-caused and will be overwhelming, they appear to be more closely related to an appraisal of the extent to which the individual is responsible for the problem and the severity of the threat associated with it.

In general, individuals, who perceive a health condition as expected, controllable, and changeable, are likely to rely on approach coping. In contrast, individuals, who perceive the condition as more severe and threatening, are likely to rely on avoidance coping. In an analysis of illness representations, individuals reporting more control over their epilepsy relied more on problem-focused coping and less on wishful thinking and other aspects of avoidance coping (Kemp et al., 1999).

Adaptive Tasks

Different health problems encompass many comparable tasks, such as managing physical impairments, accepting one's illness and personal needs, giving up ordinary activities, adapting to an altered social identity, and finding new ways to maintain social relationships (De Ridder, Schreurs, & Bensing, 1998; Heijmans et al., 2004). These tasks can be divided into seven groups: three tasks are related to the health condition and its treatment; the other four tasks are more general and apply to all types of life-crises. These seven tasks are typically encountered with all CIDs, but their relative importance varies, depending on the person, the specific health problem, and the unique set of circumstances.

Managing Symptoms

The first set of tasks is to manage the discomfort, incapacitation, and other symptoms of an ongoing health condition. This covers a range of disturbing symptoms, such as pain, weakness, dizziness, incontinence, paralysis, loss of control, the feeling of suffocation, and permanent disfigurement. Individuals with CID must learn to recognize the signs of impending crises and to control their symptoms whenever possible. For instance, individuals with chronic heart failure or renal disease must regulate their diet and daily exercise; individuals with diabetes must try to prevent potential crises caused by the complications of excess sugar or insulin shock.

Managing Treatment

A second set of tasks entails managing treatment procedures. Therapeutic measures that create special adaptive tasks include surgical procedures (e.g., mastectomy and colostomy), debridement as a treatment for burns, radiotherapy and chemotherapy with their concomitant side effects, the need to wear a cumbersome brace for certain orthopedic disorders, and long-term renal dialysis or organ transplantation. Specialized hospital environments such as operating and recovery rooms, intensive care units, premature baby nurseries, and even waiting rooms of oncology clinics also encompass significant stressors.

Forming Relationships with Health-Care Providers

This set of tasks involves developing and maintaining adequate relationships with health-care providers and other professional caregivers. Individuals with CID often experience considerable turmoil about how to express their need for more pain medication or how to manage their anger at a nurse who does not answer their call for help, how to cope with a caregiver's apparent condescension, and how to question a physician's diagnosis and ask for a second opinion or an alternate treatment. The individual's dependence and the frequent turnover of providers and specialized caregivers make this an unusually complex set of tasks.

[handwritten in left margin: Related to health condition]

Managing Emotions

The fourth set of tasks involves preserving a reasonable emotional balance by managing upsetting feelings aroused by the health crisis and its aftermath. Many disturbing emotions are associated with health crises, such as a gnawing foreboding about the unknown, long-term course of an illness or disability, a sense of alienation and isolation, and feelings of inadequacy and anger in the face of seemingly insurmountable demands. An important aspect of this task is for individuals to maintain some hope, even when its scope is sharply limited by circumstances.

[handwritten in left margin: General Crisis]

Maintaining a Positive Self-Image

The next set of tasks is to preserve a satisfactory self-image and maintain a sense of competence and mastery. Changes in physical functioning or appearance, such as permanent weakness or scarring, must be blended into a revised self-image. This "identity crisis" may require a shift in personal values as, for example, when individuals, who are burn survivors and are disfigured, play down the importance of physical attractiveness. Individuals, who rely on mechanical devices like cardiac pacemakers or renal dialysis, must come to terms with a "half-human-half-machine" body image. Other tasks in this category include changing one's values to accept a CID, defining the limits of independence, and readjusting goals and expectations in light of changes wrought by the illness (Wright, 1983).

Relating to Family Members and Friends

The sixth set of tasks includes sustaining positive relationships with family members, friends, and other members of one's social network. Serious illness can make it hard to keep communication open and accept comfort and support, just when these resources are most essential. Supportive relationships with other people can help an individual with CID obtain information that is necessary to make wise decisions about health-care, find emotional support for difficult decisions, and secure reassurance about impending problems. Open and caring relationships also enable family members and friends to prepare for the tasks that they themselves will encounter, such as the burden of care-giving and grief and anger at their altered life circumstances.

Preparing for an Uncertain Future

The final set of tasks entails preparing for an uncertain future, in which significant losses are threatened. The loss of sight, speech, hearing, a limb or breast by surgery, or life itself must be acknowledged and mourned. Ironically, new health-care procedures, which raise hope for individuals with previously incurable illnesses, may make this task more difficult. Individuals with CID must often prepare for permanent loss of function, while still preserving the belief that restoration of function may be possible. Similarly, in confronting a potentially terminal illness, individuals and their family members need to initiate the grieving process, while at the same time maintaining hope that new treatment procedures may prove to be beneficial.

Coping Skills   2 approaches

Two main approaches have been used to classify coping skills. One approach emphasizes the focus of coping: a person's orientation and activity in response to a stressor. An individual with CID can approach the problem and make active efforts to understand and resolve it, or try to avoid dealing directly with the problem and focus primarily on managing the emotions associated with it. A second approach emphasizes the method of coping; that is, whether a response entails primarily cognitive or behavioral efforts.

When these two approaches are combined, they specify four broad domains of coping: cognitive approach coping, behavioral approach coping, cognitive avoidance coping, and behavioral avoidance coping. Each of these four coping domains encompasses two subsets of conceptually related coping skills: (a) Cognitive approach coping encompasses logical analysis and the search for meaning and positive reappraisal and (b) behavioral approach coping includes seeking guidance and support and taking problem-solving action. (c) Cognitive avoidance coping is comprised of cognitive avoidance or denial, and acceptance or resignation and (d) behavioral avoidance coping covers seeking alternative rewards and emotional discharge.

Each of these coping skills is assessed by the Coping Responses Inventory (Moos, 1993) and is described below. The coping skills are comparable to aspects of coping that are assessed by other commonly used coping measures, and are compatible with existing models of stress and coping processes (e.g., Lazarus, 1991; Lazarus & Folkman, 1984; Parker & Endler, 1996) and of coping in the context of CID (e.g., Katz, Ritvo, Irvine, & Jackson, 1996). They are also applicable to cognitive and behavioral interventions, which are oriented toward helping individuals with CID manage their distress and engage in more positive thinking and problem-solving (Radnitz, 2001; Sharoff, 2004).

Eight Categories of Coping Skills

Logical Analysis and the Search for Meaning

This set of skills entails paying attention to one aspect of a crisis at a time, breaking a seemingly overwhelming problem into manageable parts, drawing on past experiences, mentally rehearsing potential actions and their probable consequences, and bolstering one's confidence by reminding oneself of previous successes in handling difficult problems. These skills encompass individuals' efforts to learn more about their condition, its likely course, and what they can do through medical intervention and lifestyle change to influence prognosis and symptoms. On a broader scale, they encompass the search for a pattern of meaning in the course of events and the anticipatory mourning process, in which losses or death are acknowledged beforehand.

Positive Reappraisal

This category covers cognitive strategies, by which an individual with CID accepts the basic reality of a situation but restructures it in a more favorable light. Such strategies include: reminding oneself that things could be worse, thinking of oneself as well-off compared to other people, altering values and priorities in line with changing reality, and focusing on that something good that might emerge from a health problem. For instance, a woman with breast cancer may compare herself favorably to someone who has more serious problems, while some individuals may come to see a cardiac arrest as having a positive value, because it helped them redirect their life.

Seeking Guidance and Support

This set of skills covers obtaining information about a health condition and alternative treatment-procedures and their probable outcomes. These skills are often used in combination with logical analysis, as individuals with CID try to restore a sense of control, by learning about demands that might be made on them and mentally preparing themselves to overcome expected problems by thinking through the steps involved. A related set of coping skills entails seeking emotional reassurance and tangible support from family, friends, and caregivers. Religious coping behavior, such as seeking guidance and support from a Higher Power and trying to obtain solace from religious beliefs, also falls into this category.

Taking Problem-Solving Action

This group of skills involves taking action to deal directly with a situation by, for example, learning specific health-care procedures, such as giving oneself insulin injections or using a home dialysis-machine. These skills include learning how to control symptoms by such techniques as sitting in medically contoured chairs, planning changes in daily regimens to minimize the appearance and/or effects of potentially painful symptoms, and physically reorganizing or redesigning a home to accommodate declining mobility. They also encompass the strategy of "progressive desensitization," whereby amputees or individuals with severe disfiguration gradually "expose" themselves socially, in order to dull their sensitivity to their own and others' reactions.

(5) Cognitive Avoidance or Denial *only good for Temporary*

avoidance

This category encompasses responses aimed at denying or minimizing the seriousness of a crisis. These strategies may be directed at the illness itself (e.g., an individual with a myocardial infarction maintains that "it was just severe indigestion"). Or, after the diagnosis, the strategies may be aimed at the significance of an illness (e.g., an individual with a fatal condition consults doctor after doctor looking for an alternate diagnosis). Cognitive avoidance can also involve the potential consequences of an illness, such as the initial denial that often occurs after diagnosis of a stroke. These self-protective responses can temporarily protect an individual from feeling overwhelmed emotionally and can provide time to garner other personal coping resources.

(6) Acceptance and Resignation

This category addresses coming to terms with the reality of a health condition and prognosis and acknowledging that the overall circumstances cannot be altered. Acceptance may involve admitting an ongoing health problem, giving up unproductive efforts to control symptoms, and committing oneself to living as satisfying a life as possible. Rapid changes in a disability may make it hard to strike a reasonable balance between acceptance with continued hope and acceptance with resignation. As death approaches, a conscious decision to accept the inevitable helps to mitigate distress and free the individual with CID to search for deeper meaning in their circumstances.

(7) Seeking Alternative Rewards *Setting new goals*

These skills encompass attempts to replace the losses, which are involved in a health condition, by changing one's activities and creating new sources of satisfaction. Such coping responses entail redirecting one's energies toward a new goal, when an original goal becomes unattainable. For example, after undergoing surgery for breast cancer, a woman might redirect her activities toward helping others with the same disorder by sharing information, acting as a role model, or raising funds to find a cure. These activities give individuals with CID a constructive involvement to look forward to and provide a realistic opportunity to achieve a goal they consider meaningful.

(8) Emotional Discharge

This set of responses includes openly venting one's feelings of anger or despair, crying or screaming in protest at news of a fateful prognosis, and using jokes and gallows' humor to help allay distress. It also entails "acting out" by not complying with a treatment regimen, as well as behavior that may temporarily reduce tension, such as when an individual on dialysis goes on eating binges. Such behavior may involve a temporary failure of affective regulation, as individuals alternate between emotional control and emotional discharge.

These eight categories cover the most common types of coping skills, which are employed to deal with the tasks that are involved in managing health crises. Such skills are seldom used singly or exclusively. An individual with CID may deny or minimize the seriousness of a crisis when talking to a family member, may seek information about a prognosis from a physician, and may openly vent anger and despair to a friend. An ongoing health condition presents a variety of related tasks and requires a combination or sequence of coping skills.

Health-Related Outcomes

Approach coping generally has adaptive advantages over avoidance coping in managing CID. Ultimately, however, coping choices must match the task requirements of the specific health crisis.

Approach vs. Avoidance

Although there are some important exceptions, research findings on coping with CID (Horgan & MacLachlan, 2004; Livneh & Antonak, 1997; Penley, Tomaka, & Wiebe, 2002) generally indicate that approach-coping strategies are associated with fewer symptoms, less distress, and more well-being. Findings are clearest for the adaptive advantages of positive reappraisal, seeking guidance and support, and problem-solving. In contrast, avoidance-coping strategies, especially cognitive avoidance and emotional discharge, tend to be associated with poorer psychosocial outcomes.

Avoidance coping also can affect health-related outcomes (Roesch et al., 2005). Reliance on behavioral disengagement and resignation has been associated with a higher likelihood of mortality from chronic heart failure (Murberg & Bru, 2001). Lack of adherence to treatment recommendations is one key reason that avoidance coping is linked to poorer health-related outcomes. In a study of individuals with hypertension, diabetes, chronic heart disease, or depression, those who relied more on avoidance coping at baseline were less likely to adhere to treatment recommendations over a subsequent two-year follow-up (Sherbourne, Hays, Ordway, DiMatteo, & Kravitz, 1992).

Coping as a Mediator

Findings on health-related outcomes are consistent with our conceptualization that coping skills mediate the influence of personal, health-related, environmental, appraisal, and task factors on health outcomes. For example, in a study of bone-marrow transplantation, individuals low in social support and high in avoidance coping prior to the transplant had the most severe PTSD symptoms after the transplant. These results fit a model in which supportive social relationships encourage individuals, who might otherwise rely on avoidance coping, to cognitively process and habituate to trauma-related thoughts and memories (Jacobsen et al., 2003).

Similarly, among individuals with insulin-dependent diabetes, Turan and colleagues (2003) found that a dismissive attachment style, characterized by a tendency to avoid other people, predicted poor adjustment, as well as poor adherence to blood tests and insulin injections. The association between a dismissing attachment-style and poor health outcomes was mediated by avoidance-coping strategies. Among women with breast cancer, cognitive avoidance mediated the association between lack of optimism and negative emotions during the pre-biopsy period (Stanton & Snider, 1993). Further, in a longitudinal study of women with early-stage breast cancer, avoidance coping mediated the link between a partner's unsupportive behavior and subsequent emotional distress (Manne, Ostroff, Winkel, Grana, & Fox, 2005).

We examined the conceptual framework, which was outlined in this chapter, in a four-year follow-up of individuals with cardiac illnesses (Holahan, Moos, Holahan, & Brennan, 1997). Although individuals with cardiac illnesses reported more depressive symptoms on average than did persons free of illness, more social resources at baseline predicted fewer depressive symptoms among individuals with cardiac problems. Consistent with the proposed model, adaptive coping strategies operated as a mechanism, through which social resources were linked to psychological adjustment. Positive aspects of relationships enhanced adaptive coping efforts and, in turn, promoted better psychological adjustment. Negative aspects of relationships, such as conflict and criticism from family members and friends, eroded adaptive coping and were linked to poorer psychological adjustment.

Task-Coping Match

More reliance on approach coping and less reliance on avoidance coping tend to be associated with better outcomes; however, there are important exceptions due to the match or mismatch between specific adaptive tasks and particular coping responses.

Temporary Benefits of Cognitive Avoidance

Denial may help regulate mood when it is used in the early stages after an especially traumatic event (Goldbeck, 1997). Individuals relying on denial in the immediate aftermath of a myocardial infarction or coronary bypass surgery typically spend fewer days in intensive care and have fewer signs of cardiac dysfunction. However, in the following year, these individuals seem to be less compliant with the treatment regimen and more likely to require re-hospitalization. Among individuals with spinal cord injury, temporary denial has been associated with a strengthened sense of coherence, the belief that post-injury stressors will be manageable, and the motivation to pursue efforts to resolve them (Lustig, 2005).

Denial may also be beneficial in dealing with aspects of health problems that are unalterable. In coping with the physical problems associated with multiple sclerosis, wishful thinking or denial has been related to better perceived health status; however, when coping with associated psychosocial problems, wishful thinking was unrelated to health status. Wishful thinking may help some individuals reframe their physical problems in a more positive light, but it may not help re-appraise relationship or employment issues (Pakenham, Stewart, & Rogers, 1997). Emotional blunting may also be beneficial after treatment is accepted and the task involves enduring necessary, but difficult, procedures. For example, among women with breast cancer, seeking support was more closely related to well-being in the hospitalization stage, whereas denial and diversion were more associated with well-being in the chemotherapy stage (Heim, Valach, & Schaffner, 1997).

Detrimental Aspects of Approach Coping

Attempts to gain active control, in situations that an individual with CID cannot change, can arouse feelings of undue personal responsibility, blame, and guilt. As a case in point, compared to women with breast cancer who always insisted on control, women yielding control when appropriate and accepting the situation without resignation or helplessness were better adjusted at an eight-month follow-up (Astin et al., 1999).

In home-based treatments for end-stage renal disease (ESRD), individuals are expected to self-administer treatment through continuous peritoneal dialysis (CAPD). However, this procedure can be an unwanted burden when individuals with ESRD think that they may be blamed for relapses, or for not implementing the treatment adequately. In fact, when disease severity is high, the control and responsibility associated with CAPD can add to the burden of illness and impair individuals' quality of life (Eitel, Hatchett, Friend, Griffin, & Wadhwa, 1995).

The match between the perceived controllability of a stressor and coping is also important. For example, when individuals on dialysis experienced relatively controllable stressors (problems with fluid intake), their problem-solving efforts were associated with better treatment adherence. For uncontrollable stressors (a problem with the dialysis procedure), however, efforts involving logical analysis and emotional self-control were associated with better adherence, whereas seeking information was linked to poorer adherence. When trying to manage an uncontrollable treatment-related stressor, obtaining more information may lead to rumination and unproductive attempts to change the situation, whereas understanding the problem as it is and controlling one's feelings is more likely to favor continued cooperation with the treatment regimen. In general, a more vigilant and active coping style was associated with more favorable adherence only for individuals with ESRD undergoing patient-directed, home-based dialysis.

Among individuals receiving hospital-based, provider-controlled treatment, a less vigilant or more passive coping style was associated with more favorable adherence (Christensen, 2000).

Crisis Growth Growing as a person

The traumatic aspects of CID cannot be denied. Yet, individuals often emerge from the onset of a CID with new coping skills, closer relationships with family and friends, broader priorities, and a richer appreciation of life. Adaptive coping is central to psychological growth in the context of health crises. Positive feedback from successful coping experiences strengthens resources under adaptive challenge. Resilience develops from confronting stressful experiences and coping with them effectively; novel crisis situations promote new coping skills, which can lead to new personal and social resources (Schaefer & Moos, 1998).

The approach-coping skills of positive reappraisal and taking problem-solving action are important for such growth. For example, Urcuyo and colleagues (2005) found that women with breast cancer, who relied on positive reframing, also had an ability to perceive benefits from their illness. Further, among individuals with cancer undergoing bone-marrow transplantation, coping strategies of positive reinterpretation and problem-solving, as well as seeking alternative rewards, predicted psychological growth during the post-transplant period (Widows, Jacobsen, Booth-Jones, & Fields, 2005). Coping mediation also may play a role in psychological growth in the context of health crises. Among individuals with heart disease, Sheikh (2004) found that problem-focused coping partially mediated the relationship between extraversion and psychological growth.

Future Directions

Several key issues remain to be addressed in this area. At the personal level, models need to consider the co-occurrence of medical and psychological disorders: health crises often evolve in the context of emotional problems. At the societal level, models need to reflect the changing landscape of health-care, with growing institutional bureaucracy on one hand, and an active self-help movement on the other.

Mental-Health Disorders and Coping with Medical Problems

About 25% of individuals who have ongoing health problems may have diagnosable psychiatric disorders or serious mental-health problems, such as depression, PTSD, or substance use disorders that can impair their self-efficacy and coping abilities (Frayne et al., 2005; Holbrook et al., 2005; Spindler & Pedersen, 2005). These disorders may reflect pre-existing problems that are exacerbated by a health trauma, or they may be an outgrowth of a severe CID. Individuals, who have both medical and mental-health problems, tend to experience less assertive treatment and poorer proximal outcomes, such as lower rates of cardiac catheterization after myocardial infarction and poorer glycemic and lipemic control among patients with diabetes (Druss, Bradford, Rosenheck, Radford, & Krumholz, 2000; Frayne et al., 2005).

More information is needed about the reasons for these disparities in treatment and outcome. Individuals with mental-health conditions may delay help-seeking, establish less trusting relationships with providers, be less likely to adhere to treatment regimens, have less social support, and/or use less effective coping skills. For example, individuals who have cardiac problems and PTSD are more likely to rely on cognitive avoidance or denial, which is associated with non-adherence to medication and lifestyle change and with a higher risk of morbidity and mortality (Tedstone & Tarrier, 2003). Individuals, who are pessimistic or depressed, are more likely to ruminate about their problems and less likely to confront them; individuals with substance-use disorders tend to rely on avoidance strategies and to self-medicate with alcohol to reduce tension (Maisto, Carey, & Bradizza, 1999; Nolen-Hoeksema, 1998; Scheier, Carver, & Bridges, 2002). Individuals with these types of problems present special challenges for health-care providers and should be screened and targeted for preventive interventions, in order to increase their health-related self-efficacy and coping skills.

The Context of Health-Care

The growing complexity and bureaucracy of the health-care system, including restrictive managed-care policies, individuals who limit access to specialty care (i.e., gatekeepers), constant provider turnover, and confusing insurance and benefit plans, cause individuals a bewildering array of problems. In fact, individuals with CID frequently report issues in interactions with providers, including lack of information about their health conditions and treatment options, inability to obtain timely refills of medications, lack of access to specialists, and little attention to their most pressing concerns (Parchman, Noel, & Lee, 2005).

The tasks and effective coping skills, which are involved in managing these and related aspects of the health-care context, need to be conceptualized. It is also important to develop measures of the proximal outcomes of these tasks, such as individuals' beliefs in the justice of health-care decision-making and the extent to which they think that providers and health-plan representatives treat them with trust and impartiality and enable them to participate in health-care decisions (Fondacaro, Frogner, & Moos, 2005). Positive interaction with the health-care context can contribute to better treatment adherence and health outcomes (Safran, 2003).

Mutual Help Groups and Communal Coping

Self-help and mutual support groups exist for individuals with almost every type of disorder and disability. However, relatively little is known about the "active ingredients," whereby these groups enhance individuals' self-efficacy, coping skills, social integration, and personal growth. Studies of Alcoholics Anonymous (AA) have shown that members teach each other specific problem-solving skills, enhance each other's self-efficacy, provide general social support, and engage in a reciprocal learning process that involves sharing information and role-modeling (Humphreys, 2004).

By participating in mutual help groups, individuals with CID and their family members can enhance their self-efficacy and coping skills. Moreover, in cohesive and well-organized groups, coping may reflect a communal problem-solving process, in which the trauma and associated adaptive tasks elicit cooperative action. As Lyons and colleagues (1998) have noted, coping can become a relationship-focused process that expands individuals' resources to confront adversity and enhances family cohesion and social integration. Communal coping may also contribute to altruistic behavior, such as volunteering to raise money to find a cure for breast cancer, becoming a transplant advocate who meets individuals pre-operatively and shares experiences with them, or participating in an AIDS walk-a-thon. Through helping others, individuals with CID can engender a sense of purpose or gratification that can improve their well-being and, perhaps, experience an epiphany that changes their life for the better.

Conclusion

A focus on coping skills and associated coping resources encourages a competence-enhancing view of individuals' adaptive potential in the face of adversity. Moreover, the model detailed here can guide intervention efforts to enhance individuals' coping strengths in a broad range of health crises. Each path in the conceptual framework (Figure 6.1) identifies a general process that is potentially alterable.

Although disorder-specific research is useful, there is a need for a more integrated understanding of the common adaptive tasks and the role of coping in managing CID. Diverse health conditions involve common adaptive challenges and common coping requirements. It is hoped that this model will contribute to developing a broad understanding of people's adaptive strengths and capacity for personal growth, in the context of a wide spectrum of health crises[1].

---

[1] *Acknowledgments:* Preparation of the chapter was supported in part by Department of Veterans Affairs Health Services Research and Development Service funds. Bernice Moos compiled the references and assisted in preparation of the manuscript. The opinions expressed here are the authors' and do not necessarily represent the views of the Department of Veterans Affairs.

References

Alonzo, A. A. (2000). The experience of chronic illness and post-traumatic stress disorder: The consequences of cumulative adversity. *Social Science and Medicine, 50*, 1475–1484.

Angyal, A. (1941). *Foundations for a science of personality.* New York: Commonwealth Fund.

Astin, J., Anton-Culver, H., Schwartz, C., Shapiro, D., McQaude, J., Breuer, A., et al. (1999). Sense of control and adjustment to breast cancer: The importance of balancing control coping styles. *Journal of Behavioral Medicine, 25*, 101–109.

Backus, F. I., & Dudley, D. L. (1974). Observations of psychosocial factors and their relationship to organic disease. *International Journal of Psychiatry in Medicine, 5*, 499–515.

Bandura, A. (1977). Self-efficacy: Toward a unifying theory of behavioral change. *Psychological Review, 84*, 191–215.

Caplan, G. (1964). *Principles of preventive psychiatry.* New York: Basic Books.

Christensen, A. J. (2000). Patient-by treatment context interaction in chronic disease: A conceptual framework for the study of patient adherence. *Psychosomatic Medicine, 62*, 435–443.

De Ridder, D., & Schreurs, K. M. G. (1996). Coping, social support and chronic disease: A research agenda. *Psychology, Health, & Medicine, 1*, 71–82.

De Ridder, D., Schreurs, K. M. G., & Bensing, J. M. (1998). Adaptive tasks, coping and quality of life of chronically ill patients. The cases of Parkinson's disease and the chronic fatigue syndrome. *Journal of Health Psychology, 3*, 87–101.

Druss, B. G., Bradford, D. W., Rosenheck, R. A., Radford, M. J., & Krumholz, H. M. (2000). Mental disorders and use of cardiovascular procedures after myocardial infarction. *Journal of the American Medical Association, 283*, 506–511.

Eitel, P., Hatchett, L., Friend, R., Griffin, K., & Wadhwa, N. (1995). Burden of self-care in seriously ill patients: Impact on adjustment. *Health Psychology, 14*, 457–463.

Erikson, E. (1963). *Childhood and society* (2nd ed.). New York: Norton.

Feifel, H., Strack, S., & Nagy, V. T. (1987). Degree of life threat and differential use of coping modes. *Journal of Psychosomatic Research, 31*, 91–99.

Fondacaro, M., Frogner, B., & Moos, R. (2005). Justice in health care decision-making: Patients' appraisals of health care providers and health plan representatives. *Social Justice Research, 18*, 63–81.

Frayne, S., Halanych, J., Miller, D., Wang, F., Lin, H., Pogach, L., et al. (2005). Disparities in diabetes care: Impact of mental illness. *Archives of Internal Medicine, 165*, 2631–2638.

Goldbeck, R. (1997). Denial in physical illness. *Journal of Psychosomatic Research, 43*, 575–593.

Groves, M. S., & Muskin, P. R. (2005). Psychological responses to illness. In J. E. Levenson (Ed.), *American psychiatric textbook of psychosomatic medicine* (pp. 67–88). Washington, DC: American Psychiatric Publishing.

Haan, N. (1977). *Coping and defending: Processes of self-environment organization.* New York: Academic Press.

Hartmann, H. (1950). Comments on the psychoanalytic theory of the ego. *Psychoanalytic Study of the Child, 5*, 74–95.

Heijmans, M., Rijken, M., Foets, M., De Ridder, D., Schreurs, K., & Bensing, J. (2004). The stress of being chronically ill: From disease-specific to task-specific aspects. *Journal of Behavioral Medicine, 27*, 255–271.

Heim, E., Valach, L., & Schaffner, L. (1997). Coping and psychological adaptation: longitudinal effects over time and stage in breast cancer. *Psychosomatic Medicine, 59,* 408–418.

Holahan, C. J., Moos, R., Holahan, C. K., & Brennan, P. L. (1997). Social context, coping strategies, and depressive symptoms: An expanded model with cardiac patients. *Journal of Personality and Social Psychology, 72,* 918–928.

Holbrook, T. L., Hoyt, D. B., Coimbra, R., Potenza, B., Sise, M., & Anderson, J. P. (2005). Long-term posttraumatic stress disorder persists after major trauma in adolescents: New data on risk factors and functional outcome. *The Journal of Trauma Injury, Infection, and Critical Care, 58,* 764–771.

Horgan, O., & MacLachlan, M. (2004). Psychosocial adjustment to lower-limb amputation: A review. *Disability and Rehabilitation, 26,* 837–850.

Humphreys, K. (2004). *Circles of recovery: Self-help organizations for addictions.* Cambridge, UK: Cambridge University Press.

Jacobsen, P. B., Sadler, I. J., Booth-Jones, M., Soety, E., Weitzner, M. A., & Fields, K. K. (2003). Predictors of posttraumatic stress disorder symptomatology following bone marrow transplantation for cancer. *Journal of Consulting and Clinical Psychology, 70,* 235–240.

Katz, J., Ritvo, P., Irvine, M. J., & Jackson, M. (1996). Coping with chronic pain. In M. Zeidner & N. Endler (Eds.), *Handbook of coping: Research, theory, and applications* (pp. 252–278). New York: Wiley.

Kemp, S., Morley, S., & Anderson, E. (1999). Coping with epilepsy: Do illness representations play a role? *British Journal of Clinical Psychology, 38,* 43–58.

Krantz, D. S., & McCeney, M. K. (2002). Effects of psychological and social factors on organic disease: A critical assessment of research on coronary heart disease. *Annual Review of Psychology, 53,* 341–369.

Lazarus, R. (1991). *Emotion and Adaptation.* New York: Oxford.

Lazarus, R., & Folkman, S. (1984). *Stress, Appraisal, and Coping.* New York: Springer.

Leigh, H., & Reiser, M. (1992). *The patient: Biological, psychological, and social dimensions of medical practice* (3rd ed.). New York: Plenum.

Levenson, J. L. (Ed.). (2005). *Textbook of psychosomatic medicine.* Washington, DC: American Psychiatric Publishing.

Lindemann, E., & Lindemann, E. (1979). *Beyond grief: Studies in crisis intervention.* New York: Aronson.

Livneh, H., & Antonak, R. F. (1997). *Psychosocial adaptation to chronic illness and disability.* Gaithersburg, MD: Aspen Publishers.

Livneh, H., & Parker, R. M. (2005). Psychosocial adaptation to disability: Perspectives from chaos and complexity theory. *Rehabilitation Counseling Bulletin, 49,* 17–28.

Lustig, D. C. (2005). The adjustment process for individuals with spinal cord injury: The effect of perceived premorbid sense of coherence. *Rehabilitation Counseling Bulletin, 48,* 146–156.

Lyons, R. F., Mickelson, K. D., Sullivan, M. J., & Coyne, J. C. (1998). Coping as a communal process. *Journal of Personal and Social Relationships, 15,* 579–605.

Maisto, S. S., Carey, K. B., & Bradizza, C. (1999). Social learning theory. In K. E. Leonard & H. T. Blane (Eds.), *Psychological theories of drinking and alcoholism* (pp. 106–163). New York: Guilford.

Manne, S. L., & Glassman, M. (2000). Perceived control, coping efficacy, and avoidance coping as mediators between spouse unsupportive behaviors and cancer patients' psychological distress. *Health Psychology, 19,* 155–164.

Manne, S. L., Ostroff, J., Winkel, G., Grana, G., & Fox, K. (2005). Partner unsupportive responses, avoidant coping, and distress among women with early stage breast cancer: Patient and partner perspectives. *Health Psychology, 24*, 635–641.

McCaul, K. D., Sandgren, A. K., King, B., O'Donnell, S., Branstetter, A., & Foreman, G. (1999). Coping and adjustment to breast cancer. *Psycho-Oncology, 8*, 230–236.

Moos, R. (1993). *Coping Responses Inventory Adult Form Professional Manual*. Odessa, FL: Psychological Assessment Resources.

Moos, R., & Holahan, C. J. (2003). Dispositional and contextual perspectives on coping: Toward an integrative framework. *Journal of Clinical Psychology, 59*, 1387–1403.

Murberg, T. A., & Bru, E. (2001). Coping and mortality among patients with congestive heart failure. *International Journal of Behavioral Medicine, 8*, 66–79.

Nolen-Hoeksema, S. (1998). The other end of the continuum: The costs of rumination. *Psychological Inquiry, 9*, 216–219.

Norton, T. R., Manne, S. L., Rubin, S., Hernandez, E., Carlson, J., Bergman, C., et al. (2005). Ovarian cancer patients' psychological distress: The role of physical impairment, perceived unsupportive family and friend behaviors, perceived control, and self-esteem. *Health Psychology, 24*, 143–152.

Pakenham, K. I., Stewart, C. A., & Rogers, A. (1997). The role of coping in adjustment to multiple sclerosis-related adaptive demands. *Psychology, Health, & Medicine, 2*, 197–211.

Parchman, M. L., Noel, P. H., & Lee, S. (2005). Primary care attributes, health care system hassles, and chronic illness. *Medical Care, 43*, 1123–1129.

Parker, J. D., & Endler, N. S. (1996). Coping and defense: A historical overview. M. Zeidner & N. Endler (Eds.), *Handbook of Coping: Theory, Research, Applications* (pp. 3–13). New York: Wiley.

Penley, J. A., Tomaka, J., & Wiebe, J. S. (2002). The association of coping to physical and psychological health outcomes: A meta-analytic review. *Journal of Behavioral Medicine, 25*, 551–603.

Radnitz, C. L. (Ed.). (2001). *Cognitive behavioral therapy for persons with disabilities*. Northvale, NJ: Jason Aronson.

Roberts, A. R. (2000). *Crisis intervention handbook: Assessment, treatment, and research*. New York: Oxford University Press.

Roesch, S. C., Adams, L., Hines, A., Palmores, A., Vyas, P., Tran, C., et al. (2005). Coping with prostate cancer: A meta-analytic review. *Journal of Behavioral Medicine, 28*, 281–293.

Rohrbaugh, M., Shoham, V., Coyne, J. C., Cranford, J. A., Sonnega, J. S., & Nicklas, J. M. (2004). Beyond the "self" in self-efficacy: Spouse confidence predicts patient survival following heart failure. *Journal of Family Psychology, 18*, 184–193.

Safran, D. G. (2003). Defining the future of primary care: What can we learn from patients? *Annals from Internal Medicine, 138*, 248–255.

Schaefer, J. A., & Moos, R. H. (1998). The context for personal growth: Life crises, individual and social resources, and coping. In R. Tedeschi, C. Park, & L. Calhoun (Eds.), *Posttraumatic growth: Positive change in the aftermath of crisis*. Mahueah NJ: Erlbaum.

Scharloo, M., & Kaptein, A. (1997). Measurement of illness perceptions in patients with chronic somatic illness: A review. In K. J. Petrie & J. A. Weinman (Eds.), *Perceptions of health and illness: Current research and applications* (pp. 103–154). Amsterdam: Harwood Academic Publishers.

Scheier, M. F., & Carver, C. S. (1987). Dispositional optimism and physical well-being: The influence of generalized outcome expectancies on health. *Journal of Personality, 55*, 169–210.

Scheier, M. F., Carver, C. S., & Bridges, M. W. (2002). Optimism, pessimism, and psychological well-being. In E. C. Chang (Ed.), *Optimism & pessimism: Implications for theory, research, and practice* (pp. 189–216). Washington, DC: American Psychological Association.

Selye, H. (1956). *The stress of life.* New York: McGraw Hill.

Sharoff, K. (2004). *Coping skills therapy for managing chronic and terminal illness.* New York: Springer Publishing.

Sheikh, A. I. (2004). Posttraumatic growth in the context of heart disease. *Journal of Clinical Psychology in Medical Settings, 11*, 265–273.

Sherbourne, C. D., Hays, R. D., Ordway, L., DiMatteo, M. R., & Kravitz, R. L. (1992). Antecedents of adherence to medical recommendations: Results from the Medical Outcomes Study. *Journal of Behavioral Medicine, 15*, 447–468.

Spindler, H., & Pedersen, S. S. (2005). Posttraumatic stress disorder in the wake of heart disease: Prevalence, risk factors, and future research directions. *Psychosomatic Medicine, 67*, 715–723.

Stanton, A. L., & Snider, P.R. (1993). Coping with a breast cancer diagnosis: A prospective study. *Health Psychology, 12*, 16–23.

Tedstone, J. E., & Tarrier, N. (2003). Posttraumatic stress disorder following medical illness and treatment. *Clinical Psychology Review, 23*, 409–448.

Turan, B., Osar, Z., Turan, J. M., Ilkova, H., & Damci, T. (2003). Dismissing attachment and outcome in diabetes: The mediating role of coping. *Journal of Social & Clinical Psychology, 22*, 607–626.

Urcuyo, K. R., Boyers, A. E., Carver, C. S., & Antoni, M. H. (2005). Finding benefit in breast cancer: Relations with personality, coping, and concurrent well-being. *Psychology & Health, 20*, 175–192.

Walker, J. G., Jackson, H. J., & Littlejohn, G. O. (2004). Models of adjustment to chronic illness: Using the example of rheumatoid arthritis. *Clinical Psychology Review, 24*, 461–488.

Widows, M. R., Jacobsen, P. B., Booth-Jones, M., & Fields, K. K. (2005). Predictors of posttraumatic growth following bone marrow transplantation for cancer. *Health Psychology, 24*, 266–273.

Wright, B. (1983). *Physical disability: A psychological approach* (2nd ed.). New York: Harper Collins.

Part II

7
Coping with AIDS: The Challenges of an Evolving Disease

James Walkup and Laura Cramer-Berness

Introduction

The story of Acquired Immunodeficiency Syndrome (AIDS) – the search for its cause, the struggle to prevent its spread, the yet unsuccessful search for effective vaccines and cures– is a social drama with few parallels in the history of medicine. Several elements in this story set it apart from most other medical conditions, and give a distinctive cast to many of the issues associated with coping (Epstein, 1998). It appeared out of nowhere, spread with blazing speed, and awakened a massive political and scientific response.

As has happened with some past epidemics, the AIDS epidemic was associated in the public mind with stigmatized behaviors and social groups. In contrast to prior epidemics, one of the stigmatized groups was newly empowered by the gay rights movement and thus, its members were able to marshal social and legal resources. Already existing social networks could thus be mobilized in efforts to resist anticipated use of legal sanctions by public health authorities; in community-based efforts to curtail disease-spread, and provide resources and support for those already infected; and in pressuring federal agencies and drug manufacturers. Political lobbying for specific chronic illnesses and disabilities (CID) was not new, but AIDS advocacy, in particular, has produced a high-visibility confrontational style, mass mobilization, and close involvement with the details of research and drug production.

This chapter selectively reviews research relevant specifically to coping. It also builds on and updates material from several useful chapters on this topic (Antoni, Esterling, Lutgendorf, Fletcher, & Schneiderman, 1995; Folkman & Chesney, 1995; Satriano, Riemen, & Berkman, 2004; Schneiderman & Antoni, 2003). Particular attention is given to the close relationship between coping demands and specific disease characteristics and evolving treatments. As dramatic shifts have occurred in the disease epidemiology, incidence, prevalence, course, and outcome, the stressors and coping needs have changed. Yet, research findings can quickly become dated and inapplicable (e.g., the demands of pregnancy, for example, have been utterly transformed by the virtual elimination in the U.S. of mother-to-infant transmission of the disease). To cover the topic within the limited space available, this chapter will focus on the research from the past decade, and, almost exclusively, on research related to the Human Immunodeficiency Virus (HIV) epidemic in the U.S.

Incidence and Prevalence of HIV/AIDS

HIV can be transmitted when blood or body fluids that contain HIV somehow contact the bloodstream or mucosal tissue of the uninfected person, typically through unprotected sex or contact with infected blood (e.g., by needle-sharing); but it can also be transmitted to infants perinatally or by nursing. The world-wide prevalence of HIV/AIDS is approximately 38.6 million individuals, according to 2005 data, and there is an estimated incidence of 4.1 million new cases a year (UNAIDS, 2006). In the United States, figures from the end of 2005 estimate 215,039 persons living with HIV (not AIDS) and 437,982 persons living with AIDS in the 50 states and U.S. dependencies (Centers for Disease Control & Prevention 2006). Estimates indicate that approximately a quarter of those infected with HIV in the United States are not aware of their status, with higher unawareness noted among some subgroups (Centers for Disease Control & Prevention, 2003).

Socio-demographic facts show cases are clustered in several respects (Kaiser Family Foundation, November, 2005). More than four of five reported AIDS cases are found in large metropolitan areas, with 10 metropolitan areas accounting for 42% of all reported cases. Minorities, particularly African Americans, are disproportionately impacted. African Americans make up approximately 12–13% of the U.S. population, but constitute almost half (47%) of those living with AIDS and more than half (55%) of the deaths due to HIV in 2002. In 2004, the AIDS case rate per 100,000 for African Americans adults/adolescents was almost 10.2 times that of whites (Kaiser Family Foundation, February, 2006).

Several observations can be made regarding disease dynamics. First, developments in treatment technologies have had a dramatic impact on epidemiology. The striking, stop-the-presses example is the rapid decline in perinatal HIV transmission by more than 90% between 1992 and 2003. As will be discussed in a later section, the 1996 introduction of effective antiviral therapies quickly began to affect two facts that have had wide-ranging impact on the epidemic. Survival time increased and new AIDS cases dropped. This drop in AIDS cases subsequently leveled off and then increased slightly (Kaiser Family Foundation, June, 2006).

Quantitatively, the logic of epidemiology dictates that when any decrease in mortality is combined with stable disease incidence (number of new cases in a population), the result is an increase in disease prevalence (number of cases in a population). That is, better treatment means more people are living with HIV. In one sense, successful antiretroviral treatments have increased the disease burden for a population; but an offsetting influence comes from decreases in average disease-severity occasioned by delaying the AIDS-onset.

Evidence indicates that symptom profiles (Zingmond, Kilbourne, Justice, Wenger, & Rodriguez-Barradas, 2003), medication response (Wellons et al., 2002), and disease progression (Zingmond et al., 2001) differ in the era of improved antiretroviral care. In addition, because individuals are living longer and reaching ages not previously reached in large numbers, they must face complications of long-term use of medication and the physical and psychological challenges of aging itself (Goodroad, 2003). A longer life also means a host of life-span developmental challenges are framed in the context of viral suppression and continuing disease (e.g., long-term partnership/marriage, parenthood, career development). Implications of these challenges for coping have been explored, and interventions developed (Heckman et al., 2001).

Testing

Forty-eight percent of U.S. adults surveyed in 2004 report they have been tested for HIV (Kaiser Family Foundation, June 2005). Socio-demographic character-istics predict testing, with higher rates reported by those under age 65, African Americans, and Latinos (Kaiser Family Foundation, June 2005). HIV testing can be anonymous or confidential, and has historically been accompanied by counseling regarding HIV risk, testing, and treatment. Reporting of HIV and AIDS cases is now required in all states and territories, although some base reporting on a code, rather than a name.

Existing data regarding testing suggest that many people with HIV miss the opportunity to benefit from early treatment or prophylaxis. At CDC-funded sites, 31% of those testing positive in 2000 failed to return for test results (CDC, 2003). Examination of four states' Medicaid claims files for individuals diagnosed with conditions indicative of high risk (i.e., gonorrhea or chlamydia) found that only 15% had been tested for HIV (Rust, 2003). Both site-based (Samet et al., 1998) and national data (Bozzette et al., 1998) have found evidence that testing occurs late in disease development. The CDC (2005) reports that 39% of those diagnosed in 2002 received an AIDS diagnosis within a year of a positive test.

Treatment

Twenty-one medications are currently approved by the Food and Drug Admin-istration for treatment of HIV. These fall into four drug classes: Nonnucleoside Reverse Transcriptase Inhibitors (NNRTIs), Nucleoside Reverse Transcriptase Inhibitors (NRTIs), Protease Inhibitors (PIs), and Fusion Inhibitors. Highly Active Anti-retroviral Therapy (HAART) combines three or more medications, because a viral load decrease as a result of one or two medicines almost always proves temporary. To put HAART in proper context requires recognition, first, that it has dramatically transformed life for most people with HIV in the U.S. and, second, that increasing experience with HAART has brought to light its many limitations.

According to the two most direct measures – delayed onset of AIDS among those with HIV, and reduced AIDS-related mortality – HAART soon provided evidence of success (Carpenter et al., 1997; Fauci, 1996; Hogg et al., 1998; Lee, Karon, Selik, Neal, & Fleming, 2001; Palella et al., 1998). After rising steadily throughout the epidemic, HIV mortality rates peaked in 1995 in the U.S., then went into a steep decline, leveling off somewhat in recent years (Karon, Fleming, Steketee, & de Cock, 2001). One observational study tracked a large cohort ($N = 3724$) after initiating HAART and found that HIV-related deaths declined from 3.8 to 0.7 per 100 person-years in the period between 1996 and 2000 (van Sighem et al., 2003). Overall, U.S. age-adjusted death rates dropped 70% between 1995 and 2002. The impact of this mortality reduction can be observed in the net increase in persons living with AIDS. Despite slowed progression to AIDS of those with HIV, the number of those living with AIDS increased from 333,1512 in 2001 to 425,910 at end of 2005[1] (CDC, 2005).

HAART's success in clinical practice falls short of what might be hoped. Reports from the late 1990s indicated that HAART sometimes "failed" in one way or another for more than half of seropositive individuals who started it (Valdez et al., 1999). A number of factors seem to be at work. Achieving maximum benefit from HAART is not easy. HAART is unusually unforgiving of adherence lapses, with some reports that viral suppression drops off drastically when patient adherence is below 95% (Paterson et al., 2000). Dosing has historically been quite complex, particularly in the early days, with some combinations requiring up to two dozen pills a day plus dietary and fluid restrictions; but regimens recently have become simpler. Side effects can be intrusive, medically serious, or both. They include: insomnia, fatigue, nausea, diarrhea, taste alterations, various liver problems, pancreatitis, diabetes, abnormal fat distribution, decreased bone density, skin rash (which can be quite severe), high cholesterol, and neuropathy. The challenge posed to adherence by difficult dosing and serious side effects is compounded because inconsistent HAART use can produce viral resistance and treatment failure for the patient (Gifford et al., 2000; Press, Tyndall, Wood, Hogg, & Montaner, 2002), and can heighten the risk of producing drug-resistant strains of the virus, which can be transmitted into the population by risky behavior (Boden et al., 1999; Hecht et al., 1998).

Even with ideal adherence, HAART is not the hoped-for cure. Some had initially believed that starting HAART as soon as possible – using it to "hit early and hit hard" – might drastically curtail the long term viability of the virus. Bolstering this optimism were findings from polymerase chain reaction (PCR) assays that the amount of virus was so low it could not be detected. But it now appears undetectable levels of HIV persist in sanctuary sites (Zhang et al.,

---

[1] It should be noted that the improved disease course now experienced in the U.S. has also been affected by the contribution of better prophylaxis for the prevention of opportunistic infections.

1999), spreading rapidly when HAART is discontinued, and making it difficult to regain pre-interruption CD4 T-cell count levels (Mata et al., 2005). At the end of 2004, the "hit early and hit hard" approach was replaced by one that advocates the following HAART treatment: monitoring for individuals' CD4 count below 350 (unless viral load is elevated), offered to those with 200–350, and definitely started for those below 200 (Panel for Clinical Practices, 2005).

Coping with HIV

Depression, Distress, and Coping with HIV

Given the complexity of this disease and its widespread effects on individuals' lives, it is not surprising that it is a disease that may lead to significant psychological distress. The presence of HIV has been associated with experiences liable to make a person feel depressed. These include unsupportive interactions (Ingram, Jones, Fass, Neidig, & Song, 1999), bereavement (Folkman, Chesney, Collette, Boccellari, & Cooke, 1996; Kemeny & Dean, 1995; Kemeny et al., 1994), and trauma (Simoni & Ng, 2000). Under some circumstances, situationally-triggered depression (e.g., post-bereavement) negatively impacted coping (Folkman et al., 1996).

Most studies report higher rates of current and lifetime depression in individuals with HIV/AIDS (Asch, et al., 2003; Bing, et al., 2001; Rabkin, 1996; Rabkin & Ferrando, 1997; Stober et al., 1997) than found in the general population (Kessler et al., 1994). Because many of the groups that are at highest risk of infection also have elevated depression rates, it is unclear whether HIV confers an additional risk for depression (and may directly or indirectly contribute to mood symptoms). While many identified cases may be relapses of prior depression history (Rosenberger et al., 1993), two types of studies have demonstrated that more factors are at work. First, comparisons of the occurrence of depression have been made between HIV (+) and HIV (−) individuals. A recent meta-analysis of these studies indicates major depression occurs at almost twice the rate among those with HIV (Ciesla & Roberts, 2001). Second, longitudinal work has followed individuals over time and found HIV infection is associated with new cases of major depression (Dew et al., 1997). Depression may or may not be linked to progression of HIV disease, a topic treated in more detail in a recent literature review (see Leserman, 2003).

Examination of mutual influences at work between psychiatric symptoms and physical Health Related Quality of Life (HRQOL) requires sophisticated designs. In a large ($N = 2431$) longitudinal study, differences between depression and anxiety were found. At eight-month follow-up, depressive symptoms were predicted by baseline general health and physical functioning, while anxiety symptoms were predicted by baseline general health and lack of pain (Orlando, Tucker, Sherbourne, & Burnam, 2005). Further complexity is added by the common presence of co-occurring conditions. For example, both posttraumatic stress disorder and depression symptoms predicted lower medication adherence. Yet, only depression symptoms were associated with lower CD4 counts and presence of detectable levels of viral load (Boarts, Sledjeski, Bogart, & Delahunty, 2006; Sledjeski, Delahanty, & Bogart, 2005). Data from the longitudinal Coping in Health and Illness Project[2] have offered the opportunity to examine the effects of chronic depression. With data from this study, depression can be treated as a time-dependent variable, using cumulative depression to predict immune markers and progression to AIDS (Leserman et al., 1999, 2002).

In addition to studies examining specific psychological disorders such as depression, psychological distress in general has been linked to the progression of the HIV disease. The link between perceived stress and diminished antiretroviral adherence has been established (French et al., 2005). For example, individuals who exhibited the highest levels of distress and denial of their illness immediately following their diagnosis of HIV were found to have poorer immune functioning and subsequently a quicker progression to AIDS (Ironson et al., 1994). Given that this hastened path to AIDS results in shortened lives, it is of utmost importance to consider how individuals may improve the ways in which they effectively cope with this disease, and subsequently diminish their levels of distress.

The Challenges of Conducting Research on Coping

Lazarus and Folkman (1984) have described coping as "constantly changing cognitive and behavioral efforts to manage specific external and/or internal demands that are appraised as taxing or exceeding the resources of the person" (p. 141). In this model, the appraisal process consists of primary appraisal, focused on assessing the personal threat of the significance of a stressor, such as a challenge or harm/loss that has occurred (or threatens to occur); and secondary appraisal, which is the assessment of the available options for coping, including estimation of the extent to which the person can affect the stressful situation.

Further, coping responses can be seen as "transactions" between the individual and the environment: attempts to actively alter the environment (problem-focused coping) or to regulate internal states (emotion-focused coping). At the most basic level, problem-focused coping involves individuals engaging in efforts to reduce or remove sources of distress through planning and other methods, while emotion-focused coping involves individuals trying to disengage themselves from distress through tactics such as minimization of the problem and distraction from it. However, as will be discussed, the classification of different coping strategies has been greatly expanded, and there are various subtypes that have yielded different outcomes in individuals with HIV.

---

[2] The Coping in Health and Illness Project is a federally funded research project that examines how multiple variables are related to the progression of disease in men with HIV. Specifically, it focuses on how psychological, psychosocial, and physiological factors influence the progression of HIV in this population.

Types of Coping in Individuals with HIV

Some coping research that focuses on individuals with HIV classifies coping into problem-focused and emotion-focused. For example, Pakenham and Rinaldis (2001) found that HIV-infected homosexual or bisexual men, who were better adjusted to their illness, were more likely to engage in problem-focused coping, as opposed to emotion-focused coping. This finding that problem-focused coping is related to better adjustment in individuals with HIV has been supported across other studies as well (e.g., Leserman, Perkins, & Evans, 1992). More active coping strategies also appear to be associated with future-oriented psychological states, such as optimism (Rogers, Hansen, Levy, Tate, & Sikkema, 2005).

Results from research on emotion-focused coping are more complex. Both negative and positive outcomes have been found, depending on the type of emotion-focused coping utilized. For example, findings from one study (Fleishman & Fogel, 1994) indicated that avoidant emotion-focused coping is related to greater distress, while active emotion-focused coping is related to improved adjustment to HIV.

Recent literature on individuals with HIV has expanded upon the traditional classifications of problem-focused and emotion-focused in order to examine the configurations of coping that individuals with HIV utilize. This is based on the rationale that individuals tend to use multiple strategies when they cope, as opposed to using one specific type only. In one study of 2864 individuals with HIV, four patterns of coping were identified (Fleishman et al., 2003). The most frequent configuration utilized was labeled as distancing coping. Individuals who utilized this strategy reported trying not to think about AIDS or letting it bother them. Two other configurations, blame-withdrawal coping and active-approach coping, were utilized with almost identical frequency. In blame-withdrawal coping, individuals reported avoiding interactions with people and criticizing themselves. In active-approach coping, individuals endorsed items, such as talking to others about their feelings regarding their HIV status, or engaging in volunteer work.

Fleishman and colleagues (2003) also identified a fourth coping configuration that they labeled as passive coping. Individuals identified as engaging in passive coping were not likely to endorse any of the aforementioned coping approaches. Further analyses indicated that individuals in the passive coping configuration were more likely to report positive factors, such as social support and emotional well-being. This suggests that they may not have engaged in other coping mechanisms, because there simply was no need. However, individuals who engaged in blame-withdrawal coping reported more negative factors, such as more symptoms of HIV.

Turner-Cobb et al. (2002) examined the relationship between coping strategies, social support, attachment style, and adjustment in individuals with HIV. Individuals who reported more positive mood were more likely to express satisfaction with their social support and have more secure attachment in their relationships. More positive mood also was associated with a decrease in behavioral disengagement as a coping strategy. As behavioral disengagement has been identified as a negative coping strategy for dealing with a chronic illness that requires active management, these findings indicated the importance of factors, such as positive mood, social support, and secure relationships, for engaging in effective coping.

Coping and Stress

Individuals with HIV confront various sources of stress. Many have faced multiple losses to HIV of friends, intimate partners, and family members (Ickovics, Druley, Morril, Grigoronko, & Rodin, 1998; Kemeny & Dean, 1995). They have the chronic stress of coping with a serious illness on a daily basis. In addition to the health-related stressors, HIV affects everything from parenting abilities to romantic relationships to employment. While positive HIV serostatus is certainly a stressor for lower SES populations, it increases both the stress experienced in multiple, already burdensome areas of life and depression levels in these individuals (Gurung, Taylor, Kemeny, & Myers, 2004).

The long-term presence of multiple life stressors on individuals with HIV has been shown to hasten their progression to AIDS and ultimately death (Leserman et al., 1999). For instance, Leserman et al. followed a group of HIV-infected homosexual men over several years and found that individuals, who scored above the median on a measure of stress (indicating high stress), were two to three times more likely to develop AIDS than were individuals who scored below the median. Thus, it is critical to understand the presence of stress in the lives of individuals with HIV and how it interacts with their ability to cope with their disease effectively.

The recent advances in medication, such as the use of HAART, have extended the lives of individuals with HIV and helped HIV evolve into a chronic illness rather than a terminal one. It generally was hoped that in addition to the medical benefits of HAART, individuals receiving this treatment would experience improved quality of lives overall. It, therefore, might be expected that individuals receiving HAART would experience less stress than their predecessors did prior to its inception. However, contrary to these expectations, it has been found that individuals receiving HAART may experience more psychosocial stressors.

Siegel and Schrimshaw (2005) compared matched samples of women with HIV prior to and after the start of HAART. They found that women receiving HAART reported more stress related to HIV-stigma and to the disclosure of their HIV status. Women receiving HAART perceived their health status more negatively than did women in the pre-HAART group. Women receiving HAART also were more likely to utilize negative forms of coping, such as escape-avoidant coping. Again, this is contrary to the problem-solving coping strategies that were anticipated within the HAART group. This provides evidence that despite what many perceive as improvements in the physical health status of individuals with

HIV, the psychosocial stressors related to the illness have not subsided, and in fact have increased. This also further establishes the link between reports of stressors and engagement in non-adaptive coping strategies.

Coping and Social Support

As is the case for people in a variety of populations (Avlund, Damsgaard, & Holstein, 1998; Gallant, 2003), an "individual with HIV/AIDSs' relationship" to his or her social environment has been associated with functionally-important mood states, various aspects of self-care, including medical care, and ultimately, to health-related outcomes. Social isolation in individuals with HIV has been linked to increased negative mood and decreased positive mood (Fleishman et al., 2000).

However, these findings do not mean that all types of social interactions ensure enhanced mood. The quality of the social support is important. Individuals who report conflictual social interactions (e.g., arguments, inappropriate demands by others) resemble those who are socially isolated in that they are more likely to report a negative mood (Fleishman et al. 2000). As negative mood has been linked to engaging in negative coping strategies, such as isolation and anger (Fleishman et al. 2000), and positive mood has been linked to decreases in negative coping strategies (Turner-Cobb et al., 2002), this suggests that helping individuals with HIV achieve more positive mood through high quality, beneficial social relationships is important.

Though there is strong evidence that high-quality social interactions play an important role in utilizing appropriate coping strategies, attaining such social interactions may sometimes be challenging for individuals with HIV. The positive link between symptoms associated with HIV and conflictual social interactions (Fleishman et al., 2000) suggests that as HIV becomes more severe, individuals may experience more conflictual social interactions when they are most in need of positive, supportive social relationships. The negative relationship between physical limitations brought forth by HIV and perceived social support further supports this point (Fleishman et al. 2000).

Poor medication adherence may play a role in the association between a lack of positive social support and faster progression to AIDS (Leserman et al., 1999). Low levels of perceived social support also have been linked to increased utilization of avoidance-oriented (i.e., negative) coping strategies (Weaver et al., 2005). While it also may be possible that individuals who utilize avoidant coping strategies also "avoid" social support available to them, a relationship has been found between having limited social support and subsequently engaging in avoidant coping strategies with negative consequences. For example, the utilization of avoidance-oriented coping strategies has been associated with poorer medication adherence and a higher viral load, thus negatively affecting the progression of HIV (Halkitis, Parsons, Wolitski, & Remien, 2003; Ironson et al., 2005; Weaver et al., 2005).

Physical and Psychosocial/Behavioral Interventions to Increase Coping

Treating Depression

As with the depression accompanying other medical conditions, standard treatments are efficacious including older (Rabkin, Rabkin, Harrison, & Wagner, 1994) and new generation antidepressants (Elliott et al., 1998; Fernandez & Levy, 1991; Hintz, Kuck, Peterkin, Volk, & Zisook, 1990; Zisook et al., 1998), as well as psychotherapy (Markowitz et al., 1995). Psychosocial functioning, including health-related quality of life, appears to benefit from treatment of depression (Elliott, Russo, & Roy-Byrne, 2002).

The impact of depression treatment on HAART adherence may be complex. One multi-site prospective study found that, among depressed individuals with HIV/AIDS, HAART utilization was superior for those receiving mental health therapy plus antidepressant treatment, or mental health therapy alone, compared to the untreated depression group; however, no such benefit was found for antidepressant treatment alone (Cook et al., 2006). It has been suggested that HAART regimens themselves may exert some beneficial impact on depression (Brechtl, Breitbart, Galietta, Krivo, & Rosenfeld, 2001; Judd et al., 2000; Low-Beer, 2000).

Interventions to Improve Coping in Individuals with HIV

As previously discussed, research indicates that high levels of stress and limited social support are strongly related to physical health outcomes and to whether or not individuals utilize effective coping strategies. As such, it is critical to develop ways to help individuals with HIV address these issues. The approaches that have been developed to help individuals with HIV cope with their diagnosis and illness typically encompass several components which are aimed at addressing the different ways that HIV affects the lives of individuals.

Cognitive Behavioral Stress Management

One of the most studied interventions to help individuals manage the stress associated with HIV is cognitive-behavioral stress management (CBSM). In a CBSM intervention, individuals are taught a combination of relaxation and stress management techniques, which typically include cognitive restructuring, relaxation training, and social skills training (Lichtstein, 1988). CBSM interventions with individuals with health conditions also may include didactic training on how stress functions and its effects on emotions and physical health.

The initial application of CBSM to individuals with HIV was conducted by Antoni et al. (1991). Prior to the notification of their HIV status, individuals were assigned to either an assessment-only group or to a CBSM group, which included group training in progressive muscle relaxation, cognitive restructuring, assertiveness, behavior-modification techniques, and didactic information on topics such as stress and health issues related to HIV. While individuals in the control group exhibited increases in depression and minimal immunological changes after their diagnosis of HIV, individuals in the CBSM group did not exhibit increases in depression and actually showed significant improvements in their immunological functioning, such as increases in helper-inducer (CD4) and natural killer (CD56) cell counts, after their notification of the positive HIV status. This study showed clear evidence that psychosocial interventions could play a critical role in better coping with the distress associated with a diagnosis of HIV, while concurrently improving immunological functioning.

In another study of CBSM (Lutgendorf et al., 1997), homosexual men, who were HIV-positive and experiencing HIV-related symptoms (but who had not yet developed AIDS), were provided with a 10-week intervention. The CBSM intervention included weekly stress management and relaxation, with instructions to practice relaxation two times a day. Participants also received information on such topics as how to identify and utilize social supports, and the link between stress and immune functioning. Compared to the wait-list control condition, individuals in the intervention group exhibited decreases in anxiety and dysphoria. This is consistent with more recent research that has found CBSM effective in decreasing psychological distress amongst men with HIV (Creuss, Antoni, Schneiderman, et al., 2000). There also was a positive immunological benefit in the intervention group of decreased herpes simplex virus antibodies. This same physiological benefit has been replicated in other research as well (Creuss, Antoni, Schneiderman, et al., 2000).

Research has integrated CBSM with additional interventions. For example, Jones et al. (2003) combined CBSM with expressive supportive therapy to help "... make the intervention less didactic and to provide an opportunity for greater emotional expressiveness..." (p. 467). Results indicated that women with AIDS, who had low medication adherence and who were in the intervention group, increased their medication adherence and decreased their utilization of denial coping strategies. In a recent study, Antoni et al. (2006) combined CBSM with training on medication adherence to examine their joint effect on HIV-positive homosexual men. Results indicated that over a fifteen-month period, men who received the combined treatment of medication adherence and CBSM exhibited decreases in their HIV viral loads, while the group that received only the medication-adherence training exhibited no change in their HIV viral loads. Participants in the combined intervention group also reported significantly lower levels of depression than did participants in the medication-adherence only group, which helps explain the discrepancy in viral loads. Again, this provides ongoing support for the use of CBSM, in conjunction with other interventions, to maximize beneficial outcomes in a high-risk population.

Collectively, these and other research findings indicate that CBSM is a well-supported intervention that serves many purposes (see Schneiderman & Antoni, 2003). CBSM can assist individuals with HIV/AIDS in coping with their stress, can diminish distress related to symptoms, and can improve immunological functioning. Though the recent study by Antoni et al. provides important long-term data, more longitudinal studies of the efficacy of CBSM are needed in order to better understand the role of CBSM and where it can be used most effectively.

Coping Effectiveness Training

Given the variety of severe stressors that confront individuals with HIV, it is not surprising that many individuals have difficulty coping with all of them effectively. Individuals may use any combination of coping techniques. The type of coping an individual utilizes is largely influenced by the stressor itself (e.g., Is the stressor something over which the individual has control?). Coping effectiveness training (CET) takes this into account. Its goal is to train individuals with HIV to choose the most appropriate type of coping for a particular stressor.

In a preliminary study of CET (Chesney, Folkman, & Chambers, 1996), individuals with HIV were trained to use the emotion-focused and problem-focused coping strategies that were most adaptive to the individual's situation. They also were taught how to utilize social support effectively and how to maintain improvements in overall functioning. The results were very promising: individuals who participated in CET exhibited improvements in their coping skills, less stress, and less emotional distress.

In a more recent study of HIV-positive homosexual/bisexual men (Chesney, Chambers, Taylor, Johnson, & Folkman, 2003), CET was compared to an active informational (HIV information) control group, and to a wait-list control group. The findings indicated that individuals in the CET group exhibited significant decreases in perceived stress and burnout compared to both control groups, and decreases in anxiety and improvements in positive states of mind, compared to the wait-list control group. The CET group maintained its improvements in positive states of mind at six- and 12-months follow-up. These findings indicate that CET is successful in providing individuals with the tools to use appropriate coping skills that subsequently lead to improved psychological well-being.

While CET and CBST have different components within their treatments, they share an important commonality – they typically are administered in group settings. As previously discussed, high-quality social support helps individuals with HIV more effectively cope with the chronic stressors that accompany the disease. Thus, it seems logical that group settings may be beneficial when conducting therapeutic interventions with this population. Such groups foster a supportive environment that individuals with HIV may not otherwise have.

While interventions often conceptualize the individual as the locus of coping, suggestive data have been collected on an intervention that targets the couple as the unit, such as the Sharing Medical Adherence Responsibilities Together (SMART) Couples Study (Remien et al., 2005). Delivered to heterosexual and homosexual serodiscordant couples ($N = 215$) in a randomized controlled trial, this intervention used four 45–60 minutes sessions delivered over five weeks to boost support for partner adherence and increase communication, problem-solving skills, and intimacy. Compared to individuals receiving usual care, treated couples showed higher mean medication adherence on a range of measures at week eight, although differences declined over time, which may suggest the probable need for booster sessions. Taken together, these studies indicate that coping strategies can be improved in individual with HIV/AIDS, using diverse methodology and settings.

Vocational and Social Implications

Improved disease management and psychosocial coping can improve quality of life, but access to valued social roles must also confront at least two sorts of social barriers: stigma and work-related discrimination. Stigma research has faced challenges which are attributable to the statistical clustering of HIV in subgroups that are already subject to social discrimination and virus transmission via proscribed or stigmatized behaviors. Multiple studies by Herek and colleagues have isolated two stigma types. The first, instrumental stigma, is constituted around specific fears directly linked to HIV-disease characteristics, such as trans-missibility, severity, and visibility. The second, symbolic stigma, is expressive, inasmuch as the response to HIV expresses negative cultural responses toward negatively-viewed associated groups and practices, such as homosexual sex and drug use.

Further refinements to the basic model of stigma have been advocated by those who focus on what McBride (1998) refers to as the "layering" of stigma produced by membership in multiple stigmatized groups. A conceptual model and quantitative measurement strategy has recently been proposed by Reidpath and Chan (2005). They distinguish four components: a first stigma source; a second stigma source; the shared stigma (the combined stigma of the stigma sources); and what they term a "synergistic" stigma, conceptualized as stigma in excess of that predicted by the addition of the two sources independently.

Another strategy can be found in a vignette study by the authors (Walkup, Cramer, & Yeras, 2004), which was motivated by the spread of HIV among people with severe mental illness. While the Reidpath and Chan framework was not used in the study design, the research question introduced a compli-cation that was not explicitly considered in the framework. Specifically, since the 1980s, evidence has mounted that stigma may be associated with an individual's perceived responsibility for infection (McBride, 1998; Weiner, Perry, & Magnusson, 1988). For example, early on, distinctions were noted between so-called "innocent" victims of AIDS, who acquired the virus through prenatal infection or blood transfusion, and those who acquired it through unpro-tected sex or intravenous drug use. A person who is blamed for his or her illness seems to be an object of greater stigmatization (Leiker, Taub, & Gast, 1995).

Therefore, we wondered whether the presence of mental illness would add to the stigma of HIV, or somehow reduce perceived responsibility by causing respondents to see the person as less responsible for their infection. We found that the presence of mental illness did not significantly reduce HIV stigma; rather, the level of stigma attached to mental illness was so high that the addition of HIV did not significantly raise stigma ratings (Walkup et al., 2004). Despite the ongoing challenge to quantify and conceptualize clearly HIV-related stigma and to understand its relationship with other typically stigmatized conditions, it is clear HIV is a highly stigmatized condition.

Work

Individuals with HIV have high rates of unemployment, worry about the types of jobs that may or may not be suitable for them, and experience anxiety about their employers' attitudes towards them (Dray-Spira & Lert, 2003). In addition, HAART-related preservation, or recovery, of health and functioning has forced reexamination of the significance of HIV/AIDS for work. Sheer numbers make this an important policy dilemma for federal disability programs, such as Social Security Disability Insurance (SSDI) or Supplemental Security Income (SSI), that are based on an impairment-related inability to work.

Negotiating return to work poses numerous challenges, whether or not one is receiving disability compensation (World Institute on Disability, 1994). Many people consider returning to work when improved health and increased activity are combined with a desire for more income and to return to a more "normal" life that includes work (Ferrier & Lavis, 2003). Qualitative research in the U.S. (Brooks & Klosinski, 1999) and in Canada (Ferrier & Lavis, 2003) has documented concerns regarding loss of income or benefits and workplace discrimination. Martin and colleagues (2003) reported on an extensive survey regarding areas of concern about workforce reentry. Disease acuity predicted greater concern across a range of topic areas. Factor analysis identified six areas of concern: benefits-loss, work-related health, job skills, discrimination, personal health-care, and workplace accommodations.

The 1990 Americans with Disabilities Act (ADA; US Department of Justice, 1992) covers individual with HIV/AIDS, as it does other citizens with qualified disability status. In a practical sense, some issues may have particular importance for individual with HIV/AIDS, both because the underlying disease has distinctive features and because public attitudes have historically reflected misconceptions about disease features.[3] No public entity and no private employer with more than 14 employees may discriminate in employment practices. Prior to a job offer, the employer may not inquire about a disability (although inquiries about specific job functions are allowed), nor may they require a medical examination (although the job offer may be conditional on satisfactory result of a post-offer medical exam, if this is required of all entering employees in

---

[3] Chapter text here draws directly from material of the U.S. Department of Justice, Civil Rights Division, Disability Rights Section, found at http://www.usdoj.gov/crt/ada/pubs/hivqanda.text (Accessed January 10, 2006).

that category). Disability status or illness alone may not be the grounds for a subsequent withdrawal of a job offer (or subsequent decision not to retain an employee). The employee must be unable to perform core job duties, even if reasonable accommodation is provided. Only current ability to perform may be considered; fear of future medical decline may not figure in the decision.

Once the person is hired, HIV/AIDS in and of itself may not be the basis of job assignment, wages, promotions, or benefits (including health insurance). An employee's disclosure of disability status obligates the employer to make reasonable accommodations. While it may be technically sufficient to disclose only that one has an illness or disability covered by the ADA, and that one wants an accommodation to help with some problem, the employer has a right to require medical documentation regarding the condition and the limitations it imposes.

Using a national database of HIV discrimination cases filed between the implementation of the ADA through 1999, Studdert (2002) reported 18.0% were found to have merit and 14.1% received monetary compensation. Results of a multivariate analysis were interpreted to suggest that there might be "underclaiming" by young workers. In one study ($N = 84$) of individuals with HIV/AIDS, more than half had used some form of accommodation at work. A minority of those using accommodations reported they could not work without them (14%), and a somewhat larger group said they were unsure (34%) (Conyers & Boomer, 2005)[4].

Conclusions

There undoubtedly has been progress made in the development of medical treatments for HIV and AIDS. However, while developments of medical approaches, such as HAART, have extended the life expectancy of individuals with HIV/AIDS, these developments do not automatically translate into improved quality of life. Individuals with HIV/AIDS must juggle a strict medical regimen, symptoms of their disease, stigma from others, and numerous other stressors. It is quite logical then that coping effectively with the multiple aspects of HIV/AIDS often can be extremely difficult.

Further research is needed to better understand the types of coping that may occur under the umbrellas of these different classifications of coping, and why some coping types may be more beneficial than others in certain circumstances. Simply grouping and labeling different coping approaches does not automatically

---

[4] Interested readers may want to consult an associated special issue of *Journal of Vocational Rehabilitation,* resulting from work done in connection with an April 2003 multidisciplinary gathering of stakeholders, called the Working Positive Summit, which was organized by the Matrix Research Institute, and was devoted to what they described as the "emergent disability" status of HIV/AIDS (Conyers, 2005, p. 67). This meeting led to establishment of the National Working Positive Coalition (NWPC), chaired by Liza Marie Conyers at Pennsylvania State University.

facilitate better understanding of their efficacy. This is especially critical when coping strategies may affect physical health outcomes or medication adherence, as is the case with individuals with HIV (Bianchi, Zea, Poppen, Reisen, & Echeverry, 2004; Stein & Rotheram-Borus, 2004).

While part of the dilemma that pervades the coping literature is identifying what type of coping mechanisms individuals utilize and how effective such approaches are in different circumstances for individuals with HIV/AIDS, the complexity of HIV/AIDS and its many consequences make developing and implementing effective coping strategies even more difficult. Significant progress has been made, particularly in development of techniques such as cognitive behavioral stress management and coping effectiveness training that benefit psychological, social, and medical outcomes. Yet challenges remain. First, these coping interventions need to be disseminated to a much larger percentage of individual with HIV/AIDS, and as early on in the course of the disease as possible. Second, people with HIV/AIDS should be included in intervention research and dissemination. Third, additional studies that follow individuals over a longer course of time are needed to determine at what points coping interventions are most effective, and whether they need to be constantly implemented, or if "booster" interventions will suffice.

Taking steps, such as the ones outlined above, will not cure HIV/AIDS. However, they can be used in conjunction with appropriate medical treatment to ensure that individual with HIV/AIDS learn to effectively cope and to enhance their quality of life. Because psychological problems, such as depression, are associated with poorer health outcomes, providing coping training in conjunction with medical treatment can help improve a person's overall psychological and medical condition. This is a crucial combination for managing a very difficult disease.

References

Antoni, M. H., Baggett, L., Ironson, G., LaPerriere, A., August, S., Klimas, N., et al. (1991). Cognitive-behavioral stress management intervention buffers distress responses and immunological changes following notification of HIV-1 seropositivity. *Journal of Consulting and Clinical Psychology, 59,* 906–915.

Antoni, M.H., Carrico, A.W., Duran, R.E., Spitzer, S., Penedo, F., Ironson, G., et al. (2006). Randomized clinical trial of cognitive behavioral stress management on human immunodeficiency virus viral load in gay men treated with highly active antiretroviral therapy. *Psychosomatic Medicine, 68,* 143–151.

Antoni, M.H., Esterling B.A., Lutgendorf, S., Fletcher, M.A., & Schneiderman N. (1995). Psychosocial stressors, herpes virus reactivation, and HIV-1 infection. In M. Stein & A. Baum (Eds.), *Chronic diseases: Perspectives in behavioral medicine* (pp. 135–168). Hillsdale, NJ: Lawrence Erlbaum Associates.

Asch, S. M., Kilbourne, A. M., Gifford, A. L., Burnam, M. A., Turner, B., Shapiro, M. F., et al. (2003). For the HCSUS Consortium – Underdiagnosis of depression in HIV: Who are we missing? *Journal of General Internal Medicine, 6,* 450–460.

Avlund, A., Damsgaard, M. T., & Holstein, B. E. (1998). Social relations and mortality: An eleven-year follow-up study of 70-year old men and women in Denmark. *Social Science & Medicine, 47,* 645–643.

Bianchi, F. T., Zea, M. C., Poppen, P. J., Reisen, C. A., & Echeverry, J. J. (2004). Coping as a mediator of the impact of sociocultural factors on health behavior among HIV-positive Latino gay men. *Psychology and Health, 19,* 89–101.

Bing, E. G., Burnam, M. A., Longshore, D., Fleishman J. A., Sherbourne C. D., London, A. S., et al. (2001). Psychiatric disorders and drug use among human immunodeficiency virus-infected adults in the United States. *Archives of General Psychiatry, 58,* 721–728.

Boarts, J., Sledjeski, E., Bogart, L., & Delahunty, D. L. (2006). The differential impact of PTSD and depression on HIV disease markers and adherence to HAART in people living with HIV. *AIDS and Behavior.* Accessed from http://springerlink.com/lh4plt3ecnalnt3d5cqxv155)/app/home/contribution.asp?referrer+parent&backto=issue, 13,22;linkingpublicationresults.1:104828.1

Boden, D., Hurley, A., Zhang, L., Cao, Y., Guo, Y., Jones, E., et al. (1999). HIV-1 drug resistance in newly infected individuals. *Journal of the American Medical Association 282,* 1135–1141.

Bozzette, S.A., Berry, S.H., Duan, N., Frankel, M.R., Leibowitz, A.A., Lefkowitz, D., et al. (1998). The care of HIV infected adults in the United States. HIV cost and services utilization study consortium. *The New England Journal of Medicine, 339,* 1897–1904.

Brechtl, J. R., Breitbart, W., Galietta, M., Krivo, S. & Rosenfeld, B. (2001). The use of highly active antiretroviral therapy (HAART) in patients with advanced HIV infection: Impact on medical, palliative care, and quality of life outcomes. *Journal of Pain & Symptom Management, 21,* 41–51.

Brooks, R. A., & Klosinski, L. E. (1999). Assisting persons living with HIV/AIDS to return to work: Programmatic steps for AIDS service organizations. *AIDS Education and Prevention, 11*(3), 212–223.

Carpenter, C. C., Fischl, M. A., Hammer, S. M., Hirsch, M. S., Jacobsen, D. M., Katzenstein, D. A., et al. (1997). Antiretroviral therapy for HIV infection in 1997. Updated recommendations of the International AIDS Society-USA panel. *Journal of the American Medical Association, 277,* 1962–1969.

Centers for Disease Control and Prevention (2003). Advancing HIV prevention: new strategies for a changing epidemic – United States, 2003. Atlanta: U.S. Department of Health and Human Services, Centers for Disease Control and Prevention. Retrieved July 23, 2006, from http://www.cdc.gov/mmwr/preview/mmwrhtml/mm5215a1.htm.

Centers for Disease Control and Prevention (2005). *HIV surveillance report, 2005* Vol. 17. Retrieved February 1 2007 from http://www.cdc.gov/hiv/topics/surveillance/resources/reports/2005report/coverhtm.

Chesney, M. A., Chambers, D. B., Taylor, J. M., Johnson, L. M., & Folkman, S. (2003). Coping effectiveness training for men living with HIV: Results from a randomized clinical trial testing a group-based intervention. *Psychosomatic Medicine, 65,* 1038–1046.

Chesney, M., Folkman, S., & Chambers, D. (1996). Coping effectiveness training for men living with HIV: Preliminary findings. *International Journal of STD & AIDS, 7*(2), 75–82.

Ciesla, J. A., & Roberts, J. E. (2001). Meta-analysis of the relationship between HIV infection and risk for depressive disorders. *American Journal of Psychiatry, 158,* 725–730.

Conyers, L. M. (2005). HIV/AIDS as an emergent disability: The response of vocational rehabilitation. *Journal of Vocational Rehabilitation, 22*(2), 67–73.

Conyers, L., & Boomer K. B. (2005). Factors associated with disclosure of HIV/AIDS to employers among individuals who use job accommodations and those who do not. *Journal of Vocational Rehabilitation, 22,* 189–196.

Cook, J. A., Grey, D., Burke-Miller, M. H., Cohen, M. H., Anastos, K., Ghandi, M., et al. (2006) Effects of treated and untreated depressive symptoms on highly active antiretroviral therapy use in a US multi-site cohort of HIV-positive women. *AIDS Care, 18,* 93–100.

Creuss, S., Antoni, M., Creuss, D., Fletcher, M. A., Ironson, G., Kumar, M., et al. (2000). Reductions in herpes simplex virus type 2 antibody titers after cognitive behavioral stress management and relationships with neuroendocrine function, relaxation skills, and social support in HIV-positive men. *Psychosomatic Medicine, 62,* 828–837.

Creuss, D. G., Antoni, M. H., Schneiderman, N., Ironson, G., McCabe, P., Fernandez, J. B., et al. (2000). Cognitive-behavioral stress management increases free testosterone and decreases psychological distress in HIV-seropositive men. *Health Psychology, 19,* 12–20.

Dew, M. A., Becker, J. T., Sanchez, J., Caldararo, R., Lopez, O. L., Wess, J., et al. (1997). Prevalence and predictors of depressive, anxiety and substance use disorders in HIV-infected and uninfected men: A longitudinal evaluation. *Psychological Medicine, 27,* 395–409.

Dray-Spira, R., & Lert, F. (2003). Social health inequalities during the course of chronic HIV disease in the era of highly active antiretroviral therapy. *AIDS, 17,* 283–290.

Elliott, A., Russo, J., & Roy-Byrne, P. (2002). The effect of changes in depression on health-related quality of life in HIV infections. *General Hospital Psychiatry, 24,* 43–47.

Elliott, A.J., Uldall, K.K., Bergam, K., Russo, J., Claypoole, K., & Roy-Byrne, P.P. (1998). Randomized, placebo-controlled trial of paroxetine versus imipramine in depressed HIV-positive outpatients. *American Journal of Psychiatry, 155,* 367–372.

Epstein, S. (1998). *Impure Science: AIDS, activism, and the politics of knowledge.* Berkeley, California: University of California Press.

Fauci, A. S. (1996). Host factors and the pathogenesis of HIV-induced disease. *Nature, 384,* 529–534.

Fernandez, F., & Levy, J. K. (1991). Psychopharmacotherapy of psychiatric syndromes in asymptomatic and symptomatic HIV infection. *Psychological Medicine, 9,* 377–394.

Ferrier, S. E., & Lavis, J. N. (2003). With health comes work? People living with HIV/AIDS consider returning to work. *AIDS Care, 15*(3), 423–435.

Fleishman, J.A., & Fogel, B. (1994). Coping and depressive symptoms among people with AIDS. *Health Psychology, 13,* 156–169.

Fleishman, J. A., Sherbourne, C. D., Cleary, P. D., Wu, A. W., Crystal, S., & Hays, R. D. (2003). Patterns of coping among persons with HIV infection: Configurations, correlates, and change. *American Journal of Community Psychology, 32,* 187–204.

Fleishman, J. A., Sherbourne, C. D., Crystal, S., Collins, R., Collins, R. L., Marshall, G. N., et al. (2000). Coping, conflictual social interactions, social support, and mood among HIV-infected persons. *American Journal of Community Psychology, 28,* 421–453.

Folkman, S., & Chesney, M. (1995). Coping with HIV infection. In M. Stein & A. Baum (Eds.), *Chronic diseases: Perspectives in behavioral medicine* (pp. 115–133). Hillsdale, NJ: Lawrence Erlbaum Associates.

Folkman, S., Chesney, M., Collette, L., Boccellari, A., & Cooke, M. (1996). Post-bereavement depressive mood and its prebereavement predictors in HIV+ and HIV− gay men. *Journal of Personal and Social Psychology, 70,* 336–348.

French, T., Weiss, L., Waters, M., Tesoriero, J., Finkelstein, R., & Agins, B. (2005). Correlation of a brief perceived stress measure with nonadherence to antiretroviral therapy over time. *Journal of Acquired Immune Deficiency Syndrome, 38,* 590–597.

Gallant, M. P. (2003). The influence of social support on chronic illness self-management: A review and directions for research. *Health Education & Behavior, 30,* 170–195.

Gifford, A. L., Bormann, J. E., Shively, M. J., Wright, B. C., Richman, D. D., & Bozzette, S. A. (2000). Predictors of self-reported adherence and plasma HIV concentrations in patients on multidrug antiretroviral regimens. *Journal of Acquired Immunodeficiency Syndrome, 23,* 386–395.

Goodroad, B. K. (2003). HIV and AIDS in people over 50. A continuing concern. *Journal of Gerontology Nursing, 29*(4), 18–24.

Gurung, R. R., Taylor, S., Kemeny, M., & Myers, H. (2004). "HIV is not my biggest problem": The impact of HIV and chronic burden on depression in women at risk for AIDS. *Journal of Social and Clinical Psychology, 23,* 490–511.

Halkitis, P. N., Parsons, J. T., Wolitski, R. J., Remien, R. H. (2003). Characteristics of HIV antiretroviral treatments, access and adherence in an ethnically diverse sample of men who have sex with men. *AIDS Care, 15,* 89–102.

Hecht, F. M., Grant, R. M., Petropoulos, C. J., Dillon, B, Chesney, M. A., Tian, H., et al. (1998). Sexual transmission of an HIV-1 variant resistant to multiple reverse-transcriptase and protease inhibitors. *New England Journal of Medicine, 339,* 307–311.

Heckman, T. G., Kochman, A., Sikkema, K. J., Kalichman, S. C., Masten, J., Bergholte, J., & Catz, S. (2001). A pilot coping improvement intervention for late middle-aged and older adults living with HIV/AIDS in the USA. *AIDS Care, 13,* 129–139.

Hintz, S., Kuck, J., Peterkin, J. J., Volk, D. M., & Zisook, S. (1990). Depression in the context of human immunodeficiency virus infection: implications for treatment. *Journal of Clinical Psychiatry, 51,* 497–501.

Hogg, R. S., Heath, K. V., Yip, B., Kraib, K. G., O'Shaughnessey, M. V., Schechter, M. T., et al. (1998). Improved survival among HIV-infected individuals following initiation of antiretroviral therapy. *Journal of the American Medical Association, 279,* 450–454.

Ickovics, J. R., Druley, J., Morrill, A. C., Grigoronko, E., & Rodin, J. (1998). A grief observed: The experience of HIV-related Illness and death among women in a clinic-based sample in New Haven, CT. *Journal of Consulting and Clinical Psychology, 66,* 958–966.

Ingram, K. M., Jones, D. A., Fass, R. J., Neidig, J. L., & Song, Y.S. (1999). Social support and unsupportive social interactions: Their association with depression among people living with HIV. *AIDS Care, 11,* 313–329.

Ironson, G., Friedman, A., Klimas, N., Antoni, M., Fletcher, M. A., LaPerriere, A., et al. (1994). Distress, denial, and low adherence to behavioral interventions predict faster disease progression in HIV-1 infected gay men. *International Journal of Medicine, 1,* 90–105.

Ironson, G., O'Cleirigh, C., Fletcher, M. A., Laurenceau, J. P., Balbin, E., Klemas, N., et al. (2005). Psychosocial factors predict CD4 and viral load change in men and women with human immunodeficiency virus in the era of highly active antiretroviral treatment. *Psychosomatic Medicine, 67,* 1013–1021.

Jones, D. L., Ishii, M., LaPerriere, A., Stanley, H., Antoni, M., Ironson, G., et al. (2003). Influencing medication adherence among women with AIDS. *AIDS Care, 15*, 463–474.

Judd, A., Stimson, G. V., Hickman, M., Hunter, G. M., Jones, S., Parry, J. V., et al. (2000). Prevalence of HIV infection in a multi-site sample of injecting drug users not in contact with treatment services in England. *AIDS, 14*, 2413–2415.

Kaiser Family Foundation (June, 2005). *Fact Sheet: HIV Testing in the United States.* Retrieved April 11, 2006, from http://www.kff.org/hivaids/6094.cfm.

Kaiser Family Foundation (November, 2005). *Fact sheet: The HIV/AIDS epidemic in the United States.* Retrieved July 31, 2006, from http://www.kff.org/hivaids/upload/3029-06.pdf.

Kaiser Family Foundation (February, 2006). *Fact Sheet: African–American and HIV.* Retrieved April 22, 2006, from http://www.kff.org/hivaids/6089.cfm.

Kaiser Family Foundation (June, 2006) *Chart Pack: AIDS at 25.* Retrieved July 30, 2006, from http://www.kff.org/hivaids/upload/7525.pdf.

Karon, J. M., Fleming, P. L., Steketee, R. W., & de Cock, K. M. (2001). HIV in the United States at the turn of the century: An epidemic in transition. *American Journal of Public Health, 91*, 1060–1068.

Kemeny, M. E., & Dean, L. (1995). Effects of AIDS-related bereavement on HIV progression among New York City gay men. *AIDS Education and Prevention, 7*(Suppl.), 36–47.

Kemeny, M. E., Weiner, H., Taylor, S. E., Schneider, S., Visscher, B., Fahey, J. L. (1994). Repeated bereavement, depressed mood, and immune parameters in HIV seropostive andseronegative gay men. *Health Psychology, 13*, 14–24.

Kessler, R., McGonagle, K., Zhao, S., Nelson, C., Hughes, M., Eshlman, S., et al. (1994). Lifetime and 12-month prevalence of DSM II-R psychiatric disorders in the United States. Results from the National Comorbidity Study. *Archives of General Psychiatry, 51*, 8–19.

Lazarus, R. S., & Folkman, S. (1984). *Stress, appraisal, and coping.* Springer Publishing Company: New York.

Lee, L. M., Karon, J. M, Selik R., Newal, J. J., & Fleming, P. L. (2001). Survival after AIDS diagnosis in adolescents and adults during the treatment era, United States, 1984–1997. *Journal of the American Medical Association, 285*, 1308–1315.

Leiker, J. J., Taub, D. E., & Gast, J. (1995). The stigma of AIDS: Persons with AIDS and social distance. *Deviant Behavior: An Interdisciplinary Journal, 16*, 333–351.

Leserman J. (2003). HIV disease progression: Depression, stress, and possible mechanisms. *Biological Psychiatry, 54*, 295–306.

Leserman, J., Jackson, E. D., Petitto, J. M., Golden, R. N., Silva, S. G., Perkins, D. O., et al. (1999). Progression to AIDS: The effects of stress, depressive symptoms, and social support. *Psychosomatic Medicine, 61*, 397–406.

Leserman, J., Perkins, D.O., & Evans, D.L. (1992). Coping with the threat of AIDS: The role of social support. *American Journal of Psychiatry, 149*, 1514–1520.

Leserman, J., Petitto, J. M., Gu, H., Gaynes, B. N., Barroso, J., Golden, R. N., et al. (2002). Progression to AIDS, a clinical AIDS condition and mortality: Psychosocial and physiological predictors. *Psychological Medicine, 32*, 1059–1073.

Lichstein, K. (1988). *Clinical relaxation strategies.* New York: Wiley.

Low-Beer, S. (2000). Depressive symptoms decline among persons on HIV protease inhibitors. *Journal of Acquired Immune Deficiency Syndrome, 23*, 295–301.

Lutgendorf, S. K., Antoni, M. H., Ironson, G., Klimas, N., Kumar, M., Starr, K., et al. (1997). Cognitive-behavioral stress management decreases dysphoric mood and herpes simplex virus-type 2 antibody titers in symptomatic HIV-seropositive gay men. *Journal of Consulting and Clinical Psychology, 65*, 31–43.

Markowitz, J. C., Klerman, G. L., Clougherty, K. F., Spielman, L. A., Jacobsberg, L. B., Fishman, B., et al. (1995). Individual psychotherapies for depressed HIV-positive patients. *American Journal of Psychiatry, 152*, 1504–1509.

Martin, D. J., Brooks, R. A., Ortiz, D. J., & Veniegas, R. C. (2003). Perceived employment barriers and their relation to workforce-entry intent among people with HIV/AIDS. *Journal of Occupational Health Psychology, 8*, 181–194.

Mata, R.C., Viciana, P., De Alarcon, A., Lopez-Cortes, L. F., Gomez-Vera, J., Trastoy, M., et al. (2005). Discontinuation of antiretroviral therapy in patients with chronic HIV infection: Clinical, virologic, and immunologic consequences. *AIDS Patient Care and STDs, 19*, 550–562.

McBride, C. A. (1998). The discounting principle and attitudes toward victims of HIV infection. *Journal of Applied Social Psychology, 28*, 595–608.

Orlando, M., Tucker, J. S., Sherbourne, C. D., & Burnam, M. A. (2005). A cross-lagged model of psychiatric problems and health-related quality of life among a national sample of HIV-positive adults. *Medical Care, 43*, 21–27.

Pakenham, K. I., & Rinaldis, M. (2001). The role of illness, resources, appraisal, and coping strategies in adjustment to HIV/AIDS: The direct and buffering effects. *Journal of Behavioral Medicine, 24*, 259–279.

Palella, F. J., Jr., Delaney, K. M., Moorman, A. C., Loveless, M. O., Fuhrer, J., Satten, G. A., et al. (1998). Declining morbidity and mortality among patients with advanced human immunodeficiency virus infection. Outpatient Study Investigators. *New England Journal of Medicine, 338*, 853–860.

Panel for Clinical Practices for Treatment of HIV Infection of the US Department of Health and Human Services and the Henry J. Kaiser Foundation (2005). Retrieved April 11, 2006, from http://www.hivatis.org.

Paterson, D. L., Swindells, S., Mohr, J., Brester, M., Vergis, E. N., Squier, C., et al. (2000). Adherence to protease inhibitor therapy and outcomes in patients with HIV infection. *Annals Internal Medicine, 133*, 21–30.

Press, N., Tyndall, M. W., Wood, E., Hogg, R. S., Montaner, J. S. (2002). Virologic and immunologic response, clinical progression, and highly active antiretroviral therapy adherence. *Journal of Acquired Immune Deficiency Syndrome, 15, 31*(Suppl, 3), S112–S117.

Rabkin, J. G. (1996). Prevalence of psychiatric disorders in HIV illness. *International Review of Psychiatry, 8*(2–3), 157–166.

Rabkin, J. G., & Ferrando, S. (1997). A "second life" agenda: Psychiatric research issues raised by protease inhibitor treatments for people with human deficiency virus or acquired immunodeficiency syndrome. *Archives of General Psychiatry, 54*, 1049–1053.

Rabkin, J. G., Rabkin, R., Harrison, W., & Wagner, G. (1994). Effect of Imipramine on mood and enumerative measures of immune status in depressed patients with HIV illness. *American Journal of Psychiatry, 151*, 516–523.

Reidpath, D. D., & Chan, K. Y. (2005). A method for the quantitative analysis of the layering of HIV-related stigma. *AIDS Care, 17*(4), 425–432.

Remien, R. H., Stirratt, M., Dolezal, C., Dognin J. S., Wagner, G. J., & Carballo-Dieguez, A. (2005). Couple focused support to improve HIV medication adherence: A randomized controlled trial. *AIDS, 19*, 807–814.

Rogers, M. E., Hansen, N. B., Levy, B. R., Tate, D. C., & Sikkema, K. J. (2005). Optimism and coping with loss in bereaved HIV-infected men and women. *Journal of Social and Clinical Psychology, 24,* 341–360.

Rosenberger, P. H., Bornstein, R. A., Nasrallah, H. A., Para, M. F., Whitaker, C. C., Fass, R. J., et al. (1993). Psychopathology in Human Immunodeficiency Virus infection: Lifetime and current assessment. *Comprehensive Psychiatry, 34,* 150–158.

Rust, G. (2003). Do clinicians screen Medicaid patients for syphilis or HIV when they diagnose other sexually transmitted diseases? *Sexually Transmitted Diseases, 30,* 723–727.

Samet, J. H., Freedberg, K. A., Stein, M. D., Lewis, R., Savetsky, J., Sullivan, L., et al. (1998). Trillion virion delay: Time from testing positive for HIV to presentation for primary care. *Archives of Internal Medicine, 158*(7), 734–740.

Satriano, S., Remien, R., & Berkman, A. (2004). Acquired Immune Deficiency Syndrome and Human Immunodeficiency Virus. In H. Zaretsky, E. Richter, & M. Eisenberg (Eds.) *Medical aspects of disability: A handbook for the rehabilitation professional* (Springer Series on Rehabilitation) (pp. 59–78). New York: Springer Publishing.

Schneiderman, N., & Antoni, M. (2003). Learning to cope with HIV/AIDS. In F. Kessel, P. Rosenfield, & N. Anderson (Eds.), *Expanding the boundaries of health and social science: Case studies in interdisciplinary innovation* (pp. 316–347). New York: Oxford University Press.

Siegel, K., & Schrimshaw, E. W. (2005). Stress, appraisal, and coping: A comparison of HIV-infected women in the pre-HAART and HAART eras. *Journal of Psychosomatic Research, 58,* 225–233.

Simoni, J. M., & Ng, M. T. (2000). Trauma, coping, and depression among women with HIV/AIDS in New York City. *AIDS Care, 12*(5), 567–580.

Sledjeski, E. M., Delahanty, D. L., & Bogart, L. (2005). Incidence and impact of posttraumatic stress disorder and comorbid depression on adherence to HAART and CD4+ counts in people living with HIV. *AIDS Patient Care and STDs, 19,* 728–736.

Stein, J. A., & Rotheram-Borus, M. (2004). Cross-sectional and longitudinal associations in coping strategies and physical health outcomes among HIV-positive youth. *Psychology and Health, 19,* 321–326.

Stober, D. R., Schwartz, J. A. J., McDaniel, J. S., & Abrams, R. F. (1997). Depression and HIV disease: prevalence, correlates and treatment. *Psychiatric Annals, 27*(5), 372–377.

Studdert, D. M. (2002). Charges of human immunodeficiency virus discrimination in the workplace: The American with Disabilities Act in action. *American Journal of Epidemiology, 156,* 219–229.

Turner-Cobb, J. M., Gore-Felton, C. G., Marouf, F., Koopman, C., Kim, R., Israelski, D., & Spiegel, D. (2002). Coping, social support, and attachment style as psychosocial correlates of adjustment in men and women with HIV/AIDS. *Journal of Behavioral Medicine, 25,* 337–353.

UNAIDS (2006). 2006 Report on the global AIDS epidemic. Retrieved July 17, 2006, from http://www.unaids.org/en/HIVdata/2006GlobalReport/default.asp

US Department of Justice *Questions & Answers: The Americans with Disabilities Act and Persons with HIV/AIDS* (1992). Retrieved April 15, 2006, from http://www.usdoj.gov/crt/ada/pubs/hivquanda

Valdez, H., Lederman, M. M., Woolley, I., Walker, C. J., Vernon, L. T., Hise, A., et al. (1999). Human immunodeficiency virus 1 protease inhibitors in clinical practice: predictors of virological outcome. *Archives of Internal Medicine, 159,* 1771–1776.

Van Sighem, A. I., De Wiel, M. A., Ghani, A. C., Jambroes, M., Reiss, P., Gyssens, I. C., et al. (2003). Mortality and progression to AIDS after starting highly active antiretroviral therapy. *AIDS, 17*, 2227–2236.

Walkup, J., Cramer, L., & Yeras, J. (2004). Serious mental illness and HIV: How are stigma judgments affected by the "layering" of stigmatized conditions? *Psychological Reports, 95*, 771–779.

Weaver, K. E., Liabre, M. M., Duran, R. E., Antoni, M. H., Ironson, G., Penedo, F.J., et al. (2005). A stress and coping model of medication adherence and viral load in HIV-positive men and women on highly active antiretroviral therapy (HAART). *Health Psychology, 24*, 385–392.

Weiner, B., Perry, R. P., & Magnusson, J. (1988). An attributional analysis of reactions to stigmas. *Journal of Personality and Social Psychology, 55*, 738–748.

Wellons, M. F., Sanders, L., Edwards, L. J., Bartlett, J. A., Heald, A. E., & Schmader, K. E. (2002). HIV infection: Treatment outcomes in older and younger adults. *Journal of the American Geriatric Society, 50*, 603–607.

World Institute on Disability (1994). *Vocational rehabilitation and HIV/AIDS: A resource and training manual.* Oakland, CA: Author.

Zhang, L., Ramratnum, B., Tenner-Racz, K., He, Y., Besanen M., Leceun, S., et al. (1999). Quantifying residual HIV-1 transcription in peripheral blood mononuclear cells in patients receiving potent antiretroviral therapy. *New England Journal of Medicine, 340*, 1614–1622.

Zingmond, D. S., Kilbourne, A. M., Justice, A. C., Wenger, N. S., & Rodriguez-Barradas, M. (2003). Differences in symptom expression in older HIV-positive patients: The Veterans Aging Cohort & Site Study and HIV cost and service utilization study experience. *Journal of Acquired Immunodeficiency Syndrome, 33*(Suppl, 2), S84–S92.

Zingmond, D. S., Wenger, N. S., Crystal, S., Joyce, G.F., Liu, H., Sambamoorthi, U., et al. (2001). Circumstances at HIV diagnosis and progression of disease in older HIV-infected Americans. *American Journal of Public Health, 91*, 1117–1120.

Zisook, S., Peterkin, J., Goggin, K. J., Sledge, P., Atkinson, J. H., & Grant I. (1998). Treatment of major depression in HIV-seropositive men. HIV Neurobehavioral Research Center Group. *Journal of Clinical Psychiatry, 59*, 217–224.

8
Coping with Arthritis: From Vulnerability to Resilience

Bruce W. Smith and Jeanne Dalen

"Now that I've gone full circle, I can see the story from another side, flipped around. Isn't this finally the new view I've been looking for all along? To know a life as it is, and what it would miss ... without RA."

Mary Felstiner (2005, p. 202) – person with rheumatoid arthritis (RA)

Arthritis is a collection of chronic conditions that damage the health of the joints. The word arthritis is from the Greek "arthro" for joint and "itis" for inflammation. It has been estimated that as many as one-third of all Americans suffer from some form of arthritis (Arthritis Foundation, 2005a). Arthritis and related conditions cost the U.S. economy nearly $86 billion in medical costs and indirect expenses each year (Arthritis Foundation, 2005a). The most common problems caused by arthritis are pain in the affected joints and disability resulting from the inability to fully use these joints.

The story of learning to cope with arthritis is largely that of a journey from vulnerability to resilience. The pain and disability associated with arthritis bring increased vulnerability to personal, social, and vocational stress and increased psychological distress. Coping with arthritis may mean developing resilience in the face of these potential stressors and distress. Learning to cope may make the difference between surviving and actually thriving with arthritis.

This chapter will present an overview of what is known about the potential of coping for improving the lives of those with arthritis. It will begin by presenting a picture of the two major types of arthritis, the typical medical treatments, and the need for a biopsychosocial approach to treating arthritis. It will proceed by examining what research has taught us about coping with arthritis and the kinds of interventions that may enhance coping. It will conclude by presenting some implications of these findings and mapping out some promising new directions for enabling people with arthritis to move from vulnerability to resilience.

Major Types of Arthritis

While arthritis can be broadly defined as a condition that involves damage to the joints, there are over 100 different types of arthritis. Of these, the most common are osteoarthritis and rheumatoid arthritis. This chapter will focus on these two forms of arthritis for several reasons: because they are the most common forms of arthritis, provide an interesting contrast in terms of their etiology and effects, and have been the target of most studies seeking to understand coping.

Osteoarthritis (OA) is the most common type of arthritis and affects an estimated 21 million people in the U.S. (Arthritis Foundation, 2005b). OA primarily affects the cartilage, which is the slippery tissue that covers the ends of the bones in a joint. The primary joints affected include the knees, hips, hands, lower back, and neck. In OA, the top layer of the cartilage wears away and allows the bones under the cartilage to rub together. This results in stiffness, pain, and loss of movement in the joint. OA is often called a "wear and tear" disease. It usually begins after age 40 and progresses slowly. It may affect over 50% of people above age 70 (Arthritis Foundation, 2005b). While the causes of OA are not fully understood, risk factors for developing it include joint injury or overuse, aging, obesity, heredity, nerve injury, and lack of physical activity (Arthritis Foundation, 2005b).

The type of medical treatments that are prescribed for people with OA vary with the symptoms and focus on decreasing pain and/or increasing mobility (Arthritis Foundation, 2005b). The treatments can include more passive approaches such as medication, rest, and joint protection, or more active approaches such as exercise, physical therapy, and occupational therapy. Pain medications, such as acetaminophen and non-steroidal anti-inflammatory drugs (NSAIDS), help reduce joint pain, stiffness, and swelling. Joint protection can prevent stress or prevent strain on affected joints, while exercise can help by increasing range of motion and increasing muscle strength. Corticosteroids can be injected into joints that are not responsive to other treatments. Hip or knee replacement surgery is often a treatment of last resort for those with the most extensive joint damage.

Rheumatoid arthritis (RA) is the second most common form of arthritis and affects 2.1 million Americans (Arthritis Foundation, 2005c). While the cause of RA is not known, it is an autoimmune disorder in which joint damage results from the immune system attacking the joints. RA is characterized by inflammation of the lining of the joints, resulting in pain, swelling, stiffness, and loss of function in the joints. The inflammation most often affects joints in the hands and feet on both sides of the body. While OA affects a nearly equal proportion of men and women, RA is 2.5 times more common in women (Arthritis Foundation, 2005c). The onset of RA usually occurs in middle-age, but can occur in the 20s and 30s. Also, in contrast to OA, RA is a systemic disease that can affect bodily tissue other than joints, including the skin, blood vessels, heart, lungs, and muscles.

The goals of the medical treatment of RA are to reduce joint pain, swelling, and stiffness and to prevent joint damage (Arthritis Foundation, 2005c). As with

OA, this treatment can include a combination of passive and active approaches including rest, exercise, the use of heat and cold, and physical or occupational therapy. Like people with OA, people with RA often use NSAIDs, or in more severe cases, corticosteroids to reduce joint pain, swelling, and stiffness.

However, in contrast to OA, people with RA often are prescribed disease-modifying anti-rheumatic drugs (DMARDS). Biologic response modifiers (BRMS) are also used to reduce inflammation and joint damage by inhibiting cytokine production, a protein involved in regulating inflammation. Finally, either arthroscopic or joint-replacement surgery is sometimes performed on the most severely damaged joints.

Biopsychosocial Approach to Arthritis

Although the standard regimens for treating OA and RA have been rooted in a biomedical model of illness, the significance of coping may only fully be appreciated in the context of a biopsychosocial approach (Engel, 1977). The biomedical approach has emphasized the importance of understanding the underlying biology and physiology of arthritis. In addition, it has often assumed a direct causal relationship between these biological factors and the pain and disability experienced by those with OA, RA, and other forms of arthritis (Sokka, Kankainen, & Hannonen, 2000). Consequently, the biomedical approach has fostered the use of medical and surgical treatments that attempt to directly treat the underlying physiological pathology (Coulter, Entwistle, & Gilbert, 1998).

In contrast, a biopsychosocial model of arthritis recognizes the possibility that psychological and social factors are related to and may even influence arthritis pain and disability (Keefe et al., 2002). There are several reasons for including psychological and social factors. First, objective markers of disease activity of arthritis have not been able to fully account for the pain and disability that people with OA and RA report (Keefe et al., 1987; Sokka et al., 2000). Second, pain is a primary symptom of arthritis; theories of pain have shown how psychosocial factors may influence pain perception and reports (Melzack, 1999; Melzack & Wall, 1965). Third, research has increasingly shown that psychosocial factors are related to arthritis pain and disability, and may even influence disease activity (Schoenfeld-Smith et al., 1996; Zautra, Hamilton, Potter, & Smith, 1999).

The "gate-control theory" (Melzack & Wall, 1965) provides a biological explanation of how psychosocial factors may influence the experience of pain. The gate-control theory asserts that pain is not just a sensory experience influenced by tissue damage. Rather, pain is a multidimensional experience including sensory, affective, and evaluative components, which can be influenced by psychological processes occurring in the brain. The gate-control theory proposes that there are descending systems, through which the brain can increase or decrease the pain signals that originate in the periphery, by the brain's influence on a gating mechanism in the spinal cord. In support of this theory, behavioral and functional neuro-imaging experiments have shown that cognitive and affective factors may affect the report and experience of pain (Meagher, Arnau, & Rhudy, 2001; Petrovic & Ingvar, 2002). The implication for those with arthritis is that how they think and feel may directly influence the pain and associated disability that they experience.

There is also a large body of research suggesting a link between psychosocial factors and arthritis-related pain and disability. Aside from coping, factors that have been most consistently identified as important include: stress, depression, self-efficacy, helplessness, and social relationships. Stress and depression may both be a consequence of having arthritis and may themselves lead to exacerbations of disease activity (Smith & Zautra, 2002; Zautra & Smith, 2001; Zautra et al., 2004). Self-efficacy, helplessness, and social relationships have been related to pain and disability in people with arthritis and may also have important implications for coping (Lefebvre et al., 1999; Manne & Zautra, 1989; Schoenfeld-Smith et al., 1996). In addition, there is reason to suspect that less-examined factors, such as anxiety and positive affect, may also be important for those with arthritis (Newman & Mulligan, 2000; Zautra, Johnson, & Davis, 2005). While there has been an over-reliance on observational rather than experimental studies, the consistent associations found between these variables and important disease-related outcomes support the inclusion of psychosocial factors in a comprehensive model of arthritis.

Research on Coping with Arthritis

While many psychosocial factors are important for people with arthritis, coping may have a central place in a biopsychosocial model of arthritis. There is a substantial literature showing that various coping styles and strategies are related to important arthritis outcomes.

Coping Measures

Research examining coping with arthritis has focused on both broad coping styles and more specific strategies. The general styles examined have included the dichotomy of problem-focused vs. emotion-focused coping (Lazarus & Folkman, 1984) and of an active vs. passive (e.g., avoidant) coping (Brown & Nicassio, 1987). In addition, arthritis researchers have often used measures that examine a variety of specific coping strategies for coping with pain and other stressors.

The vast majority of studies examining coping in RA and OA have used questionnaires designed to assess strategies for coping with chronic pain. One of the most widely used scales has been the Coping Strategies Questionnaire (CSQ; Rosenstiel & Keefe, 1983). The strategies assessed have included diverting attention, reinterpreting pain sensations, coping self-statements, ignoring pain sensations, praying and hoping, increasing activity level, and catastrophizing. At the end of the questionnaire, there are two additional items where participants rate how much control they have over pain and how much they are able to decrease it. Factor analyses of the CSQ have resulted in a "coping attempts" factor, which consists of all subscales except catastrophizing, and a "pain-control and rational thinking" (PCRT) factor, which consists of two coping-efficacy items and catastrophizing that has been reverse-coded (Keefe et al., 1987; Parker et al., 1989).

Another frequently used questionnaire has been the Vanderbilt Multidimensional Pain Coping Inventory (VMPCI; Smith, Wallston, Dwyer, & Dowdy, 1997). The VMPCI consists of 11 subscales, including problem-solving, positive reappraisal, distraction, confrontative coping, distancing or denial, stoicism, use of religion, self-blame, self-isolation, wishful thinking, and disengagement.

Predictors of Coping

Several variables have been found to predict the choice of coping styles and strategies. Psychosocial factors that have been associated with the use of coping strategies in RA or OA include self-efficacy, optimism, and spousal relations. Lefebvre et al. (1999) found that self-efficacy was related to the daily use and effectiveness of pain-coping strategies in people with RA. Brenner, Melamed, and Panush (1994) found that optimism predicted increased problem-focused coping 16 months later in RA. Finally, Manne and Zautra (1989) found that spousal support predicted information seeking/cognitive restructuring coping and that spousal criticism predicted wishful thinking for women with RA.

Gender, socioeconomic status, and ethnicity have also predicted coping choice. Affleck et al. (1999) examined people with RA and OA and found that women used more emotion-focused coping than men, regardless of their disease and after controlling for level of pain. Similarly, France et al. (2004) found that women with OA were more likely than men to use emotion-focused strategies. Downe-Wamboldt and Melanson (1995) examined socioeconomic status in men and women with RA and found that higher socioeconomic status was related to a greater use of confrontative coping strategies. Among women with RA, Jordan, Lumley, and Leisen (1998) found that African-Americans used more diverting attention, praying, and hoping, while European–Americans used more ignoring of pain.

Coping Styles and Outcomes

There are a large number of studies that have examined the use of general coping strategies according to the problem vs. emotion-focused, and active vs. passive coping dichotomies. As with the literature regarding other kinds of stressors, problem-focused coping has generally been related to better outcomes in individuals with arthritis. Brenner et al. (1994) found that problem-focused coping was related to higher life-satisfaction in people with RA. In daily diary studies, Affleck, Urrows, Tennen, and Higgins (1992) and Keefe et al. (1997)

found that problem-focused strategies were related to improved, next-day pain and mood in people with RA.

In contrast to problem-solving, emotion-focused coping has generally been related to poorer outcomes. Lambert (1985) found that emotion-focused coping was related to poorer well-being in women with OA. France et al. (2004) found that emotion-focused coping was related to more arthritis pain and lower pain-tolerance for laboratory-induced pain.

Similar results have been obtained in examining the active vs. passive (e. g., avoidant) dichotomy of coping styles. Brown and Nicassio (1987) examined people with RA and found that active coping was related to less depression, pain, and functional impairment, while passive coping was related to more depression, pain, and functional impairment. Similarly, Hampson, Glasgow, and Zeiss (1996) found that active coping, when used by people with OA, was related to less depression, while passive coping was related to greater negative mood. Further, in a weekly diary study, Smith (2002) found that active coping was related to more positive affect (but unrelated to negative affect), while avoidant coping was related to more negative affect (but unrelated to positive affect) in women with RA or OA.

Coping Strategies and Outcomes

Several specific coping strategies appear to be generally related to better or worse outcomes. One of the most consistently useful coping approaches appears to be tapped by the pain control and rational thinking (PCRT) factor, which was derived from the CSQ (Rosenstiel & Keefe, 1983) and discussed previously in the coping measures section. Keefe et al. (1987) found that among people with OA of the knee, PCRT was related to lower pain and less physical and psychological disability, even when controlling for objective ratings of joint damage in X-rays. Parker et al. (1989) studied people with RA and found that the PCRT was related to improvements in pain, psychological status, and health status. Parker et al. (2005) also examined people with RA and found that the PCRT mediated the relationship between health status and depression for those who were moderately depressed.

As noted in the coping measures section, the PCRT consists of items representing the lack of catastrophizing and coping efficacy. The individual items assessing catastrophizing and those assessing coping efficacy have also been studied separately. Catastrophizing has been consistently related to worse outcomes. Keefe, Brown, Wallston, and Caldwell (1989) studied people with RA and found that catastrophizing was related to increased pain, functional disability, and depression six months later. Keefe et al. (2000) examined people with OA of the knee and found that catastrophizing was related to more pain and disability. France et al. (2004) examined people with OA and found that catastrophizing was related to greater arthritis pain and lower levels of pain threshold and pain tolerance. In contrast to catastrophizing, coping efficacy has been related to better outcomes. Keefe et al. (1997) had people with RA complete a daily diary. They found that daily coping efficacy was related to less same-day pain and negative mood and less next-day pain.

The other specific coping approaches that appear to affect arthritis-related outcomes include wishful thinking, the ability to find benefits in stressful situations, and the use of religion and spirituality. Manne and Zautra (1989) found that wishful thinking was related to poorer psychological adjustment in a path model, which included coping, social support, and adjustment. Parker et al. (1988) found that wishful thinking was related to more depression, daily stress, psychological distress, and helplessness in people with RA. Smith et al. (1997) found that wishful thinking was related to more pain concurrently, as well as to more negative affect 18 months later.

The developing literature on what has been called "posttraumatic growth" or "finding benefits" in stressful situations suggests that such perspectives may be useful ways of coping with stress (Tedeschi, Park, & Calhoun, 1998). Tennen, Affleck, Urrows, Higgins, and Mendola (1992) examined the effects of finding benefits among people with RA and found that it was related to better daily mood. Abraido-Lanza, Guier, and Colon (1998) examined finding benefits (which they called "thriving") in Latina women, 70% of whom had RA or OA. They found that the ability to find benefits was strongly related to more positive affect and less negative affect. Most recently, Danoff-Burg and Revenson (2005) found that finding interpersonal benefits predicted less disability 12 months later in women with RA.

The use of religion and spirituality in coping with arthritis has been studied, utilizing different measurement approaches. Smith et al. (1997) incorporated a "use of religion" subscale and found that it was concurrently related to more pain in people with RA. In this study, the use of religion may be related to more pain, because religion may be mobilized to help people cope with their pain. In studies where religious coping is positively related to undesirable outcomes (e.g., pain), it is important to consider the possibility that a third variable (e.g., the stress of having a chronic illness) may lead to increases in both religious coping and undesirable outcomes (Pargament, 1997). In these instances, controlling for the third variable and examining the prospective relationship between religious coping and undesirable outcomes may reveal a more accurate picture regarding the influence of religion on these outcomes.

Using a different approach, Keefe et al. (2001) examined the role of positive and negative religious/spiritual pain-coping and religious/spiritual coping-efficacy in a daily diary study in people with RA. Positive religious/spiritual pain-coping was related to a more positive mood, while negative religious/spiritual pain-coping was related to a less positive mood. In addition, the efficacy of religious/spiritual pain-coping was related to less pain and negative mood and more positive mood and social support.

Many of the other strategies included on the CSQ, VMPCI, and other coping inventories have only shown weak or inconsistent relationships with arthritis-related outcomes. For example, the "coping attempts" factor of the CSQ, which includes all of the subscales except catastrophizing and coping efficacy, has not consistently been related to outcomes (Keefe et al., 1987). Jordan et al. (1998) found that the relationship between praying/hoping and reinterpreting pain sensations and adjustment in people with RA varied by ethnicity. Similar inconsistencies have been found in examining the effects of attempts to distance or divert attention away from pain (Jordan et al., 1998; Smith et al., 1997).

Research on Interventions for Coping

There is a growing literature on the effects of psychosocial and self-management interventions in the lives of people with arthritis. These interventions are important for understanding coping, because they indirectly involve coping or incorporate ways of improving coping. Some target coping directly and try to determine whether it mediates changes.

Self-Management Interventions

Recent literature reviews of self-management and psychological interventions provide a broad context for understanding how interventions may impact coping. Newman, Steed, and Mulligan (2004) reviewed a large number of self-management interventions, including 24 studies with individuals with arthritis. Sixty-seven percent of the interventions for individuals with arthritis were conducted in a group setting. The interventions generally relied on cognitive-behavioral, social learning, or educational principles. Those that included cognitive-behavioral interventions were usually based on a stress and coping model and targeted coping skills. Approximately 40% of the interventions showed improvement on measures of self-reported symptoms and disability. Six of 10 studies, which measured psychological well-being, showed improvements; five of these studies used cognitive-behavioral techniques. Twelve studies assessed change in self-management behaviors, such as diet, exercise, and coping; 10 of the 12 demonstrated positive changes.

The self-management studies showed that exercise may be important for those with OA (e.g., Thomas et al., 2002) Astin, Beckner, Soeken, Hochberg, and Berman (2002) conducted a meta-analysis of 25 studies with RA patients, comparing psychological interventions to non-intervention controls (e.g., wait list, usual care, or attention placebo). The interventions included some psychological component beyond simply providing education (e.g., relaxation, biofeedback, or cognitive-behavioral therapy). Their findings regarding coping provide strong evidence that psychological interventions can impact coping in individuals with arthritis. They found significant pooled effect sizes for coping (0.46), as well as for pain (0.22), functional disability (0.27), depression (0.15), and self-efficacy (0.35). At follow-ups averaging 8.5 months, they found significant effects for coping (0.52), tender joints (0.33), and depression (0.30). All of the studies that found changes in coping used either behavioral or cognitive techniques.

Coping Skills Interventions

One of the most useful ways to understand the relationship between research that examines the most effective coping approaches and the interventions that may improve coping, is to examine the interventions that specifically target coping. Two prime examples are the "coping skills training," developed by Keefe and colleagues (Keefe et al., 1990a, 1990b), and the stress management program, developed by Parker and colleagues (Parker et al., 1995). Both of these programs have directly focused on bolstering the coping of individuals in the lives of patients with OA or RA.

Coping Skills Training (CST) is based on a cognitive-behavioral model of pain and involves teaching cognitive and behavioral skills for managing pain (Keefe et al., 1990a, 1990b; Keefe, Abernathy, & Campbell, 2005). It includes 10 group-sessions, in which patients learn three sets of coping skills, after being taught the gate-control theory of how psychological factors can influence pain. The first set of skills involves learning attention-diversion strategies for controlling pain, including progressive relaxation, guided imagery, and distraction techniques. The second set of skills involves learning to alter activity patterns, including activity-pacing, goal-setting, and pleasant activity-scheduling. The third set of skills involves learning to control pain by identifying negative and distorted thoughts and replacing them with more adaptive thoughts. CST also includes homework, involving the practice of specific skills and a maintenance plan.

The CST studies conducted by Keefe and colleagues have found that it has improved disease-related outcomes, coping, and provided evidence of coping as a mediator of the beneficial effects on disease-related outcomes. In one study, people with OA were randomized into CST, an arthritis-education control, or standard-care groups (Keefe et al., 1990a). Those receiving CST had lower levels of pain and psychological disability, relative to the control groups. In addition, the PCRT factor of the CSQ (Rosenstiel & Keefe, 1983) indicated that increases in the PCRT were related to reduced pain, pain behavior, and physical disability at six months (Keefe et al., 1990b). In more recent studies, CST has been combined with spouse-assisted CST (Keefe et al., 1999) and with exercise training (Keefe et al., 2004) and has shown beneficial effects.

Parker and colleagues have taken a somewhat different approach in the development of their stress-management program for people with arthritis (Parker et al., 1995). Rather than focusing primarily on coping with pain, they developed a protocol to help people with RA manage a full range of stressors that may be related to their disease. Their program is comprehensive in that it teaches skills for coping with emotions and interpersonal stressors, as well as pain. There are also components for identifying the stressors that people with RA experience and methods for identifying life goals.

In a test of the stress-management intervention, Parker et al. (1995) randomized people with RA to stress management, attention control, and standard-care control groups. The stress-management group improved on measures of coping, self-efficacy, helplessness, pain, and health status. A later study examined the data from the stress-management and standard-care groups, attempting to determine the mechanism for the positive changes in the stress-management group (Rhee et al., 2000). They found that decreased pain and depression were mediated by increases in coping strategies (e.g., confidence in the ability to manage pain) and self-efficacy, and by a decrease in helplessness.

Other researchers have tested similar interventions and arrived at comparable results. Leibing, Pfingsten, Bartmann, Rueger, and Schuessler (1999) randomized people with RA into a Cognitive Behavioral Therapy (CBT) intervention group that taught coping skills or a standard-care control group. They found that CBT reduced anxiety, depression, affective pain, and improved coping. Kraaimaat, Brons, Geenen, and Bijlsma (1995) randomized RA patients into a CBT group, an occupational therapy (OT) group, and a waiting-list control group. CBT resulted in changes in pain-coping behavior, and both CBT and OT resulted in increased knowledge of RA. Sinclair, Wallston, Dwyer, Blackburn, and Fuchs (1998) examined the effects of a nurse-led CBT group among women with RA. Although there was no control group, the interventions resulted in improved coping, psychological well-being, and reduced pain and fatigue; further, improved coping predicted the other outcomes (Sinclair & Wallston, 2001). Finally, van Lankveld, van Helmond, Naring, de Rooij, and van den Hoogen (2004) randomized people with RA to spouse-assisted CBT and non-spouse-assisted CBT groups. Both groups showed improvements in coping, disease activity, and physical and psychological functioning.

Emotional Disclosure

While the great majority of interventions targeting coping in arthritis have been based on cognitive and behavioral techniques, there is evidence that a very different kind of intervention may also improve coping and health-related outcomes for people with arthritis. Pennebaker (1997) developed an emotional-disclosure paradigm that has shown beneficial effects on a variety of outcomes. This paradigm involves having participants write about the most traumatic experience of their lives for 15–30 minutes for three to four days.

Two studies have used variations of this paradigm in people with RA. Kelley, Lumley, and Leisen (1997) randomly assigned patients with RA to either talk privately about stressful events or to talk about trivial events. They found that talking about stressful events was related to less affective disturbance and better physical functioning three months later. Similarly, Smyth, Stone, Hurewitz, and Kaell (1999) randomly assigned patients with RA to either write privately about their most stressful experience or to write about their plans for the day. Neither group received feedback concerning their writing assignments. They found that writing about traumatic stressors was related to improvements in health status and disease activity four months later.

Implications of Coping and Interventions

The research on coping and interventions has important clinical, social, vocational, and societal implications. While it is difficult to recommend specific coping strategies for all people in all situations, research suggests that a more active and problem-focused approach may generally be more helpful than one that involves passivity or avoidance in the face of arthritis-related stressors (Brown & Nicassio, 1987). Also, research indicates that reducing the tendency to catastrophize and increasing the sense that one can cope with the disease is important (Keefe et al., 1987). In addition, wishful thinking appears to be harmful, while finding benefits in the stresses of having arthritis may be helpful.

Further, the use of religion or spirituality may have differential effects on arthritis-related outcomes, depending on how these approaches are used. With regard to intervention research, it is still unclear just what specific components may be most helpful, because most intervention studies have included many different components that assess multiple outcomes. Thus, teaching a broad array of behavioral and cognitive strategies for coping with the stresses of arthritis may be most advisable at this point. This could include the kinds of skills that are the focus of Keefe's Cognitive Skills Training (CST) (Keefe et al., 2005), as well as broader skills for dealing with stressors other than pain (Parker et al., 1995).

The social implications of the arthritis-related research on coping and interventions are that the support or lack of support offered by significant others may be very important in shaping coping responses and their effectiveness. The work of Manne and Zautra (1989) demonstrated that spousal support or lack of support may directly impact coping choice, and that this may also have implications for psychological adjustment. Likewise, the work of Keefe et al. (1999) showed that including spouses in a coping-intervention group can improve arthritis-related outcomes. However, there is much research to be done, in order to understand the role that social relationships play in how individuals with arthritis cope with their disease. It is also very likely that the improvements in coping experienced by individuals with arthritis would have an impact on their social relationships. While much of this impact may be positive, family-systems theories would suggest that such changes could alter the system, in ways that could have both positive and negative consequences.

Finally, improved coping in people with arthritis may have benefits for the broader society. As stated above, it has been estimated that as many as one-third of all Americans may experience, during their lifetime, some form of arthritis, and that arthritis and related disorders may account for $86 billion in medical costs annually (Murphy, Cisternas, Yelin, Trupin, & Helmick, 2004). Health-care cost and utilization studies have already shown that interventions, which address coping in individuals with arthritis, can have a positive impact (Weinberger, Tierney, Cowper, Katz, & Booher, 1993; Young, Bradley, & Turner, 1995). An increase in productivity in such a large portion of society, and the accompanying decrease in medical expenses, could have a profound impact on the national and world economy. Reducing the problems experienced by people with arthritis could also have beneficial effects in decreasing the care-giving burden of significant others. Finally, those who successfully cope with arthritis could become an example of how to face adversity and still make a meaningful contribution to society.

Limitations and Future Directions

Despite these potential implications, there are several important limitations that need to be addressed before we can fully realize the potential of improved coping in people with arthritis. These involve the breadth of issues addressed in coping research, the use of interventions, and the theories that inform coping and interventions.

Although research has made progress in identifying what may generally be the more helpful and harmful coping styles and strategies for dealing with arthritis, there has been a lack of focus on other important issues in an arthritis stress and coping model. First, there should be a greater emphasis on what kinds of appraisals may be most useful in conjunction with specific types of coping strategies. Second, more research needs to be conducted on how various personal, social, and economic resources influence the ability to cope with arthritis and the choice of effective coping strategies. Third and most importantly, there needs to be more careful work on how to best match coping resources, appraisals, and particular strategies to specific kinds of people and stressors.

Next, there are several important issues that need to be addressed in the development of coping-based interventions. One issue is how to prevent relapse and maintain treatment gains (Keefe & Van Horn, 1993). Another issue, which has begun to be addressed, is comparing coping interventions with other standard forms of treatment for individuals with arthritis (Keefe et al., 2004; Kraaimaat et al., 1995). Another important issue involves testing different and potentially more cost-effective ways of delivering interventions. While group interventions for individuals with arthritis have been the norm, the telephone, the internet, and telemedicine may offer other effective, and perhaps more efficient ways to reach more people (Weinberger et al., 1993).

There is an even greater lack of understanding in the application of our evolving understanding of coping and coping interventions within the realm of work lives of those with arthritis. Potter, Smith, Strobel, and Zautra (2002) found that workplace stressors can impact both the psychological and the physical well-being of people with RA or OA. Blalock, deVellis, Holt, and Hahn (1993) found that people use many of the same cognitive and behavioral strategies in attempting to cope with problems at work, as they do with problems in leisure or other daily activities. Others have begun to examine how to prevent workplace disability in those with arthritis (Varekamp, Haafkens, Detaille, Tak, & van Dijk, 2005). However, there has been a lack of studies that have attempted to test coping-skills interventions that are tailored for the workplace. As with the social implications of coping, it is likely that improved coping will have a positive impact on vocational functioning. However, financial, vocational, and health-care incentives against becoming more healthy may also present obstacles to effective coping in the workplace.

Although there have been clear demonstrations that group cognitive-behavioral interventions can help individuals with arthritis under ideal circumstances, more research is needed to test and disseminate these interventions in real-world settings. Lorig's work regarding the development and testing of lay-led, self-management interventions for individuals with arthritis has been a step in the right direction (Lorig, Ritter, & Plant, 2005). These types of programs could better integrate the research regarding coping and more directly address the most effective coping strategies. In a similar vein, it is essential in today's managed-care environment to demonstrate the cost-effectiveness of interventions and to advocate for integrating them into a more comprehensive and biopsychosocial approach to arthritis (Young et al., 1995).

Finally, while past research has been unified around a cognitive-behavioral approach, there is a pressing need to refine the theoretical understanding of the mechanisms of action for coping and to consider a broader array of theories about how to enhance coping. With regard to effective mechanisms, the aspects of coping that have received the strongest support have been active, problem-focused approaches (Brenner et al., 1994; Brown & Nicassio, 1987), and specifically the pain control and rational thinking (PCRT) factor of the CSQ (Keefe et al., 1987; Parker et al., 1989). However, the active and problem-focused measures have been composites of a variety of coping strategies, while the PCRT may be more a measure of appraisal or coping efficacy than of specific strategies. A question that needs scientific exploration is: How much is effective coping the result of using a particular strategy, versus a belief about a stressor or one's ability to cope with it? Theoretical clarity on this issue is critical for knowing what to best target in interventions. Careful experimental and observational studies need to be done to better distinguish appraisals, coping efficacy, and specific coping strategies and their effects on arthritis-related outcomes.

One important limitation regarding theories on coping with arthritis is the focus on changing rather than accepting the pain. McCracken (1998) has done pioneering work regarding acceptance with regard to chronic pain. His understanding of acceptance is rooted in the Relational Frame Theory (RFT; Hayes, Barnes-Holmes, & Roche, 2001). He has developed a measure of pain acceptance and found it was related to less pain, disability, and depression in chronic pain patients after controlling for traditional coping measures (McCracken & Eccleston, 2003). Moreover, a recent intervention based on an acceptance-based approach (Acceptance and Commitment Therapy; Hayes, Jacobson, Follette, & Dougher, 1994) found significant pre-post improvements in pain, disability, and depression in chronic pain patients (McCracken, Vowles, & Eccleston, 2005). Mindfulness-Based Stress Reduction (Kabat-Zinn, 1990) is another acceptance-based approach that has shown promise in helping chronic pain patients (Goldenberg et al., 1994).

Finally, perhaps the greatest theoretical limitation of stress and coping models and cognitive-behavioral constructs has been the focus on reducing vulnerability to the negative effects of immediate stressors, rather than improving well-being and building resources for increasing resilience (Zautra et al., 2005). There is a strong need to incorporate recent research and theory regarding the value of positive emotions into the literature on coping with arthritis. Fredrickson (1998) has developed a "broaden-and-build" model of positive emotions, based on evidence that positive emotions can expand and build resources for resilience in coping with stress. Zautra et al. (2005) has developed a "dynamic model of affect," based on evidence that the presence of positive emotions may be critical for preserving well-being in times of stress. Zautra and colleagues have conducted studies showing that positive affect and psychological well-being can be resources for resilience in coping in people with RA or OA (Smith & Zautra, 2004; Zautra, Smith, Affleck, & Tennen, 2001a).

Summary and Conclusion

Arthritis is a collection of diseases that can severely damage joints, can cause great suffering in those who have it, and can have a profound negative impact on the broader society, including the financial liability placed on the health-care system, the burden placed on caregivers, and productivity lost in the workplace. Research on coping with arthritis and interventions that may enhance coping offer a beacon of hope to people with arthritis, in addition to society as a whole. Basic coping research has revealed that taking an active approach, believing in one's ability to cope, and possibly even finding benefits in the stresses of arthritis may be fruitful for people with arthritis.

Further, intervention research has shown that it is possible to enhance the coping of people with arthritis and that enhanced coping does seem to make a difference. Even with these hopeful beginnings, there are many questions that remain, much research yet to be done, and other forms of coping that may be helpful and thus, need to be explored. Learning to accept the inevitable pains and stressors of arthritis may complement the ability to actively cope and problem-solve when change is possible. Positive emotions and psychological well-being may build coping resources and provide meaning and joy, in the midst of the pain and stress of having arthritis. Continuing to investigate the role of coping in arthritis can help those who suffer from it to find a clearer and surer path on their journey from vulnerability to resilience.

References

Abraido-Lanza, A. F., Guier, C., & Colon, R. M. (1998). Psychological thriving among Latinas with chronic illness. *Journal of Social Issues, 54*(2), 405–424.

Affleck, G., Tennen, H., Keefe, F. J., Lefebvre, J. C., Kashikar-Zuck, S., Wright, K., et al. (1999). Every day life with osteoarthritis or rheumatoid arthritis: Independent effects of disease and gender on daily pain, mood, and coping. *Pain, 83*, 601–609.

Affleck, G., Urrows, S., Tennen, H., & Higgins, P. (1992). Daily coping with pain from rheumatoid arthritis: Patterns and correlates. *Pain, 51*, 221–229.

Arthritis Foundation. (2005a). *Arthritis prevalence: A nation in pain.* p. 1. Retrieved December 21, 2005, from www.Arthritis.org/conditions/Fact_Sheets/Arthritis_Prev_Fact_Sheet.asp

Arthritis Foundation. (2005b). *Osteoarthritis fact sheet: Impact of Osteoarthritis.* p. 1. Retrieved December 21, 2005, from www.Arthritis.org/ conditions/Fact_Sheets/OA_Fact_Sheet.asp

Arthritis Foundation. (2005c). *Rheumatoid arthritis fact sheet: Impact of Rheumatoid arthritis.* p. 1. Retrieved December 21, 2005, from www.Arthritis.org/conditions/Fact_Sheets/RA_Fact_Sheet.asp

Astin, J. A., Beckner, W., Soeken, K., Hochberg, M. C., & Berman, B. (2002). Psychological interventions for rheumatoid arthritis: A meta-analysis of randomized controlled trials. *Arthritis and Rheumatism, 47*(3), 291–302.

Blalock, S. J., deVellis, B. M., Holt, K., & Hahn, P. M. (1993). Coping with rheumatoid arthritis: is one problem the same as another? *Health Education Quarterly, 20*(1), 119–132.

Brenner, G. F., Melamed, B. G., & Panush, R. S. (1994). Optimism and coping as determinants of psychosocial adjustment to rheumatoid arthritis. *Journal of Clinical Psychology in Medical Settings, 1*(2), 115–134.

Brown, G. K., & Nicassio, P.M. (1987). Development of a questionnaire for the assessment of active and passive coping strategies in chronic pain patients. *Pain, 31*, 53–64.

Coulter, A., Entwistle, V., & Gilbert, D. (1998). *Informing patients: An assessment of the quality of patient information materials.* London: Kings Fund.

Danoff-Burg, S., & Revenson, T. A. (2005). Benefit-finding among patients with rheumatoid arthritis: Positive effects on interpersonal relationships. *Journal of Behavioral Medicine, 28*(1), 91–103.

Downe-Wamboldt, B. L., & Melanson, P. M. (1995). Emotions, coping, and psychological well-being in elderly people with arthritis. *Western Journal of Nursing Research, 17*(3), 250–265.

Engel, G. L. (1977). The need for a new medical model: A challenge for biomedicine. *Science, 196*, 129–136.

Felstiner, M. (2005). *Out of joint: A private & public story of arthritis.* Lincoln, NE: University of Nebraska Press.

France, C. R., Keefe, F. J., Emery, C. F., Affleck, G., France, J. L., Waters, S., et al. (2004). Laboratory pain perception and clinical pain in post-menopausal women and age-matched men with osteoarthritis: Relationship to pain coping and hormonal status. *Pain, 112*, 274–281.

Fredrickson, B. L. (1998). What good are positive emotions? *Review of General Psychology, 2*(3), 300–319.

Goldenberg, D. L., Kaplan, K. H., Nadeau, M. G., Brodeur, C., Smith, S., & Schmid, C. H. (1994). A controlled study of a stress-reduction, cognitive-behavioral treatment program in fibromyalgia. *Journal of Muscuoloskeletal Pain, 2*(2), 53–66.

Hampson, S. E., Glasgow, R. E., & Zeiss, A. M. (1996). Coping with osteoarthritis by older adults. *Arthritis Care and Research, 9*(2), 133–141.

Hayes, S. C., Barnes-Holmes, D., & Roche, B. (2001). *Relational frame theory: A post-Skinnerian account of human language and cognition.* New York: Kluwer/Plenum.

Hayes, S. C., Jacobson, N. S., Follette, V. M., & Dougher, M. J. (1994). *Acceptance and change: Content and context in psychotherapy.* Reno, NV: Context Press.

Jordan, M. S., Lumley, M. A., & Leisen, J. C. (1998). The relationships of cognitive coping and pain control beliefs to pain and adjustment among African-American and Caucasian women with rheumatoid arthritis. *Arthritis Care and Research, 11*, 80–88.

Kabat-Zinn, J. (1990). *Full catastrophe living: Using the wisdom of your body and mind to face stress, pain, and illness.* New York: Delacorte.

Keefe, F. J., Abernathy, A. P., & Campbell, L. C. (2005). Psychological approaches to understanding and treating disease-related pain. *Annual Review of Psychology, 56*, 601–630.

Keefe, F. J., Affleck, G., Lefebvre, J. C., Starr, K., Caldwell, D. S., & Tennen, H. (1997). Pain coping strategies and coping efficacy in rheumatoid arthritis: A daily process analysis. *Pain, 69*, 35–42.

Keefe, F. J., Affleck, G., Lefebvre, J. C., Underwood, L., Caldwell, D. S., Drew, J., et al. (2001). Living with rheumatoid arthritis: The role of daily spirituality and daily religious and spiritual coping. *The Journal of Pain, 2*(2), 101–110.

Keefe, F. J., Blumenthal, J. A., Baucom, D., Affleck, G., Waugh, R., Caldwell, D. S., et al. (2004). Effects of spouse-assisted coping skills training and exercise training in patients with osteoarthritic knee pain: A randomized controlled study. *Pain, 110*, 539–549.

Keefe, F. J., Brown, G. K., Wallston, K. A., & Caldwell, D. S. (1989). Coping with rheumatoid arthritis pain: Catastrophizing as a maladaptive strategy. *Pain, 37*, 51–56.

Keefe, F. J., Caldwell, D. S., Baucom, D., Salley, A., Robinson, E., Timmons, K., et al. (1999). Spouse-assisted coping skills training in the management of knee pain in osteoarthritis: Long-term follow-up results. *Arthritis Care and Research, 12*(2), 101–111.

Keefe, F. J., Caldwell, D. S., Queen, K. T., Gil, K. M., Martinez, S., Crisson, J. E., et al. (1987). Pain coping strategies in osteoarthritis patients. *Journal of Consulting and Clinical Psychology, 55*(2), 208–212.

Keefe, F. J., Caldwell, D. S., Williams, D. A., Gil, K. M., Mitchell, D., Robertson, C., et al. (1990a). Pain coping skills training in the management of osteoarthritis knee pain: A comparative study. *Behavioral Therapy, 21*, 49–62.

Keefe, F. J., Caldwell, D. S., Williams, D. A., Gil, K. M., Mitchell, D., Robertson, C., et al. (1990b). Pain coping skills training in management of osteoarthritis knee pain: II. Follow-up results. *Behavioral Therapy, 21*(4), 435–447.

Keefe, F. J., Lefebvre, J. C., Egert, J., Affleck, G., Sullivan, M. J., & Caldwell, D. S. (2000). The relationship of gender to pain, pain behavior, and disability in osteoarthritis patients: The role of catastrophizing. *Pain, 87*, 325–334.

Keefe, F. J., Smith, S. J., Buffington, A. L., Gibson, J., Studts, J. L., & Caldwell, D. S. (2002). Recent advances and future directions in the biopsychosocial assessment and treatment of arthritis. *Journal of Consulting and Clinical Psychology, 70*(3), 640–655.

Keefe, F. J., & Van Horn, Y. (1993). Cognitive-behavioral treatment of rheumatoid arthritis pain: Maintaining treatment gains. *Arthritis Care and Research, 6*(4), 213–222.

Kelley, J. E., Lumley, M. A., & Leisen, J. C. (1997). Health effects of emotional disclosure in rheumatoid arthritis patients. *Health Psychologist, 16*(4), 331–340.

Kraaimaat, F. W., Brons, M. R., Geenen, R., & Bijlsma, J. W. (1995). The effect of cognitive behavioral therapy in patients with rheumatoid arthritis. *Behavioral Research and Therapy, 33*(5), 487–495.

Lambert, V. A. (1985). Study of factors associated with psychological well-being in rheumatoid arthritic women. *Journal of Nursing Scholarship, 17*(2), 50–53.

Lazarus, R. S., & Folkman, S. (1984). *Stress, appraisal, and coping.* New York: Springer Publishing Company.

Lefebvre, J. C., Keefe, F. J., Affleck, G., Raezer, L. B., Starr, K, Caldwell, D. S., et al. (1999). The relationship of arthritis self-efficacy to daily pain, daily mood, and daily pain coping in rheumatoid arthritis patients. *Pain, 80,* 425–435.

Leibing, E., Pfingsten, M., Bartmann, U., Rueger, U., & Schuessler, G. (1999). Cognitive-behavioral treatment in unselected rheumatoid arthritis outpatients. *Clinical Journal of Pain, 15*(1), 58–66.

Lorig, K., Ritter, P. L., & Plant, K. (2005). A disease-specific self-help program compared with a generalized chronic disease self-help program for arthritis patients. *Arthritis and Rheumatism, 53*(6), 950–957.

Manne, S. L, & Zautra, A. J. (1989). Spouse criticism and support: Their association with coping and psychological adjustment among women with rheumatoid arthritis. *Journal of Personality and Social Psychology, 56*(4), 608–617.

McCracken, L. M. (1998). Learning to live with the pain: Acceptance of pain predicts adjustment in persons with chronic pain. *Pain, 74,* 21–27.

McCracken, L. M., & Eccleston, C. (2003). Coping or acceptance: What to do about chronic pain? *Pain, 105,* 197–204.

McCracken, L. M., Vowles, K. E., & Eccleston, C. (2005). Acceptance-based treatment for persons with complex, long standing chronic pain: A preliminary analysis of treatment outcome in comparison to a waiting phase. *Behavior Research and Therapy, 43,* 1335–1346.

Meagher, M. W., Arnau, R. C., & Rhudy, J. L. (2001). Pain and emotion: Effects of affective picture modulation. *Psychosomatic Medicine, 63,* 79–90.

Melzack, R. (1999). From the gate to the neuromatrix. *Pain* (Suppl. 6), S121–S126.

Melzack, R., & Wall, P. D. (1965). Pain mechanism: A new theory. *Science, 150,* 971–979.

Murphy, L., Cisternas, M., Yelin, E., Trupin, L., & Helmick C. (2004). Update: Direct and indirect costs of arthritis and other rheumatic conditions-United States, 1997. *Morbidity & Mortality Weekly Report, 53*(18), 388–389.

Newman, S., & Mulligan, K. (2000). The psychology of rheumatic diseases. *Bailliere's Clinical Rheumatology, 14*(4), 773–786.

Newman, S., Steed, L., & Mulligan, K. (2004). Self-management interventions for chronic illness. *The Lancet, 364,* 1523–1537.

Pargament, K. I. (1997). *The psychology of religion and coping: Theory, research, and practice.* New York: The Guilford Press.

Parker, J. C., McRae, C., Smarr, K. L., Beck, N., Frank, R., Anderson, S., et al. (1988). Coping strategies in rheumatoid arthritis. *Journal of Rheumatology, 15,* 1376–1383.

Parker, J. C., Smarr, K. L., Buckelew, S. P., Stucky-Ropp, R. C., Hewett, J. E., Johnson, J. C., et al. (1995). Effects of stress-management on clinical outcomes in rheumatoid arthritis. *Arthritis and Rheumatism, 38*(12), 1807–1818.

Parker, J. C., Smarr, K. L., Buescher, K. L., Phillips, L. R., Frank, R. G., Beck, N. C., et al. (1989). Pain control and rational thinking: Implications for rheumatoid arthritis. *Arthritis and Rheumatism, 32*(8), 984–990.

Parker, J. C., Smarr, K. L., Hewett, J. E., Ge, B., Hanson, K. D., Slaughter, J. R., et al. (2005). Health status, cognitive coping, and depressive symptoms: Testing for a mediator effect. *Journal of Rheumatology, 32*(8), 1584–1588.

Pennebaker, J. W. (1997). *Opening up: The healing power of expressing emotions.* New York: The Guilford Press.

Petrovic, P., & Ingvar, M. (2002). Imaging cognitive modulation of pain processing. *Pain, 95,* 1–5.

Potter, P. T., Smith, B. W., Strobel, K. R., & Zautra, A. J. (2002). Interpersonal workplace stressors and well-being: A multi-wave study of employees with and without arthritis. *Journal of Applied Psychology, 87*(4), 789–796.

Rhee, S. H., Parker, J. C., Smarr, K. L., Petroski, G. F., Johnson, J. C., Hewett, J. E., et al. (2000). Stress management in rheumatoid arthritis: What is the underlying mechanism? *Arthritis Care and Research, 13*(6), 435–442.

Rosenstiel, A. K., & Keefe, F. J. (1983). The use of coping strategies in chronic low back pain patients: Relationship to patient characteristics and current adjustment. *Pain, 17,* 33–44.

Schoenfeld-Smith, K., Petroski, G. F., Hewett, J. E., Johnson, J. C., Wright, G. E., Smarr, K. L., et al. (1996). A biopsychosocial model of disability in rheumatoid arthritis. *Arthritis Care and Research, 9*(5), 368–375.

Sinclair, V. G., & Wallston, K. A. (2001). Predictors of improvement in a cognitive-behavioral intervention with rheumatoid arthritis. *Annals of Behavioral Medicine, 23*(4), 291–297.

Sinclair, V. G., Wallston, K. A., Dwyer, K. A., Blackburn, D. S., & Fuchs, H. (1998). Effects of a cognitive-behavioral intervention for women with rheumatoid arthritis. *Research in Nursing and Health, 21,* 315–326.

Smith, B. W. (2002). *Vulnerability and resilience as predictors of pain and affect in women with arthritis.* Unpublished doctoral dissertation, Arizona State University, Tempe, AZ.

Smith, B. W., & Zautra, A. J. (2002). The role of personality in exposure and reactivity to interpersonal stress in relation to arthritis disease activity and negative affect in women. *Health Psychology, 21,* 81–88.

Smith, B. W., & Zautra, A. J. (2004). The role of purpose in life in knee surgery. *International Journal of Behavioral Medicine, 11*(4), 197–202.

Smith, C. A., Wallston, K. A., Dwyer, K. A., & Dowdy, S. W. (1997). Beyond good and bad coping: A multidimensional examination of coping with pain in persons with rheumatoid arthritis. *Annals of Behavioral Medicine, 19*(1), 11–21.

Smyth, J. M., Stone, A. A., Hurewitz, A., & Kaell, A. (1999). Effects of writing about stressful experiences on symptom reduction in patients with asthma or rheumatoid arthritis: A randomized trial. *Journal of the American Medical Association, 281*(14), 1304–1309.

Sokka, T., Kankainen, A., & Hannonen, P. (2000). Scores for functional disability in patients with rheumatoid arthritis are correlated at higher levels with pain scores than with radiographic scores. *Arthritis and Rheumatism, 43*(2), 386–389.

Tedeschi, R. G., Park, C. L., & Calhoun, L. G. (1998). *Posttraumatic growth: Positive changes in the aftermath of crisis.* Mahwah, NJ: Lawrence Erlbaum Associates.

Tennen, H., Affleck, G., Urrows, S., Higgins, P., & Mendola, R. (1992). Perceiving control, construing benefits, and daily processes in rheumatoid arthritis. *Canadian Journal of Behavioural Science, 24*(2), 186–203.

Thomas, K. S., Muir, K. R., Doherty, M., Jones, A. C., O'Reilly, S. C., & Bassey, E. J. (2002). Home based exercise programme for knee pain and knee osteoarthritis: Randomized controlled trial. *British Medical Journal, 325,* 752.

Van Lankveld, W., van Helmond, T., Naring, G., de Rooij, D. J., & van den Hoogen, F. (2004). Partner participation in cognitive-behavioral self-management group treatment for patients with rheumatoid arthritis. *Journal of Rheumatology, 31*(9), 1738–1745.

Varekamp, I., Haafkens, J. A., Detaille, S. I., Tak, P. P., & van Dijk, F. J. (2005). Preventing work disability among employees with rheumatoid arthritis: What medical professionals can learn from the patients' perspective. *Arthritis and Rheumatism, 53*(6), 965–972.

Weinberger, M., Tierney, W. M., Cowper, P. A., Katz, B. P., & Booher, P. A. (1993). Cost-effectiveness of increased telephone contact for patients with osteoarthritis: A randomized, controlled trial. *Arthritis and Rheumatism, 36*(2), 243–246.

Young, L. D., Bradley, L. A., & Turner, R. A. (1995). Decreases in health care resource utilization in patients with rheumatoid arthritis following a cognitive-behavioral intervention. *Biofeedback and Self-Regulation, 20* (3), 259–268.

Zautra, A. J., Hamilton, N. A., Potter, P., & Smith, B. W. (1999). Field research on the relationships between stress and disease activity in rheumatoid arthritis: Key measurement and design components. *Annals of the New York Academy of Sciences, 876*, 397–412.

Zautra, A. J., Johnson, L., & Davis, M. E. (2005). The role of positive affect in chronic pain: Applications of a dynamic affect model. *Journal of Consulting and Clinical Psychology, 73*(2), 212–220.

Zautra, A. J. & Smith, B. W. (2001). Depression and reactivity to stress in older women with rheumatoid arthritis and osteoarthritis. *Psychosomatic Medicine, 63*, 687–696.

Zautra, A., Smith, B., Affleck, G., & Tennen, H. (2001).Examinations of chronic pain and affect relationships: Applications of a dynamic model of affect. *Journal of Consulting and Clinical Psychology, 69*(5), 786–795.

Zautra, A. J., Yocum, D. C., Villanueva, I., Smith, B. W., Davis, M. C., Attrep, J., et al. (2004). Immune activation and depression in women with rheumatoid arthritis. *Journal of Rheumatology, 31*(13), 457–463.

9
Coping with Burn Injury: Research Summary and a New Model of the Influence of Coping on Psychological Complications

James A. Fauerbach, Melissa G. Bresnick and Michael T. Smith

Physical Complications Associated with Burn Injury

Despite substantial improvements made over the last two to three decades in acute care (Munster, Meek, & Sharkey, 1994), burn injuries often involve long recovery periods and result in poor functional outcomes for many individuals (Esselman, Thombs, Magyar-Russell, & Fauerbach, 2006). There is a well-established relationship between injury severity (e.g., inhalation injury; total body surface area, TBSA) and morbidity and mortality (Renz & Sherman, 1992). Many long-term physical complications can develop secondary to a major burn injury including: Hypertrophic or keloidal scarring (Bombaro et al., 2003), limitations in range of motion across scarred joints, and impaired skin integrity and sensation (Costa et al., 2003), and damaged or amputated body parts (Herndon, 2002).

According to disability determination evaluations following the conclusion of optimal medical, surgical, and reconstructive treatment, functional impairment resulting from a major burn injury has been estimated at between 17% and 19% (Costa et al., 2003). This is likely an underestimation, as pre-burn conditions were purposely excluded from consideration, thus overlooking some common burn-related impairments (e.g., further declines in already-compromised psychological health and function). Unfortunately, a recent systematic review found that, for most psychosocial and physical rehabilitation interventions following burn injury, the evidence base is quite limited, and recommended that the field conduct more rigorous investigations, preferably using randomized controlled trials, in order to assess treatment efficacy (Esselman et al., 2006).

Major burn injuries generate vigorous responses from the adreno-cortical stress system, and other regulatory systems promote healing, infection control and thermo-regulation. The energy required to sustain these activities results in a

173

hypermetabolic response (Graves, Cioffi, McManus, Mason, & Pruitt, 1988), leading to a catabolic breakdown of body protein (muscle), and, consequently, severe deconditioning and muscle atrophy. In severe inhalation injury (Herndon, 2002), hypoxia and carbon monoxide poisoning can lead to further tissue loss and central nervous-system damage.

Deep partial thickness (involving entire epidermal layer) and full thickness (involving underlying dermis) burns damage the layer of skin, containing the nerves that provide somatosensory feedback to the brain (Herndon, 2002). Severe pain, both at rest and during procedures, is ubiquitous following acute burn injury and it is routinely managed aggressively with a variety of analgesics. Because burn injuries can involve substantial nerve damage or loss, burn clients are at elevated risk for developing chronic and disabling neuropathic pain and contracture-related pain. Physical pain and alterations in sensory experiences, mediated by the skin and related structures (e.g., pruritis, increased or diminished sensitivity, heat or cold intolerance), are some of the most pervasive problems in the first year following burn injury. Sensory problems become chronic in up to 80% of individuals surviving major burns (Malenfant et al., 1998). Chronic, disabling pain has an estimated prevalence of between 35% and 52% (Choiniere, Melzack, & Paillon, 1991; Choiniere, Melzack, Rondeau, Girard, & Paquin, 1989; Malenfant et al., 1996).

Sleep disturbance is a symptom related to many psychosomatic states, such as hypermetabolism, depression, posttraumatic stress, and pain. During the acute hospitalization phase, multiple factors interfere with sleep, including metabolic and circadian dysregulation (Rose, Sanford, Thomas, and Opp, 2001), pain (Raymond, Nielsen, Lavigne, Manzini, & Choiniere, 2001), and environmental factors that are associated with the acute care environment (noises, medical interventions, etc.) (Helton, Gordon, & Nunnery, 1980). Acute insomnia and intrusive nightmares affect between 50% and 73% of individuals hospitalized with a burn injury (Boeve et al., 2002; Lawrence, Fauerbach, Eudell, Ware, & Munster, 1998a). Individuals, who suffer serious burn injury, report chronic sleep disturbance for up to 11 years (Boeve et al., 2002; Kravitz et al., 1993; Lawrence et al., 1998a; Low et al., 2003; Raymond, Ancoli-Israel, & Choiniere, 2004; Rose et al., 2001).

Polysomnographic study has found that, relative to age-matched controls, hospitalized burn victims demonstrated significant reductions in slow wave sleep and rapid eye movement (REM) sleep, increased sleep fragmentation, and an increased percentage of the lighter stages of non-REM sleep (Gottschlich et al., 1994). These findings may have particular implications for wound-healing (Gumustekin et al., 2004) and the hypercatabolic process associated with severe burn injury, because the majority of endogenous growth-hormone secretion occurs during slow wave sleep. Growth hormone modulates the hypermetabolic effects of burn injury by inducing protein synthesis (Herndon & Tompkins, 2004; Obal & Krueger, 2004).

Burn scars develop as a result of the formation of new connective tissue, as well as from an uneven deposition of collagen in the new cells. These and other physical-healing processes produce burn scars that contract the surrounding skin in random patterns. Additionally, hypertrophic scarring, a raised, rigid scar with altered pigmentation that leads to the development of contractures and functional impairment, develops in approximately 67% of individuals hospitalized with major burns (Bombaro et al., 2003).

Following wound closure, scar maturation is prolonged, with its greatest activity at one to three months and often continuing to at least 12–13 months (Schwanholt et al., 1994). Optimizing scar appearance and functional outcomes requires intense rehabilitation procedures that are often aversive, yet unavoidable (e.g., range of motion exercises, compression garments). The challenging rehabilitation period further complicates adaptation to altered capabilities. Furthermore, although location of the scar (e.g., hands, face) can have a greater impact on psychological and social outcomes than total body surface area, both have less of an impact than that of psychological distress (e.g., depression) (Lawrence, Fauerbach, Heinberg, & Doctor, 2004).

Psychological Aspects Associated with Burn Injury

Each of the physical complications described above represents a major life stressor requiring adaptive coping, in order to facilitate assimilation of new information into existing cognitive schema, or accommodation of those schema to new perspectives about the self, others, or the world. The challenges brought on by these processes can generate considerable psychological distress in various forms and severities depending on the source, degree of threat, and potential impact.

Accumulating evidence suggests that, following major burn injury, psychological distress is among the most disabling of secondary complications (Blakeney, Fauerbach, Meyer, & Thomas, 2002; Van Loey, Maas, Faber, and Taal, 2003). Distress can be manifested in a number of specific symptoms or syndromes, including sleep disturbance (Lawrence et al., 1998a), depression (Fauerbach et al., 1997; Ptacek, Patterson, Heimbach, 2002; Wiechman et al., 2001), body-image dissatisfaction (Lawrence et al., 1998b; Thombs, Notes, Magyar-Russell, Lawrence, & Fauerbach, 2006) and posttraumatic distress (Difede et al., 2002; Ehde, Patterson, Wiechman, & Wilson, 1999; Ehde, Patterson, Wiechman, & Wilson, 2000; Fauerbach et al., 1997).

Symptoms of depression may occur when the stressor involves loss, bereavement, diminished self-efficacy, or lowered self-esteem. For example, physical threats stemming from unavoidable, painful dressing-changes and rehabilitation procedures, as well as the social threats from altered appearance and function, can result in depression and anxiety. Clinically significant symptoms of depression were reported in 22.6% of individuals with burns at two years post-burn (Wiechman et al., 2001). Additionally, the changes in appearance caused by the wound and scarring can lead to body image dissatisfaction (BID) and social avoidance, due to expectations of stigmatizing reactions from others (Fauerbach et al., 2000; Lawrence, Fauerbach, Heinberg, & Doctor, 2006).

Posttraumatic stress symptoms occur when the stressor is perceived as life-threatening and induces severe helplessness or horror. Both acute stress disorder (ASD) at one month (19%) and posttraumatic stress disorder (PTSD) at six months (36%) are quite common among adults with recent burns (Difede et al., 2002; Fauerbach et al., 1997; Powers, Cruse, Daniels, & Stevens, 1994) and children (Armstrong, Gay, & Levy, 1994; Saxe et al., 1994; Stoddard, Norman, Murphy, & Beardslee, 1989; Tarnowski, Rasnake, Gavaghan-Jones, & Smith, 1991). PTSD symptoms have a marked detrimental impact on health and function (Fauerbach, Lawrence, Munster, Palombo, & Richter, 1999).

Finally, psychological distress can be manifested as heterogeneous symptoms that do not conform to any diagnostic category, but are nonetheless enduring and disabling (Fauerbach et al., 2005; Fauerbach et al., 2006). Of note, there is a 33% prevalence of clinically significant symptoms of psychological distress from hospital discharge through at least two years post-burn, with few cases resolving over time (Fauerbach et al., 2006). This contrasts sharply with the 10% incidence of clinically significant psychological distress in an adult, non-medically ill normative sample (Derogatis & Melisaratos, 1983).

Although adjustment can be difficult even among those who functioned well prior to injury (Roca, Spence, & Munster, 1992; Stoddard et al., 1989), symptoms of psychological distress (Fauerbach et al., 2005), posttraumatic distress (Fauerbach et al., 1999), depression (Fauerbach et al., 2002b), body image dissatisfaction (Lawrence et al., 1998b), and both social discomfort and social stigmatization (Lawrence et al., 1998a; Lawrence et al., in press; Thombs et al., 2006), all have a negative and prolonged impact on physical, psychological, and social health and function (Fauerbach, Lawrence, Schmidt, Munster, & Costa, 2000; Lawrence et al., 1998a, 1998b). The effect of pre-injury psychological functioning on outcomes may, at least in part, be mediated by cognitive (Achterberg-Lawliss, 1995; Willebrand et al., 2004), behavioral (Kiecolt-Glaser & Williams, 1987), social (Beard, Herndon, & Desai, 1989; Blakeney, Portman, & Rutan, 1990; Orr, Reznikoff, & Smith, 1989), and developmental factors (Armstrong et al., 1994; Tarnowski et al., 1991), each of which can impair cognitive processing and self-regulation.

Coping with Burns: Predicting and Controlling Psychological Distress

Risk Factors and Moderators of Outcomes

Psychological Distress

When studying the prevalence, impact, and predictors of post-burn adjustment, it is important that pre-injury functioning be taken into account. Prospective, multi-variate research has consistently found that pre-injury psychiatric adjustment, social isolation, and initial symptom severity predict severe post-burn psychological distress (Patterson, Ptacek, Cromes, Fauerbach, & Engrav, 2000).

For example, the risk of post-burn PTSD is greater in those with certain personality traits (e.g., high Neuroticism, low Extraversion; Fauerbach et al., 2000; Lawrence & Fauerbach, 2003), a history of pre-trauma psychopathology (e.g., mood disorder; Fauerbach et al., 1997), and non-adaptive appraisal and coping processes (e.g., approach-avoidant coping; Fauerbach et al., 2002b).

Furthermore, data from an ongoing multi-site, prospective, cohort study (National Data Coordinating Center for the Burn Model Systems, 2004) have identified a subset of key somatic, affective, and cognitive symptoms (i.e., anxiety, depression and social alienation), which if experienced in-hospital, reliably predict clinically significant psychological distress for up to two years (Fauerbach et al., 2006). Finally, individuals with burn injuries, who frequently used both the coping methods of emotional approach (e.g., processing) and emotional avoidance (e.g., suppression) during their hospitalization, experienced more severe symptoms of depression, posttraumatic distress, and body image dissatisfaction for at least several months following discharge, compared to those using only one or neither of the coping methods (Fauerbach et al., 2002b; Fauerbach, Richter, & Lawrence, 2002d; Fauerbach et al., 2002a).

Acute and Chronic Pain

Although a systematic effort to fully understand the complex predictors of chronic pain following serious burn injury has not been undertaken, the available literature suggests that psychosocial factors, such as psychological distress, anxiety, and depression play a significant role, independent from the physical characteristics of the injury, such as burn size and need for autologous skin grafts (Choiniere et al., 1991; Choiniere et al., 1989; Malenfant et al., 1996).

Sleep disturbance, both a consequence of chronic pain and a potential risk factor for its development (Smith & Haythornthwaite, 2004), has been shown to predict next-day pain severity in hospitalized individuals with burns (Raymond et al., 2004; Raymond et al., 2001). This finding is consistent with other predictive studies of chronic pain, for which psychological distress and non-adaptive coping strategies (e.g., reacting to pain using catastrophic thought processes), increased the risk of chronic pain following surgical intervention (Boersma & Linton, 2006).

Arguably, coping with burn pain has been among the most well-studied of all burn complications. The correlational component of a recent experiment found catastrophising cognitive processing is related to more intense pain (Haythornthwaite, Lawrence, & Fauerbach, 2001). The experimental comparison of music distraction and present sensory-focusing versus usual care, revealed that, after controlling for catastrophizing, present sensory-focusing was related to better pain-relief and reduced recall of pain (Haythornthwaite et al., 2001). Interestingly, hypnosis (Patterson & Jensen, 2003) and virtual reality (Hoffman, Patterson, Carrougher, & Sharrar, 2001) have both been shown to substantially reduce the experience of pain during burn-dressing changes. Both of these methods of coping probably work by capturing attention so effectively that non-attended stimuli (i.e., painful procedure) are not registered in person's consciousness. Furthermore, inducing a hypnotic state, while the participant is engaging in a deeply involving, virtual-reality environment, is also effective and may have additional benefits over either method alone (Patterson, Wiechman, Jensen, & Sharar, 2006).

The relationship between acute sleep disturbance and the subsequent development of chronic post-burn pain is not fully understood. It has been convincingly shown that sleep disturbance in chronic pain populations is linked both to its interference with sleep, and to the autonomic and central arousal mechanisms associated with psychological distress (Pilowsky, Crettenden, & Townley, 1985; Wilson, Watson, & Currie, 1998). Several experimental studies have shown that sleep deprivation, particularly slow wave sleep loss, increases pain sensitivity and mood disturbance (Lentz, Landis, Rothermel, & Shaver, 1999; Onen, Alloui, Gross, Eschallier, & Dubray, 2001). Furthermore, sleep deprivation research suggests the possibility that disrupted sleep might impair central pain inhibitory processes (Smith et al., 2006; Lautenbacher & Rollman, 1997), which have been implicated in the development of chronic neuropathic pain following injury (Bouhassira, Danziger, Attal, & Guirimand, 2003; Witting, Svensson, Arendt-Nielsen, & Jensen, 1998).

One of the few experimental studies of coping behavior in this area used a randomized, controlled study ($N = 42$) to test the efficacy of two coping methods (sensory focusing, music distraction), in comparison to usual care in supplementing regular pharmacologic treatment for pain and distress during burn-dressing change (Haythornthwaite et al., 2001). The sensory-focusing group reported greater pain relief, compared to the music distraction group, and a greater reduction in remembered pain, compared to the usual care group – although group differences were not observed on subsequent ratings of pain intensity. This study also compared the effects of the targeted coping behaviors (i.e., focusing, distraction), and three confounding coping methods (i.e., ignoring, catastrophizing, reinterpreting), on intrusive re-experiencing symptoms related to dressing changes and perceived psycho-physiological tension (Fauerbach, Lawrence, Haythornthwaite, & Richter, 2002c). After controlling for the use of the confounding coping methods, the music-distraction group experienced significantly fewer intrusions than the attention-focus group. These results may imply that alternative coping methods can be recommended to individuals, depending on their symptom of greatest concern. That is, sensory focusing was effective in reducing pain (i.e., memory for pain, satisfaction with pain control), while music distraction was effective in reducing distress (i.e, re-experiencing symptoms).

Sleep Disturbance

Few studies have been undertaken to identify specific risk factors for chronic insomnia following burn injury. Relative to injury-severity variables and pain, in-hospital emotional distress was the strongest predictor of chronic sleep complaints two months later (Lawrence et al., 1998a). There are no

empirical investigations of effective methods of coping with sleep disturbance following burn injury. However, cognitive-behavioral conceptualizations
of insomnia posit that as insomnia transitions from an initial acute symptom
and/or stress reaction to a chronic problem, non-adaptive coping strategies and
behavioral contingencies begin to play a role in maintaining the sleep disturbance, independent from the primary medical or psychiatric disease processes
(Buysse et al., 1994).

Behavioral theories postulate that spending excessive time awake in the
bedroom, which is a particularly prevalent behavior for many individuals
with limited mobility, results in stimulus dyscontrol, whereby the bedroom
environment becomes associated with a variety of behaviors other than sleep
(Bootzin, Epstein, & Ward, 1991). Moreover, this excessive time awake is
often spent ruminating about trouble sleeping and/or the consequence of
poor sleep, establishing a classically conditioned association between the
bedroom environment and autonomic nervous system hyperarousal (Perlis, Giles,
Mendelson, Bootzin, & Wyatt, 1997).

Several studies have reported that individuals with burns engage in increased
napping behaviors both during acute hospitalization and at long-term follow
up periods (Boeve et al., 2002; Kravitz et al., 1993; Raymond et al., 2001).
Furthermore, the thickness of a burn that is so deep it requires surgical excision
and grafting, the use of avoidant coping styles, and a high degree of somatic
anxiety, are all significant risk factors for chronic nightmares (Low et al., 2003).
This suggests that behavioral coping methods that minimize naps and provide
training in stress management may be of particular benefit for individuals
with burns.

All of these considerations point towards the possibility that effective coping
with burn injuries must include ways to manage psychological distress, to
increase comfort, and to improve social competence. There are two important
goals for enhancing coping efforts in this setting: to reduce psychological distress
as a barrier to activity, and to improve self-efficacy in burn survivors who are
striving to achieve full recovery.

Etiology and Maintenance of Psychological Distress

Shortly after the 9/11 terrorist attacks in the U.S., experts asserted that some
key responses when coping with the aftermath and reminders of a traumatic
event are to disengage from the trauma reminders and to re-engage in daily
life-activities (Ledoux & Gorman, 2001; Silver, Holman, McIntosh, Poulin, &
Gil-Rivas, 2002). Doing so helps overcome the tendency to chronically oscillate
between arousal/vigilance and avoidance that, ultimately, results in a chronic
stress reaction (e.g., mood disorder, PTSD) (Marshall & Schell, 2002). In support
of this perspective, active coping predicted decreased psychological distress over
time, and, passive withdrawal coping predicted enduring distress at least as far
out as two and six months post-event (Ledoux & Gorman, 2001). Additionally,
difficulty disengaging from traumatic stimuli increased the risk of psychological

disorders (Silver et al., 2002). The implication is that teaching active coping and relaxation methods to injured trauma survivors, during their hospital stay, may effectively reduce arousal and psychological distress, as well as help to preserve or restore function.

There is a large and growing body of literature demonstrating the role of positive emotions, self-efficacy, resilience, and sleep in recovery from extreme stress (Charney, 2004), and trauma and adversity (Linley & Joseph, 2004). For example, baseline resilience (e.g., self-efficacy and active coping) significantly predicted positive treatment outcome for PTSD, and successful treatment produced global improvement, reduction in symptoms, and increased resilience (Connor & Davidson, 2003; Davidson et al., 2005). Relatedly, the setting, structure, and resources available in the acute-care center should promote compliance in practicing the skills learned in treatment, which would, in turn, help to optimize the potential benefit of a secondary prevention program (Carroll, Nich, & Ball, 2005).

Psychological Interventions

The evidence base for cognitive-behavioral therapy (CBT), although largely untested in the burn-injured population, vastly exceeds that of any other psychological or social intervention and, in most cases, equals or exceeds medical intervention for PTSD (Davidson, Stein, Shalev, & Yehuda, 2004), social anxiety (Ballenger et al., 1998), body image concerns (Cash & Pruzinsky, 2002), and depression (DeRubeis, Gelfand, Tang, & Simons; 1999). A significant body of research has shown that CBT increases self-efficacy and improves overall function and quality of life, while reducing secondary conditions such as chronic pain and depression (Jamison & Scogin, 1995; Lorig & Holman, 1993). However, CBT has not been well-studied among individuals with acute injuries, and only one study (described next) has directly tested an adaptive coping intervention in a burn-injured sample.

Adolescents who were identified as having difficulties in psychosocial adjustment following a burn injury were enrolled in an intensive, four-day, social-skills training program, which was designed to improve the social competency and comfort of adolescents with burn scars (Blakeney et al., 2005). This promising intervention for chronic social impairment and chronic body image disturbance used psycho-education, cognitive restructuring, and behavioral rehearsal to improve basic skills for coping with stigmatizing reactions of others, and enhancing the cognitive processing of burn-related changes in appearance. One year following the training program, the adolescents, who had received the treatment intervention, showed significantly fewer total behavioral problems than the control group. Specifically, treatment-group participants were less withdrawn and interacted better with others regarding their burn injury, than did those in the control group.

A New Coping and Motivation Model of Distress Etiology

Recently, a team has built upon this empirical base and clinical experience to develop and test a model of the etiology and maintenance of distress following traumatic injury (e.g., Fauerbach et al., 2002a, 2002b, 2002d). Following traumatic injury, one's goals, motivation, and method of coping are primarily determined by one's pre-injury personality structure, motivation, and coping dispositions. These dispositional factors directly influence the prognosis for chronic psychological distress. Two of the most common methods of coping that have been observed clinically following trauma and traumatic injury are emotional expression (processing) and distraction (suppression), both of which are thought to be equally important in determining intrusive symptoms (Salkovskis & Campbell, 1994).

Previously, investigators suggested that ineffective distracters may explain why suppressed material later returns more frequently to awareness (Wenzlaff & Wegner, 2000). This contention is supported by studies of coping with burn pain, which found that music distraction (lower salience) had little effect on pain (Haythornthwaite et al., 2001), while hypnosis and virtual reality (higher salience) had a strong effect (Patterson et al., 2006). Barlow (2002) posits that, in addition to stress reactivity, poor coping, and poor social support, the perception that negative events and or their associated cues are unpredictable or uncontrollable is fundamental to the development of anxious apprehension. Relatedly, Salkovskis & Campbell (1994) suggest that motivated monitoring of mental content may be as important as suppression in determining the frequency and aversiveness of intrusive thoughts. Consistent with this are the observations that the incompatibility of goals (e.g., an approach–avoidance conflict) is an aversive motivational state; conflict between goals induces motivational vacillation (Van Hook & Higgins, 1988).

In this new model (e.g., Fauerbach et al., 2002b), the desire to enhance control over symptoms or stressors motivates the use of cognitive and behavioral avoidance through passive coping (e.g., emotional-avoidance coping). Furthermore, we posit that the desire to increase the predictability of symptoms or stressors motivates the use of cognitive and behavioral approach through active coping (e.g., emotional-approach coping). We suggest that ambivalence between these two motivational sets (i.e., whether to enhance controllability or to increase predictability of distressing symptoms) may lead to worsened symptoms.

The *predictability motive* strives to reduce the likelihood that threat-relevant information will be overlooked or that one will be unprepared for the information when it is elaborated in consciousness. As conceived by Gray (1982), activity in the Behavioral Inhibition System (BIS) increases nonspecific arousal and allocates attention to "the maximum possible analysis of current environmental stimuli, especially novel ones" (p. 13). When the predictability motive is foremost, one copes by approaching threat-related material with the goal of preventing it from suddenly and unexpectedly emerging into consciousness. Threat-irrelevant information is also brought to attention so it can be suppressed from consciousness, enabling one to refocus on threat-related thoughts. Presumably, when this approach is successful, the system continually processes threat-related stimuli, with the result that one habituates to the aversive memory.

The *controllability motive* attempts to cope with distressing thoughts by preventing them from reaching conscious awareness. Intrusive or ruminative symptoms may arise in the presence of reminders, or, when the cognitive-processing system scans for and suppresses trauma- or loss-related stimuli. That is, intrusive thoughts originate when one scans for threat-related information, in order to more fully suppress it. When the controllability motive is foremost, the operating system seeks threat-related material so that it can be suppressed, in order to prevent it from remaining in consciousness (Wegner, 1994). If one attempts to regulate emotions by suppressing information relevant to threat or loss, then one must also scan for material related to the trauma or loss approaching awareness. Presumably, over time, one is able to continue suppressing threat-cues, ultimately resulting in confident mastery over the aversive memories.

Ambivalent motivation (goals to both control and predict distressing memories) leads to an approach–avoidance coping conflict. This phenomenon closely resembles the cyclic alternation between rumination and suppression in depression, and between intrusive and avoidance phenomena in PTSD (Horowitz, 1986). Indeed, participants in recent studies who reported engaging both in frequent processing (predictability motive) and frequent suppression (controllability motive), relative to those who used only processing or only suppression, experienced the highest levels of depression and PTSD symptoms and body image dissatisfaction (Fauerbach et al., 2002a, 2002b, 2002d).

The proposed motivational formulation, suggests that it is precisely individuals, who are ambivalent about their motivation (i.e., whether to prevent/control distress), are the ones whom experience the greatest distress. Ambivalence between the controllability and predictability motives leads to alternating between an emotional-approach and emotional-avoidance coping style. This "switch hitting" coping style then continues to reinforce the cycle of intrusiveness and avoidance. That is, motivational ambivalence triggers a conflicted approach-avoidant coping style that leads to the cyclic alternation of intrusive and avoidance symptoms.

Furthermore, inconsistent switching between these coping methods ensures the incomplete processing, or, the incomplete suppression, of relevant stimuli and associated symptoms. This promotes increased sensitization to threat stimuli and chronic perpetuation of distress responding, and makes symptoms even more resistant to extinction. Consistent with this formulation is the observation that rape survivors with PTSD report less control and more distress from intrusive thoughts when trying to suppress them (Shipherd & Beck, 1999), and the suggestion that the motivation to monitor one's obsessive thoughts (i.e., process them) may contribute to their aversiveness when trying to suppress them (Salkovskis & Campbell, 1994). Zilberg, Weiss, and Horowitz (1982) reported a posttrauma pattern of "oscillating ... between states of high intrusion and high avoidance" (p. 413) that is relevant to our model and nascent body of research.

In the proposed model, it is suggested that the ability to control intrusions, which occurs through avoidance-based coping as a function of the controllability motive, contributes to adjustment by increased mastery over responses to trauma- or loss- related cues, resulting in habituation (Fauerbach et al., 2002c). Horowitz (1986) identified several types of adaptive control: (a) Over when, how, and for how long traumatic cues are reviewed; (b) over which aspects of self-concept and world-view are related to the review; and (c) over which cues are reviewed and which are suppressed.

We suggest that, in addition to incorporating new information that is incompatible with distressing responses, reappraisal coping (i.e., predictability motive) progresses over time by desensitizing one to the cues one is processing. This occurs as a function of emotional-approach coping (e.g., processing) operating in the service of the predictability motive.

Motivation and Coping Model: Empirical Support

Studies have confirmed that, among those participants with versus without PTSD, intrusive symptoms recur more frequently after being suppressed (Shipherd & Beck, 1999). A post-suppression rebound effect has been experimentally evoked in the immediate (i.e., 5 minutes) post-suppression period in accident survivors with ASD, versus those without ASD (Harvey & Bryant, 1998). In addition, avoidant symptoms predicted higher intrusive symptoms over two months later (Lawrence, Fauerbach, & Munster, 1996). Baseline efforts to suppress traumatic memories by people diagnosed with ASD resulted in higher ratings of anxiety and more frequent trauma-related thoughts (Harvey & Bryant, 1999).

In prospective designs, ambivalent coping while in the hospital is prospectively related to distress severity. In these studies, baseline groups (i.e., in-hospital) were formed on the basis of how frequently participants used emotional approach, emotional avoidance, or both forms of coping. Symptom severity was measured both concurrently and at two-months post-discharge. On the basis of median splits, participants were assigned to one of three mutually exclusive groups if their coping behavior was above the median split: emotional approach only, emotional avoidance only, or, both emotional approach and emotional avoidance. This third group, the ambivalent coping group, experienced the greatest symptom severity at follow-up for depression, posttraumatic distress, and body image dissatisfaction (Fauerbach et al., 2002a, 2002b, 2002d). These prospective, longitudinal studies show the prolonged impact of in-hospital coping ambivalence on psychological distress.

Further support was obtained from a recent experiment where we found striking evidence for the detrimental impact of ambivalent coping. Participants were trained in two methods of coping (avoidance/suppression, approach/processing) prior to a 24-hour test period. Individuals were randomly assigned to conditions, differing only in the order of training in the two coping methods. Participants, who were trained in processing and then trained in suppressing, experienced significantly greater intrusive re-experiencing over the next 24 hours, compared to individuals who were trained first in suppressing and then in processing (Fauerbach, Richter, Lawrence, Bryant, & Richter, unpublished). Even more importantly, individuals in the Process-then-Suppress group were much more likely to develop ambivalent coping over the next 24 hours and this, in turn, led them to experience significantly greater intrusive re-experiencing symptoms.

This evidence suggests that ambivalent coping (i.e., fluctuating between emotional-approach/processing coping and emotional avoidance/suppression coping) is an important factor in the emergence and maintenance of diverse forms of psychological distress (e.g., depression, posttrauma distress, body image dissatisfaction) and related cognitions (e.g., ruminations, intrusions, worries). It remains to be seen whether the deleterious effect of alternating between these coping strategies is principally related to ambivalent motivation, greater neuroticism/negative emotionality (Fauerbach et al., 2000), or, perhaps to other factors such as the ineffective use of these coping strategies.

Summary

The level of evidence accrued to date precludes definitive recommendations. However, tentative recommendations can be offered in light of the knowledge gathered up to this point. First, the psychosocial care of individuals with burn injuries must be universally available and must incorporate routine assessment during the acute care phase. Second, assessment should include pre-injury level of health and function, history of psychological distress, and social support, as well as several indices of psychological distress (e.g., depression, posttraumatic distress, body image dissatisfaction), methods of coping with the burn injury and its complications, and, identifying health-promoting individual strengths (e.g., self-efficacy, resilience, optimism) and social resources.

Third, intervention during hospitalization (versus after discharge) is probably optimal because the distress is severe, openness to care is enhanced, concern with stigmatization is reduced, and access to services is more universal than it will ever be following discharge. Fourth, interventions that focus on enhancing coping skills and improving physical and psychological resilience/efficacy/competence are likely to be welcomed, useful, and most likely be of continued enduring benefit. Finally, in order to develop evidence-based practice, there is an urgent need for well-designed studies (e.g., randomized, controlled trials), testing such interventions in the burn-injured population.[1]

[1] Acknowledgements: This study was supported by funds from the National Institute on Disability and Rehabilitation Research in the Office of Special Education and Rehabilitative Services in the U.S. Department of Education (Dr. Fauerbach: H133A020101) and the National Institute of Neurological Disorders and Stroke (Dr. Smith: NSO47168).

References

Achterberg-Lawliss, J. (1995). Health beliefs: Predictive factors of burn rehabilitation. *Journal of Burn Care and Rehabilitation, 4*, 437–441.

Armstrong, F. D., Gay, C., & Levy, J. D. (1994). Acute reactions. In K. J. Tarnowski (Ed.), *Behavioral Aspects of Pediatric Burns* (pp. 55–75). New York: Plenum Press.

Ballenger, J. C., Davidson, J. R., Lecrubier, Y., Nutt, D. J., Bobes, J., Beidel, D. C., et al. (1998). Consensus statement on social anxiety disorder from the International Consensus Group on Depression and Anxiety. *Journal of Clinical Psychiatry, 59*(Suppl.), 54–60.

Barlow, D. H. (2002). *Anxiety and its disorders: The nature and treatment of anxiety and panic* (2nd ed.). New York: Guilford Press.

Beard, S. A., Herndon, D. N., & Desai, M. (1989). Adaptation of self-image of burn-disfigured children. *Journal of Burn Care and Rehabilitation, 10*, 550–554.

Blakeney, P. E., Fauerbach, J. A., Meyer, W. J., & Thomas, C. R. (2002). Psychosocial recovery and reintegration of clients with burn injuries. In D. Herndon (Ed.), *Total Burn Care*(2nd ed., pp. 783–798). London: Elsevier.

Blakeney, P., Portman, S., & Rutan, R. (1990). Familial values as factors influencing long-term psychological adjustment of children after severe burn injury. *Journal of Burn Care and Rehabilitation, 11*, 472–475.

Blakeney, P., Thomas, C., Holzer, C., Rose, M., Berniger, F., & Meyer, W. J. (2005). Efficacy of a short-term, intensive social skills training program for burned adolescents. *Journal of Burn Care and Rehabilitation, 26*, 546–556.

Boersma, K., & Linton, S. J. (2006). Psychological processes underlying the development of a chronic pain problem: A prospective study of the relationship between profiles of psychological variables in the fear-avoidance model and disability. *Clinical Journal of Pain, 22*, 160–166.

Boeve, S. A., Aaron, L. A., Martin-Herz, S. P., Peterson, A., Cain, V., Heimbach, D. M., et al. (2002). Sleep disturbance after burn injury. *Journal of Burn Care and Rehabilitation, 23*, 32–38.

Bombaro, K. M., Engrav, L. H., Carrougher, G. J., Wiechman, S. A., Faucher, L., Costa, B. A., et al. (2003). What is the prevalence of hypertrophic scarring following burns? *Burns, 29*, 299–302.

Bootzin, R. R., Epstein, D., & Ward, J. M. (1991). Stimulus control instructions. In P. Hauri (Ed.), *Case studies in insomnia* (pp. 19–28). New York: Plenum Press.

Bouhassira, D., Danziger, N., Attal, N., & Guirimand, F. (2003). Comparison of the pain suppressive effects of clinical and experimental painful conditioning stimuli. *Brain, 126*, 1068–1078.

Buysse, D. J., Reynolds, C. F. III, Kupfer, D. J., Thorpy, M. J., Bixler, E., Manfredi, R., et al. (1994). Clinical diagnoses in 216 insomnia clients using the International Classification of Sleep Disorders (ICSD), DSM-IV and ICD-10 categories: a report from the APA/NIMH DSM-IV Field Trial. *Sleep, 17*, 630–637.

Carroll, K. M., Nich, C., & Ball, S. A. (2005). Practice makes progress? Homework assignments and outcome in treatment of cocaine dependence. *Journal of Consulting and Clinical Psychology, 73*, 749–755.

Cash, T., & Pruzinsky, T. (Eds.) (2002). *Body Image: A handbook of theory, research and clinical practice.* New York: Guilford.

Charney, D. S. (2004). Psychobiological mechanisms of resilience and vulnerability: Implications for successful adaptation to extreme stress. *American Journal of Psychiatry, 161*, 195–216.

Choiniere, M., Melzack, R., & Papillon, J. (1991). Pain and paresthesia in clients with healed burns: An exploratory study. *Journal of Pain and Symptom Management, 6,* 437–444.

Choiniere, M., Melzack, R., Rondeau, J., Girard, N., & Paquin, M. J. (1989). The pain of burns: Characteristics and correlates. *Journal of Trauma, 29,* 1531–1539.

Connor, K. M., & Davidson, J. R. (2003). Development of a new resilience scale: The Connor-Davidson Resilience Scale (CD-RISC). *Depression and Anxiety, 18,* 76–82.

Costa, B. A., Engrav, L. H., Holavanahalli, R., Lezotte, D. C., Patterson, D. R., Kowalske, K. J., et al. (2003). Impairment after burns: a two-center, prospective report. *Burns, 29,* 71–75.

Davidson, J. R., Payne, V. M., Connor, K. M., Foa, E. B., Rothbaum, B. O., Hertzberg, M. A., et al. (2005). Trauma, resilience and saliostasis: Effects of treatment in post-traumatic stress disorder. *International Journal of Clinical Psychopharmacology, 20,* 43–48.

Davidson, J. R., Stein, D. J., Shalev, A. Y., & Yehuda, R. (2004). Posttraumatic stress disorder: Acquisition, recognition, course, and treatment. *Journal of Neuropsychiatry and Clinical Neurosciences, 16,* 135–147.

Derogatis, L. R., & Melisaratos, N. (1983). The Brief Symptom Inventory: An introductory report. *Psychological Medicine, 13,* 595–605.

DeRubeis, R. J., Gelfand, L. A., Tang, T. Z., & Simons, A. D. (1999). Medications versus cognitive behavior therapy for severely depressed outpatients: Meta-analysis of four randomized comparisons. *American Journal of Psychiatry, 56,* 1007–1013.

Difede, J., Ptacek, J. T., Roberts, J., Barocas, D., Rives, W., Apfeldorf, W., et al. (2002). Acute stress disorder after burn injury: A predictor of posttraumatic stress disorder? *Psychosomatic Medicine, 64,* 826–834.

Ehde, D. M., Patterson, D. R., Wiechman, S. A., & Wilson, L. G. (1999). Post-traumatic stress symptoms and distress following acute burn injury. *Burns, 25,* 587–592.

Ehde, D. M., Patterson, D. R., Wiechman, S. A., & Wilson, L. G. (2000). Post-traumatic stress symptoms and distress 1 year after burn injury. *Journal of Burn Care and Rehabilitation, 21,* 105–111.

Esselman, P. C., Thombs, B. D., Magyar-Russell, G. M., & Fauerbach, J. A. (2006). Burn rehabilitation: State of the science. *American Journal of Physical Medicine and Rehabilitation, 85,* 383–413.

Fauerbach, J. A., Heinberg, L., Lawrence, J. W., Bryant, A. G., Richter, L., & Spence, R. J. (2002a). Coping with body image changes following a disfiguring burn injury. *Health Psychology, 21,* 115–121.

Fauerbach, J., Heinberg, L., Lawrence, J., Munster, A., Palombo, D., & Richter, D. (2000). The effect of early body image dissatisfaction on subsequent psychological and physical adjustment following disfiguring injury. *Psychosomatic Medicine, 62,* 576–582.

Fauerbach, J. A., Lawrence, J. W., Bryant, A. G., & Smith, J. H. (2002b). The relationship of ambivalent coping to depression symptoms and adjustment. *Rehabilitation Psychology, 47,* 387–401.

Fauerbach, J. A., Lawrence, J. W., Haythornthwaite, J. A., & Richter, L. (2002c). Coping with the stress of a painful medical procedure. *Behavioral Research and Therapy, 40,* 1003–1015.

Fauerbach, J. A., Lawrence, J., Haythornthwaite, J., Richter, D., McGuire, M., Schmidt, C., et al. (1997). Psychiatric history affects post trauma morbidity in a burn injured adult sample. *Psychosomatics, 38,* 374–385.

Fauerbach, J. A., Lawrence, J. W., Munster, A., Palombo, D., & Richter, D. (1999). Prolonged adjustment difficulties among those with acute post trauma distress following burn injury. *Behavioral Medicine, 22*, 359–378.

Fauerbach, J. A., Lawrence, J., Schmidt, C., Munster, A., & Costa, P. (2000). Personality predictors of injury-related PTSD. *Journal of Nervous and Mental Disease, 188*, 510–517.

Fauerbach, J. A., Lezotte, D., Cromes, G. F., Kowalske, K., de Lateur, B. J., Goodwin, C. W., et al. (2005). 2004 American Burn Association Clinical Research Award. Burden of burn: A norm-based inquiry into the influence of burn size and distress on recovery of physical and psychosocial function. *Journal of Burn Care & Rehabilitation, 26*, 21–32.

Fauerbach, J. A., Richter, L., & Lawrence, J. W. (2002d). Regulating acute posttrauma distress. *Journal of Burn Care & Rehabilitation, 23*, 249–257.

Fauerbach, J. A., Richter, L., Lawrence, J. W., Bryant, A. G., & Richter, D. R. (no date). Maladaptive coping and re-experiencing symptoms: An ecologically valid experimental model. Unpublished data.

Fauerbach, J. A., Thombs, B. D., Lezotte, D., Holavanahalli, R., Wiechman, S., Engrav, L., et al. (2006). *Early predictors of long term psychological distress*. Paper presented at the Annual Meeting of the American Burn Association, Las Vegas, NV.

Gottschlich, M. M., Jenkins, M. E., Mayes, T., Khoury, J., Kramer, M., Warden, R. J., et al. (1994). The 1994 Clinical Research Award. A prospective clinical study of the polysomnographic stages of sleep after burn injury. *Journal of Burn Care and Rehabilitation, 15*, 486–492.

Graves, T. A., Cioffi, W. G., McManus, W. F., Mason, A. D., & Pruitt, B. A. (1988). Resuscitation of infants and children with massive thermal injury. *Journal of Trauma, 27*, 208–212.

Gray, J. A. (1982). *The neuropsychology of anxiety: An enquiry into the functions of the septo-hippocampal system*. New York: Oxford University Press.

Gumustekin, K., Seven, B., Karabulut, N., Aktas, O., Gursan, N., Aslan, S., et al. (2004). Effects of sleep deprivation nicotine and selenium on wound healing in rats. *International Journal of Neuroscience, 114*, 1433–1442.

Harvey, A. G., & Bryant, R. A. (1998). The effect of attempted thought suppression in acute stress disorder. *Behaviour Research and Therapy, 36*, 583–590.

Harvey, A. G., & Bryant, R. A. (1999). The relationship between acute stress disorder and post-traumatic stress disorder: A 2-year prospective evaluation. *Journal of Consulting and Clinical Psychology, 67*(6), 985–988.

Haythornthwaite, J. A., Lawrence, J. W., & Fauerbach, J. A. (2001). Brief cognitive interventions for burn pain. *Annals of Behavioral Medicine, 23*, 42–49.

Helton, M. C., Gordon, S. H., & Nunnery, S. L. (1980). The correlation between sleep deprivation and the intensive care unit syndrome. *Heart and Lung, 9*, 464–468.

Herndon D. (2002). *Total Burn Care* (2nd ed.). London: Elsevier Limited.

Herndon, D. N., & Tompkins, R. G. (2004). Support of the metabolic response to burn injury. *Lancet, 363*, 1895–1902.

Hoffman, H. G., Patterson, D. R., Carrougher, G. J., & Sharrar, S. R. (2001). Effectiveness of virtual reality-based pain control with multiple treatments. *Clinical Journal of Pain, 17*(3), 229–235.

Horowitz, M. J. (1986). Stress-response syndromes: A review of posttraumatic and adjustment disorders. *Hospital and Community Psychiatry, 37*, 241–249.

Jamison, C., & Scogin, F. (1995). The outcome of cognitive bibliotherapy with depressed adults. *Journal of Consulting and Clinical Psychology, 63*, 644–650.

Kiecolt-Glaser, J. K., & Williams, D. A. (1987). Self-blame, compliance and distress among burn patients. *Journal of Personality and Social Psychology, 53*, 187–193.

Kravitz, M., McCoy, B. J., Tompkins, D. M., Daly, W., Mulligan, J., McCauley, R. L., et al. (1993). Sleep disorders in children after burn injury. *Journal of Burn Care and Rehabilitation, 14*, 83–90.

Lautenbacher, S., & Rollman, G. B. (1997). Possible deficiencies of pain modulation in fibromyalgia. *Clinical Journal of Pain, 13*, 189–196.

Lawrence, J. W., & Fauerbach, J. A. (2003). Personality, coping, chronic stress, social support and PTSD symptoms: A path analysis. *Journal of Burn Care & Rehabilitation, 24*, 63–72.

Lawrence, J. W., Fauerbach, J., Eudell, E., Ware, L., & Munster, A. (1998a). The 1998 Clinical Research Award. Sleep disturbance after burn injury: A frequent yet understudied complication. *Journal of Burn Care and Rehabilitation, 19*, 480–486.

Lawrence, J. W., Fauerbach, J. A., Heinberg, L., & Doctor, M. (2004). American Burn Association 2003 Clinical Research Award: Visible versus hidden scars and their relation to body esteem. *Journal of Burn Care & Rehabilitation, 25*, 25–32.

Lawrence, J. W., Fauerbach, J. A., Heinberg, L. J., & Doctor, M. (2006). The reliability and validity of the Perceived Stigmatization Questionnaire (PSQ) and the Social Comfort Questionnaire (SCQ) in an adult burn survivor sample. *Psychological Assessment, 18*, 106–111.

Lawrence, J. W., Fauerbach, J., & Munster, A. (1996). Early avoidance of traumatic stimuli predicts chronicity of intrusive thoughts following burn injury. *Behaviour Research and Therapy, 34*(8), 643–646.

Lawrence, J. W., Fauerbach, J. A., Thombs, B. D. (2006). A test of the moderating role of importance of appearance in relation between perceived scar severity and body-esteem among adult burn survivors. *Body Image 3*, 101–111.

Lawrence, J. W., Heinberg, L. J., Roca, R., Munster, A., Spence, R., & Fauerbach, J. A. (1998b). Development and validation of the satisfaction with appearance scale: Assessing body image among burn-injured patients. *Psychological Assessment, 10*, 64–70.

Ledoux, J. E., & Gorman, J. M. (2001). A call to action: Overcoming anxiety through active coping. *American Journal of Psychiatry, 12*, 1953.

Lentz, M. J., Landis, C. A., Rothermel, J., & Shaver, J. L. (1999). Effects of selective slow wave sleep disruption on musculoskeletal pain and fatigue in middle aged women. *Journal of Rheumatology, 26*, 1586–1592.

Linley, P. A., & Joseph, S. (2004). Positive change following trauma and adversity: A review. *Journal of Traumatic Stress, 17*, 11–21.

Lorig, K., & Holman, H. (1993). Arthritis self-management studies: A twelve-year review. *Health Education Quarterly, 20*, 17–28.

Low, J. F., Dyster-Aas, J., Willebrand, M., Kildal, M., Gerdin, B., & Ekselius, L. (2003). Chronic nightmares after severe burns: Risk factors and implications for treatment. *Journal of Burn Care and Rehabilitation, 24*, 260–267.

Malenfant, A., Forget, R., Amsel, R., Papillon, J., Frigon, J. Y., & Choiniere, M. (1998). Tactile thermal and pain sensibility in burned clients with and without chronic pain and paresthesia problems. *Pain, 77*, 241–251.

Malenfant, A., Forget, R., Papillon, J., Amsel, R., Frigon, J. Y., & Choiniere, M. (1996). Prevalence and characteristics of chronic sensory problems in burn patients. *Pain, 67*, 493–500.

Marshall, G. N., & Schell, T. L. (2002). Reappraising the link between peritraumatic dissociation and PTSD symptom severity: evidence from a longitudinal study of community violence survivors. *Journal of Abnormal Psychology, 111*, 626–636.

Munster, A. M., Meek, M., & Sharkey, P. (1994). The effect of early surgical intervention on mortality and cost effectiveness in burn care, 1978–1991. *Burns, 20*, 61–64.

National Data Coordinating Center for the Burn Model Systems (2004). Retrieved on November 8, 2004, from *http://bms-dcc.uchsc.edu/*

Obal, F., & Krueger, J. M. (2004). GHRH and sleep. *Sleep Medicine Reviews, 8*, 367–377.

Onen, S. H., Alloui, A., Gross, A., Eschallier, A., & Dubray, C. (2001). The effects of total sleep deprivation selective sleep interruption and sleep recovery on pain tolerance thresholds in healthy subjects. *Journal of Sleep Research, 10*, 35–42.

Orr, D. A., Reznikoff, M., & Smith, G. M. (1989). Body image, self-esteem, and depression in burn-injured adolescents and young adults. *Journal of Burn Care and Rehabilitation, 10*, 454–461.

Patterson, D. R., & Jensen, M. (2003). Hypnosis and clinical pain. *Psychological Bulletin, 129*(4), 495–521.

Patterson, D. R., Ptacek, J. T., Cromes, F., Fauerbach, J. A., & Engrav, L. (2000). Describing and predicting distress and satisfaction with life for burn survivors. *Journal of Burn Care and Rehabilitation, 21*, 490–498.

Patterson, D. R., Wiechman, S. A., Jensen, M., & Sharar, S. R. (2006). Hypnosis delivered through immersive virtual reality for burn pain: A clinical case series. *International Journal of Clinical Hypnosis, 54*(2), 130–142.

Perlis, M. L., Giles, D. E., Mendelson, W. B., Bootzin, R. R., & Wyatt, J. K. (1997). Psychophysiological insomnia: The behavioural model and a neurocognitive perspective. *Journal of Sleep Research, 6*, 179–188.

Pilowsky, I., Crettenden, I., & Townley, M. (1985). Sleep disturbance in pain clinic patients. *Pain, 23*, 27–33.

Powers, P. S., Cruse, C. W., Daniels, S., & Stevens, B. (1994). Posttraumatic stress disorder in clients with burns. *Journal of Burn Care and Rehabilitation, 15*, 147–153.

Ptacek, J. T., Patterson, D. R., & Heimbach, D. M. (2002). Inpatient depression in persons with burns. *Journal of Burn Care and Rehabilitation, 23*, 1–9.

Raymond, I., Ancoli-Israel, S., & Choiniere, M. (2004). Sleep disturbances pain and analgesia in adults hospitalized for burn injuries. *Sleep Medicine, 5*, 551–559.

Raymond, I., Nielsen, T. A., Lavigne, G., Manzini, C., & Choiniere, M. (2001). Quality of sleep and its daily relationship to pain intensity in hospitalized adult burn patients. *Pain, 92*, 381–388.

Renz, B. M., & Sherman R. (1992). The burn unit experience at Grady Memorial Hospital - 884 cases. *Journal of Burn Care and Rehabilitation, 13*, 426–436.

Roca, R., Spence, R., & Munster, A. (1992). Posttraumatic adaptation and distress among adult burn survivors. *American Journal of Psychiatry, 149*, 1234–1238.

Rose, M., Sanford, A., Thomas, C., & Opp, M. R. (2001). Factors altering the sleep of burned children. *Sleep, 24*, 45–51.

Salkovskis, P. M., & Campbell, P. (1994). Thought suppression induces intrusion in naturally occurring negative intrusive thoughts. *Behaviour Research and Therapy, 32*, 1–8.

Saxe, G., Stoddard, F. J., Markey, C., Taft, C., King, D., King, L., et al. (1994). *Acute stress symptoms in burned children.* Paper presented at the 29th Annual Meeting of the American Burn Association, New York.

Schwanholt, C. A., Ridgway, C. L., Greenhalgh, D. G., Staley, M. J., Gaboury, T. J., Morress, C. et al. (1994). A prospective study of burn scar maturation in pediatrics: Does age matter? *Journal of Burn Care and Rehabilitation, 15*, 416–420.

Shipherd, J. C., & Beck, J. G. (1999). The effects of suppressing trauma-related thoughts on women with rape-related posttraumatic stress disorder. *Behavior Research and Therapy, 37*, 99–112.

Silver, R. C., Holman, E. A., McIntosh, D. N., Poulin, M., & Gil-Rivas, V. (2002). Nationwide longitudinal study of psychological responses to September 11. *Journal of the American Medical Association, 288*, 1235–1244.

Smith, M. T., & Haythornthwaite, J. A. (2004). How do sleep disturbance and chronic pain inter-relate? Insights from the longitudinal and cognitive-behavioral clinical trials literature. *Sleep Medicine Reviews, 8*, 119–132.

Smith, M. T., Kronfli, T. R., Whang, K. J., Koch, C. H., Wiley J. C., & Edwards, R. R. (2006). Effects of partial sleep deprivation on pain inhibition in healthy women. *Sleep, Abstract Supplement.*

Stoddard, F., Norman, D., Murphy, M., & Beardslee, W. (1989). Psychiatric outcome of burned children and adolescents. *Journal of the American Academy of the Child and Adolescent Psychiatry, 28*, 589–595.

Tarnowski, K. J., Rasnake, L. K., Gavaghan-Jones, M. P., & Smith, L. (1991). Psycholosocial sequelae of pediatric burn injuries: A review. *Clinical Psychology Review, 11*, 371–398.

Thombs, B. D., Notes, L. D., Magyar-Russell, G. M., Lawrence, J. W., & Fauerbach, J. A. (2006). *Body image satisfaction in burn survivors: From survival to socialization.* Paper presented at the Annual Meeting of the American Burn Association, Las Vegas, NV.

Van Hook, E., & Higgins, E. T. (1988). Self-related problems beyond the self-concept: The motivational consequences of discrepant self-guides. *Journal of Personality and Social Psychology, 55*, 625–633.

Van Loey, N. E., Maas, C. J. M., Faber, A. W., & Taal, L. A. (2003). Predictors of chronic posttraumatic stress symptoms following burn injury: Results of a longitudinal study. *Journal of Traumatic Stress, 16*, 361–369.

Wegner, D. M. (1994). Ironic processes of mental control. *Psychological Review, 101*(1), 34–52.

Wenzlaff, R. M., & Wegner, D. M. (2000). Thought suppression. *Annual Review of Psychology, 51*, 59–91.

Wiechman, S. A., Ptacek, J. T., Patterson, D. R., Gibran, N. S., Engrav, L. E., & Heimbach, D. M. (2001). Rates, trends, and severity of depression after burn injuries. *Journal of Burn Care and Rehabilitation, 22*, 417–424.

Willebrand, M., Low, A., Dyster-Aas, J., Kildol, M., Andersson, G., Ekselices, L., Gerden, B. (2004). Pruritus, personality traits and coping in long-term follow-up of burn-injured patients. *Acta Dermatologica Venereologiae, 84*, 375–380.

Wilson, K. G., Watson, S. T., & Currie, S. R. (1998). Daily diary and ambulatory activity monitoring of sleep in clients with insomnia associated with chronic musculoskeletal pain. *Pain, 75*, 75–84.

Witting, N., Svensson, P., Arendt-Nielsen, L., & Jensen, T. S. (1998). Differential effect of painful heterotopic stimulation on capsaicin-induced pain and allodynia. *Brain Research, 801*, 206–210.

Zilberg, N. J., Weiss, D. S., & Horowitz, M. J. (1982). Impact of Event Scale: A cross-validation study and some empirical evidence supporting a conceptual model of stress response syndromes. *Journal of Consulting and Clinical Psychology, 50*, 407–414.

10
Coping with Cancer: Findings of Research and Intervention Studies

Sharon L. Manne

It has been estimated that in 2006, approximately 1.3 million people will be diagnosed with some form of cancer and 570,280 people will die from this disease in the U.S. (American Cancer Society, 2005). Although cancer is a potentially life-threatening disease, recent advances in the treatment for many types of cancer have improved five-year survival rates by approximately 15% for all cancers over the course of thirty years (Edwards et al., 2005).

Despite these treatment advances, the vast majority of people still associate cancer with death; thus, for most individuals, a cancer diagnosis is an extremely upsetting life experience. In the chapter that follows, typical treatment regimens for different types of cancer will be reviewed, followed by an evaluation of the empirical literature on the association between coping and psychological adaptation. The discussion of the association of coping with psychological adjustment will be divided into disease phases: active treatment, survivorship, and recurrence/end of life. Finally, the growing literature, which evaluates psychological interventions to promote coping with cancer, will be reviewed.

Medical Treatments for Cancer

Treatment regimens for cancers depend on the type of cancer diagnosed, as well as the stage of disease at diagnosis. The stage of disease means the degree to which the cancer has spread; it is determined by the size of the tumor, how far the cancer has spread to the nearby lymph nodes, and whether the cancer has spread to other organs. Cancers are staged from I to IV, with higher numbers indicating more serious cancer. For a more detailed description of cancer treatment regimens for specific types of cancer, see the National Comprehensive Cancer Network's (NCCN) 2005 treatment guidelines. The majority of individuals, who are diagnosed with early stage, solid tumors, undergo immediate surgery to remove the tumor (e.g., breast, lung, colorectal cancers). For individuals diagnosed with some early stage cancers (e.g., melanoma), surgery is considered curative and there are no additional treatments offered. For individuals diagnosed with other types of cancer, surgery is followed by a course of adjuvant chemotherapy and/or radiation. Once these treatments are complete, some individuals are offered long-term hormone treatment (e.g., breast cancer). Many individuals with cancer are asked to choose among different treatments. For example, men, who are diagnosed with early stage prostate cancer, are offered a choice of watchful waiting, hormonal therapy, or surgery (Scardino, 2005). Women, who are diagnosed with stage I breast cancer, must typically choose between modified radical mastectomy and lumpectomy (Fisher et al., 1995).

For individuals diagnosed with advanced stages of disease, curative treatment is not possible. The goal of treatment for these individuals is to slow the cancer's progression, minimize the painful and disabling effects from the disease or its treatment, and maximize the length and quality of life. Surgery, chemotherapy and/or radiation may be offered to reduce the size of a tumor, to reduce the risk of additional disease metastasis, and to reduce pain (e.g., Engstrom et al., 2005). Because the goal is symptom control, individuals are offered palliative treatments to control pain, nausea, and other disabling symptoms.

Treatment regimens for individuals, who are diagnosed with non-solid tumor types of cancer, such as lymphoma, leukemia and myeloma, are typically not offered surgery, because these diseases are systemic. Individuals diagnosed with systemic cancers may receive chemotherapy or immunotherapy. Increasingly, stem-cell transplantation is used to treat systemic cancers. While potentially curative, transplantation is a difficult treatment with an uncertain outcome in most cases.

For most individuals diagnosed with cancer, disease recurrence is a significant threat. Treatment for recurrent disease is not considered curative, and in the vast majority of cases, treatment incorporates chemotherapy and/or radiation. As mentioned above, the goal of treatment for recurrent disease is to slow disease progression, lengthen life, and control symptoms.

Coping with Cancer

Coping is a ubiquitous term that holds a number of different meanings in the lay and empirical literature. Lazarus and Folkman's (1984) definition will be adopted for the purposes of this review; coping consists of "constantly changing cognitive and behavioral responses to demands that are appraised as taxing or exceeding the resources of a person" (p. 141). Before individuals decide what type of coping strategy to use in a particular situation, Lazarus and Folkman (1984) propose that individuals appraise the situation in terms of the controllability of the stressor, as well as the degree of challenge, harm, threat, or loss that is posed by the stressor. If the individual appraises significant harm, loss, threat, or challenge, then they will begin the coping process.

After appraising the challenge of the stressor, the person appraises the degree of control they have over the stressor. If the stressor is appraised as controllable, then the individual is more likely to use a *problem-focused coping* strategy, which is designed to manage the external demand by solving the problem. Problem-focused coping strategies include information seeking, seeking instrumental support, and problem-solving efforts. If the stressor is appraised as uncontrollable, then the individual is more likely to choose an *emotion-focused coping* strategy, which is designed to alter the person's emotional response and internal stress, rather than change the situation itself. Emotion-focused efforts include acceptance, positive reappraisal, distancing, cognitive or behavioral avoidance, and seeking emotional support. Lazarus and Folkman (1984) conceptualize coping as a process, in that individuals engage in an ongoing appraisal of the threat and controllability of the stressor, as well as the effectiveness of their coping choices. Based on these ongoing appraisals, the individual may alter the coping choices.

Although Lazarus and Folkman's problem- and emotion-focused taxonomy is the most common framework used to conceptualize coping, a second taxonomy emphasizes the degree of focus or orientation towards the problem. For example, Holahan and Moos (1987) label coping strategies that involve attention directed toward the threat as approach, and coping activity that is directed away from the threat as avoidance. Similar taxonomies have been developed by others (e.g., Roth & Cohen, 1986).

Associations between Coping and Psychological Outcomes across the Cancer Continuum

The following literature review is organized by disease site. In addition, if there is sufficient literature, studies focus on coping and adaptation to diagnosis and treatment and survivorship will be reviewed separately. Within each study, if both cross-sectional and longitudinal data are presented within a single study, then only the longitudinal results will be presented.

Breast Cancer: Diagnosis and Treatment Phase

The majority of the studies on coping with cancer have assessed the association between coping and psychological adjustment among women diagnosed with early stage breast cancer. One of the earliest published studies evaluated the association between the COPE scale and psychological distress as measured by the Profile of Mood States (POMS) (Carver et al., 1993). The study used a relatively small sample (N = 59) with early stage breast cancer, but assessed women at five time points. Prospective analyses suggested that higher levels of pre-surgery acceptance of the possibility that the participant might have cancer predicted less post-surgical distress. Although there were no associations between post-surgical coping and three-month distress, both denial and behavioral disengagement assessed at three months predicted higher distress at six months, and the use of humor at three months predicted less distress at six months. No coping reactions at six months predicted distress measured at one year.

Stanton and Snider (1993) evaluated the association between the Ways of Coping questionnaire and psychological distress. Greater pre-biopsy, cognitive, escape-avoidance coping predicted both higher post-biopsy and post-surgery negative mood, and lower pre-biopsy avoidance predicted greater post-surgery vigor. There was no relationship between the other four coping scales (positive focus, distancing, seeking social support, and behavioral escape avoidance) and post-biopsy mood.

Shapiro and colleagues (1997) evaluated the association between four coping "clusters" and total symptoms, summed across the three study assessments over seven days, among women with early stage breast cancer. Results indicated that fewer physical and psychological symptoms were associated with greater confrontive coping. The confrontive cluster was characterized by greater optimism about the future, greater seeking of information, and wanting to be more involved in treatment decisions.

Compas and colleagues (1999) assessed the association between emotional ventilation/expression, as measured by the Coping Strategies Inventory (CSI). Women were assessed at the time of diagnosis, and at three and six months post-diagnosis. Correlational analyses indicated that emotional ventilation, wishful thinking, self-criticism, and social withdrawal were predictors of greater distress at three and six months.

Epping-Jordan and colleagues (1999;) also used the CSI to assess coping, at diagnosis, three, and six months post-discharge. At diagnosis, problem-focused engagement coping was associated with less anxiety and depressive symptoms, whereas emotion-focused disengagement coping was associated with more symptoms. At three months post-diagnosis, there were no associations between coping and distress after controlling for distress at diagnosis. At six months post-diagnosis, problem-focused engagement was again associated with less distress, and emotion-focused disengagement was again associated with more distress, after controlling for distress at three months. In addition, emotion-focused engagement coping was associated with more distress, as was problem-focused disengagement coping. Among the predictors, emotion-focused disengagement had the strongest relationship with distress at six months.

Osowiecki and Compas (1999) used the CSI to assess coping with early stage breast cancer in a sample of 70 women. Participants completed the CSI at the time of diagnosis and at three and six months after diagnosis. The problem-focused engagement and problem-focused disengagement subscales of the CSI were used. The investigators evaluated whether perceived control moderated the association between coping and distress. They predicted that problem-focused engagement coping would be associated with less distress among women reporting high perceived control over the symptoms of their cancer, compared with women who reported low perceived control. In addition, they predicted that emotion-focused engagement would be associated with less distress when women reported low control over the symptoms of cancer. Thus, the match between appraisals of control and coping selection would be a primary predictor of adjustment. Results partially supported predictions at the Time 3 assessment (six month post-surgery). After controlling for Time 1 anxiety and depression, Time 3 problem-focused and emotion-focused disengagement coping predicted more anxiety and depression at Time 3, and emotion-focused engagement coping predicted less anxiety and depression at Time 3. There were no significant interaction effects with perceived control

Hack and Degner (2004) conducted a study with one of the longest follow-up assessments of coping and distress. They administered the Coping Responses Inventory (CRI) and the POMS to 55 women diagnosed with early stage breast cancer. Assessments were administered between 1.5 and 6 months post-diagnosis and three years later. The authors conducted a cluster analysis of the CRI baseline data that yielded three clusters of respondents: low cognitive avoidance and moderate approach (low avoidance), high cognitive avoidance and low approach (high avoidance), and moderate cognitive avoidance and high approach (high general coping). They evaluated cluster differences regarding three-year POMS outcomes. Significant differences were noted with regard to three of the seven POMS subscales: anxiety, vigor, and friendliness. Participants in the low avoidance cluster were less anxious than participants in the high general coping cluster. Participants in the high avoidance cluster had lower friendliness and lower vigor than participants in the high general coping cluster. Analyses were also conducted using the POMS total score, and indicated that negative affect was higher in the high avoidance cluster than in the low avoidance cluster. Longitudinal regression analyses of all CRI subscales, entered together to separately predict the POMS subscales, suggested that the most frequent significant predictor of negative mood was the acceptance/resignation scale of the CRI.

Culver, Arena, Antoni, and Carver (2002) evaluated prospective relations between the COPE and distress among an ethnically diverse sample of 131 women, diagnosed with early stage breast cancer. Longitudinal regression analyses indicated that acceptance at three months predicted lower distress at six months, and behavioral disengagement at three months predicted more distress at six months. Behavioral disengagement had stronger effects on subsequent distress among Hispanic women, compared with Caucasian women. However, no other longitudinal associations between coping and distress were significant. This study also examined the role of distress in predicting coping. Results indicated that pre-surgical distress predicted post-surgical religious coping and self-distraction. Greater post-surgical distress predicted greater acceptance at three months, and greater three-month distress predicted more venting at six months. Distress at six months predicted more venting and planning at one year.

Ben-Zur, Gilbur, and Lev (2001) used path modeling to evaluate the role played by problem- and emotion-focused strategies, as measured by the COPE inventory, in the psychological distress of 73 women diagnosed with early stage breast cancer. Women reporting greater use of emotion-focused coping (ventilation, denial, behavioral disengagement, religion, and restraint) reflected significantly more distress as measured by the Brief Symptom Inventory (BSI) and significantly lower scores on a measure of distress developed by the investigators.

Nosarti and colleauges (2002) included coping strategies in a longitudinal assessment of risk factors that are associated with the development of distress among women, who are newly diagnosed with early stage breast cancer. This study assessed psychological distress prior to breast cancer diagnosis by administering the Mental Adjustment to Cancer (MAC) Inventory and measures of distress approximately eight weeks and nine months after diagnosis. Unlike other studies, women were categorized as "cases" on the General Health Questionnaire (GHQ) measure. "Caseness" was defined as a GHQ score indicating a clinically significant level of distress. The investigators factor-analysed the MAC subscales and beliefs, and combined these factors with other measures to create four factors: (a) *Straightforward optimism:* made up of external cause beliefs, body image satisfaction and negative recovery beliefs; (b) *stoic acceptance:* consisting of MAC helplessness, MAC fatalism, and MAC anxious preoccupation, causal and recovery beliefs; (c) *faithful optimism:* comprised of MAC fighting spirit, MAC fatalism, positive recovery beliefs and religousity, and; (d) *personal responsibility/avoidance:* comprised of a mixture of MAC avoidant coping and internal positive recovery beliefs.

Breast Cancer: Survivorship Phase

Stanton, Danoff-Burg, and Huggins (2002) evaluated the association between the COPE and quality of life and distress in a sample of early stage breast cancer survivors. The initial assessment was made within 20 weeks of treatment completion and the second assessment three months later. Outcomes included the POMS and a measure of quality of life. Longitudinal regression analyses suggested that greater use of coping by emotional expression was associated with lower psychological distress three months later, whereas emotional processing (e.g., attempts to delve into and understand one's emotional responses) predicted higher distress three months later. Avoidant copers became more distressed over time. Higher acceptance was associated with higher quality of life over time. Women using spiritual coping became less distressed over time. These investigators evaluated a potential moderating factor for the effects of emotional expression, and found that emotional expression was associated with less distress among women reporting lower social constraints (hesitancy sharing concerns with others).

Stanton, Danoff-Burg, and Huggins (2002) also evaluated the role of hope as a moderator of the effects of active approach coping strategies (social support, problem-focused coping, positive reinterpretation, and active acceptance). Seventy women with early stage breast cancer were assessed at three months and one year following diagnosis. Active acceptance-coping (accepting that one had been diagnosed with cancer) predicted lower distress at one year.

An interaction effect indicated that women, who had low levels of hope at the baseline assessment and who turned to religion to cope with cancer, reported less distress at follow-up. Women, who had high levels of hope at the baseline assessment and who turned to religion to cope with cancer, demonstrated higher distress at follow-up. Findings regarding the moderating role for hope were also reported for positive reinterpretation coping and seeking-support coping; both coping strategies lead to lower distress among women reporting high levels of hope at baseline. Yet, it should be noted that these effects were for only one outcome measure, at one time-point.

Ransom and colleagues (2005) utilized the Illness Management Questionnaire (IMQ) to assess the association between coping and quality of life in a sample of women, who were completing treatment. Participants were assessed at the time of treatment completion and six months later. Separate hierarchical regression analyses were performed, using each of the four coping subscales to predict the Short Form-36 physical and mental quality of life at treatment-end, while controlling for quality of life and symptom-burden at the final treatment. Greater focus on symptoms predicted less improvement in physical and mental quality of life at follow-up. Greater information-seeking was associated with greater improvement in physical quality of life at follow-up.

Prostate Cancer

There have been relatively few studies evaluating the role of coping in the psychological adjustment of men diagnosed with prostate cancer. Perczek and colleagues (2002) conducted a longitudinal study administering the COPE and the POMS at pre-biopsy and at two weeks post-diagnosis to a sample of 101 men. Longitudinal regression, predicting POMS at two weeks, indicated that pre-biopsy avoidance coping was the only predictor of POMS distress two weeks post-diagnosis.

Green and colleagues (2002) administered the COPE to a group of 65 men with non-localized prostate cancer at two time points, spaced six month apart. Longitudinal regression analyses, predicting health-related quality of life subscales, indicated that higher emotion- or problem-focused coping was associated with more physical and urinary symptoms and lower subjective ratings of cognitive functioning.

Prostate Cancer: Survivorship Phase

The association between coping style and depressive symptoms was evaluated in a small cross-sectional sample of 30 men with prostate cancer, who were approximately six years post-diagnosis (Bjorck, Hopp, & Jones, 1999). Longitudinal regression analyses included the four MAC scales, three items assessing appraisal of cancer threat, and a measure of optimism. Given that the sample size was only 30 and that there were eight predictors included in the equation, there was likely insufficient power to detect contributions of coping to outcome. Nevertheless, emotional functioning was predicted by higher helplessness and more anxious preoccupation. Univariate regression analyses indicated that helplessness was negatively associated with self-esteem and that anxious preoccupation was associated with higher depression.

Gastrointestinal Cancer

Little is known regarding the association between coping and distress among individuals diagnosed with gastrointestinal cancer. Matsushita and colleagues (2005) studied 85 individuals diagnosed with stomach, colon, rectal, esophageal, pancreatic, or liver cancer. Participants completed the Coping Inventory for Stressful Situations (CISS), which assesses general style of coping with stressful situations and measures of distress and quality of life before surgery, before surgical discharge, and six months after discharge. The investigators conducted analyses predicting pre-discharge quality of life, controlling for relevant demographic and medical variables. Results indicated that participants reporting more emotion-oriented coping style had a lower pre-discharge quality of life. This coping style was characterized by self-blame and wishful thinking. Coping predictors of post-discharge quality of life were not evaluated.

Wasteson and colleagues (2002) used a daily assessment methodology to evaluate the relation between coping and distress among a sample of 95 individuals with gastrointestinal cancer. Participants completed the Daily Assessment of Coping (DCA) and a daily assessment of mood for one week. Correlational analyses indicated that there was a significant positive association between venting of emotions and higher depression.

Lung Cancer

One of the earliest studies of coping among individuals diagnosed with lung cancer was conducted by Akechi and colleagues (1998), who administered the MAC to a sample of 87 participants in active treatment. The results of this cross-sectional study indicated that the helplessness/hopelessness subscale of the MAC was associated with greater mood disturbance on the POMS.

Kuo and Ma (2002) administered the CSI, along with measures of mood and physical symptoms, to a sample of 73 individuals who were diagnosed with non-small cell lung cancer and who were undergoing active treatment for their disease. Results of cross-sectional regression analyses predicting psychological distress indicated that, after accounting for physical symptom distress, greater frequency of use of emotion-focused coping was associated with higher psychological distress.

Walker and colleagues (2006) evaluated a path model, in which coping was a mediator between social support and depressive symptoms. The COPE was factor-analyzed and two scales were formed: (a) adaptive coping, comprised of active coping and planning, suppression of competing activities, restraint, seeking support for emotional and instrumental reasons, positive reinterpretation and growth, and acceptance; and (b) non-adaptive coping, which was comprised of focus on and venting of emotions, denial, and behavioral and mental disengagement. A path model was tested using structural equation modeling. The final model indicated that non-direct instrumental support was associated with more adaptive coping, and direct instrumental support was associated with less adaptive coping. Higher adaptive coping and lower non-adaptive coping were significantly associated with lower depressive symptoms.

Gynecological Cancer

There has been only one published study evaluating the role of coping in adaptation to gynecological cancer. Constanzo and colleagues (2006) found that positive reframing and acceptance were associated with better functional well-being, while mental disengagement and cognitive avoidance were related to poorer emotional well-being, greater anxiety, and greater depressed mood. Behavioral disengagement was associated with poorer functional well-being and marginally with greater anxiety. Denial was also associated with greater anxiety. Active coping, seeking instrumental support, and active engagement were not significantly associated with quality of life. Additional analyses suggested that cognitive avoidance and instrumental support were more strongly associated with better quality of life among women undergoing more extensive treatment for their disease.

Head and Neck Cancer

Individuals undergoing treatment for head and neck cancer endure aggressive and prolonged treatment, which typically causes disabling and/or disfiguring side effects, such as trouble swallowing and speaking. Despite the importance of understanding the potential role of coping in adaptation to this illness, there has been relatively little attention paid to this topic. One of the first studies was conducted by Dropkin (2001), who used a prospective design to evaluate the association between the Ways of Coping Questionnaire and state anxiety. This study was unique, because the investigators rated participants' self-care and resocialization behaviors after surgery by participant observation (by the study author). Pre-operative coping, post-operative anxiety, and self-care were assessed. There was no association between pre-operative coping and either anxiety, self-care, or resocialization.

    Sherman and colleagues (2000) found that denial, behavioral disengagement, and emotional ventilation were associated with greater distress among individuals diagnosed with advanced head and neck cancer. These investigators evaluated differences in the strength of the associations between coping and distress across phases of treatment, and found that coping was least tied to distress among the participants who had completed treatment.

Psychological Interventions to Improve Coping with Cancer

Because the literature on psychological and/or behavioral interventions to improve adaptation to cancer is extensive, in the interest of space the reader is referred to a number of excellent meta-analyses of this literature (e.g., Barsevick, Swenney, Haney, & Chung 2002; Devine & Westlake, 1995; Newell, Sanson-Fisher, & Savolainen, 2002; Sheard & Maguire, 1999). Rather than provide an exhaustive review of this literature, two parameters will be set on this review.

First, cognitive-behavioral or skill-based intervention studies, which are designed to improve coping strategies that are assumed to be associated with better adaptation to cancer, will be reviewed. These interventions include active problem-solving, communication, and relaxation/stress management skills. Although it could be argued that the goal of supportive-expressive therapy and of non-directive supportive counseling approaches is to improve emotional expressivity, these interventions are not skill-based treatments, and therefore will not be included in this review. Second, the review will be limited to randomized clinical trials that were conducted during the past ten years, because the quality of work that has been conducted during this time has improved dramatically.

Breast Cancer: Treatment Phase

Women undergoing autologous bone marrow transplantation (ABMT) for treatment of stage two to four breast cancer may suffer from a number of aversive side effects, which can include pain, fatigue, and nausea, as well as from persistent distress reactions. Gaston-Johansson and colleagues (2000) developed a coping strategy program to assist women in dealing with BMT. This intervention was delivered to participants two weeks prior to ABMT, in order to prepare participants for side effects of treatment and to assist them in learning coping strategies. Education regarding pain management through the use of guided imagery relaxation, coping self-statements, and cognitive restructuring was provided. Participants were given handouts with coping self-statements and audiotaped relaxation instructions. Compared to women in the no-treatment condition, women participating in this intervention reported significantly less nausea and fatigue seven days after ABMT. There were no differences between the groups on psychological distress.

Antoni and colleagues (2001) conducted a widely-cited trial that tested the efficacy of cognitive-behavioral stress management (CBSM) for women with early stage breast cancer. This randomized clinical trial compared the treatment of ten two-hour group sessions, which focused on learning to manage stress by means of relaxation and cognitive restructuring, interpersonal problem resolution, and assertion training, with the treatment of a one-day seminar, in which participants reviewed similar material. One hundred participants completed the trial. Although results did not suggest that the CBSM had significant effects on POMS distress, CES-D, and IES scores, the prevalence of clinically-significant levels of depression was significantly lower in the CBSM group, than in the one-day seminar group. Benefit-finding was significantly higher in the CBSM group, compared with the one-day seminar group.

Andersen and colleagues' (2005) evaluated the effects of 18-session group psycho-educational intervention, compared with a usual care condition, on general quality of life and mood (as assessed by the POMS). Although basic education regarding proper diet and exercise practices was provided in four of the 18 sessions, cognitive-behavioral skills training (e.g., relaxation, coping, communication skills) was included in all 18 sessions, and thus formed a primary focus of this intervention. Scores on the POMS mood disturbance declined significantly more in the intervention group than the usual care condition, but only among those participants who reported high cancer-related stress in the beginning of the study. The psycho-educational intervention had significant effects on other measures of quality of life, including social adjustment, health behaviors, and immunity, compared with the usual care condition.

Manne and colleagues (2005) conducted a randomized clinical trial of a couple-focused group intervention for women with early stage breast cancer and their partners. Two hundred thirty eight couples were assigned to a six-session, couple-focused communication and coping skills group (CG) or to usual care (UC). Intent-to-treat analyses (ITT) suggested that women participating in the couple-focused group intervention reported significantly lower depressive symptoms. Subgroup analyses were conducted, comparing three groups: women, who were assigned to the couple-focused group intervention and who attended one or more of the group sessions (CG); women, who were assigned to the couple-focused intervention and who did not attend any group sessions (CG-attrition); and women, who were assigned to UC. These analyses evaluated whether attendance at the intervention had any effects on distress. Analyses indicated significant differences between CG and UC on all measures of distress. This study also evaluated the effects of one moderator variable: pre-intervention patient ratings of partner unsupportive behavior. Results of the ITT analyses indicated that CG had a significantly greater impact on distress and positive well-being of women, who rated their partners as unsupportive at pre-intervention, compared with women who did not rate their partners as unsupportive at pre-intervention. Similar results, but of smaller effect sizes, were reported for the subgroup analyses comparing CG, CG-attrition, and UC.

Early Stage Breast Cancer: Survivorship

Several recent RCTs have focused on facilitating re-entry into normal life after cancer treatment has been completed. Stanton and colleagues (2005) conducted an RCT comparing: a) Print material ("*Facing Forward*") (CTL); b) print material and a videotape of survivors, who described their survivorship experiences and how they coped with them (VID); and c) print material, the videotape described above, along with one individual in-person counseling session and one telephone counseling session, in which the participant identified concerns regarding re-entry into normal life and developed a plan for how to actively cope with each issue (EDU). Five hundred and fifty-eight women were randomized to a study condition, and 418 completed the six-month assessment. Results indicated that the VID intervention produced a significantly greater improvement in the Vitality scale of the SF-36, compared with the CTL condition. These interventions did not have significant effects on the IES, CES-D, or on posttraumatic growth.

Scheier and colleagues (2005) compared the impact, of four group-education sessions, four group-nutrition sessions, and usual care, on the quality of life of 250 women diagnosed with breast cancer prior to age 50. Educational topics included: stress management, developing meaning in life, regaining or maintaining relationship closeness, talking to one's children about cancer, as well as non-psychological topics. Outcome measures included: health-related quality of life, depressive symptoms (CES-D), and the COPE Scale. Repeated-measures analysis of variance indicated no treatment effects at the second assessment, but treatment effects on depressive symptoms for the nutrition intervention at the third assessment, compared with usual care. There were no treatment effects on mental health, as measured by the quality of life scale. Tests of potential mediating effects of coping on the depressive symptoms at Time 3 indicated that the educational intervention had indirect effects via intrusive thoughts, self-concept, self-efficacy, cancer concerns regarding recurrence and mortality, planning coping, and denial coping on depression. Only intrusive thoughts, self-concept, and self-efficacy remained as significant mediators when all variables were included in the analyses.

Gynecologic Cancer

Despite the poor prognosis and the difficult treatment course endured by women treated for gynecologic cancers, there has been very little empirical work evaluating the efficacy of psychological interventions for this population. The one published study evaluating the efficacy of psychological intervention did not report favorable results. Chan and colleagues (2005) enrolled 155 women, who were newly diagnosed with gynecological malignancy, in an RCT that evaluated the efficacy of an individual intervention versus a no-treatment control group. The intervention included the core components of stress management, relaxation, pain and distress management, and cognitive behavioral therapy. Unfortunately, the treatment was not standardized in terms of its content. The number of sessions conducted was unclear, as sessions were held bi-weekly during treatment, and every six weeks during follow-up. There were no significant effects of the intervention on quality of life, depressive symptoms, the IES, or self-efficacy.

Melanoma

There have been two studies evaluating the efficacy of a cognitive-behavioral intervention for individuals diagnosed with melanoma. In one study, 52 participants were randomly assigned to either a four-session individual cognitive-behavioral intervention or to usual care (Trask, Paterson, Griffith, Rib, & Schwartz, 2003). The intervention entailed relaxation, cognitive restructuring, and problem-solving. This study focused only on individuals who had significant levels of pre-intervention distress. The results suggested that the intervention did not reduce overall distress, but did show effects on anxiety and quality of life at six months post-intervention.

A second intervention study evaluated a group intervention that incorporated six sessions of psychoeducation focusing on stress management and problem-solving skills (Boesen et al., 2005). The control group received usual care. At six months post-intervention, participants in the intervention group showed less fatigue, more vigor, and lower total mood disturbance, as compared to the usual-care group participants. The intervention group utilized more active-behavioral and active-cognitive coping than the usual-care group participants. At the one-year follow-up, there were no group differences on other mood indicators, including depression, anxiety, and anger and no between-group differences on any outcome.

Prostate Cancer

The same cognitive-behavioral stress management intervention (CBSM), as has been used to assist women diagnosed with early stage breast cancer, has been evaluated among men diagnosed with early stage prostate cancer (Penedo et al., 2004). A ten-week CBSM group intervention was compared with a half-day seminar, which covered similar material. Results from the 92 participants, who had completed radiation therapy within the past 18 months, indicated those who attended the CBSM group reported significant improvements in quality of life, whereas quality of life did not change in the comparison group. Results indicated that stress-management skills mediated the effects of CBSM on quality of life.

Lepore, Helgeson, Eton, and Schulz (2003) conducted a randomized clinical trial (RCT), comparing group education, group education plus discussion, and usual care. Participants in the educational group attended six weekly lectures that included medical topics, stress-management skills, relationships, and sexuality. Men received print materials summarizing the lectures. The information was presented in a didactic format with no in-session practice or home assignments. In the education plus discussion group, participants discussed how the lecture topic was relevant to group members, following the initial lecture. There were significant improvements in quality of life reported among less-educated men, who participated in the two intervention conditions, as compared to men enrolled in the usual-care condition.

Mixed Tumor Sites

There have been a number of studies targeting individuals diagnosed with a variety of cancers. One study, which reported the strongest effects for a psychological intervention, was conducted by Nezu and colleagues (2003). The researchers conducted a RCT, evaluating the efficacy of ten sessions of problem-solving therapy alone (PST), compared with PST with a significant other (PST-SO), and a wait-list control (WL). Women with mixed types of cancer and their significant others participated. Only individuals reporting clinical levels of distress were eligible for this study. The results suggested that there was a significant effect on all multiple indicators of distress. PST and PST-SO participants reported significantly lower distress at follow-up, compared with WL participants. PST-SO outperformed PST at six months and at one year. This study is one of the few trials that reported both large effect size estimates and clinical significance.

Scott and colleagues (2004) investigated the efficacy of a couple-focused communication and coping skills intervention for women (CanCOPE) with breast or gynecological cancer and their husbands. Participants, who were assigned to the CanCOPE group, received five two-hour couple sessions at pre-surgery, one week, one month, five weeks, and three months post-surgery. The comparison group received medical information about medical care and telephone education about medical assistance for treatment side effects (MI), or basic coping and stress-management skills counseling given to the participant alone (PC). Distress outcome measures included the Psychological Distress (PD) subscale of the Psychosocial Adjustment to Illness Scale- Self-Report (PAIS-SR) and the Impact of Events scale (IES). Results demonstrated that the CanCOPE group reported lower psychological distress on the PAIS-SR PD Scale, as compared to the MI and PC groups. The CanCOPE group reported lower IES avoidance at follow-up, compared with the MI group. The PC group reported less IES avoidance at follow-up, compared with the MI group.

Several recent studies have supported the efficacy of mindfulness meditation-based stress reduction interventions. Speca and colleagues (2000) conducted a RCT testing seven sessions of mindfulness meditation, with a wait-list control, among a heterogenous sample of individuals being treated for cancer. The objectives of the mindfulness meditation program were to develop an understanding of one's responses to stress and to teach meditation as a way of managing stress. Only 43 participants completed the intervention and only 36 participants formed the wait-list control group. Participants in the mindfulness meditation program reported lower POMS mood disturbance at an immediate post-intervention follow-up than participants in the wait-list control. Between-group differences in POMS mood disturbance reductions were striking (65% vs 12%). These differences were maintained at a six-month follow-up (Carlson, Ursuliak, Goodey, Angen, & Speca, 2001). Similar results were reported for an eight-week mindfulness-based stress reduction intervention for participants with early stage breast or prostate cancer, with effects also noted on sleep quality (Carlson & Garland, 2005).

A number of studies have evaluated stress-management techniques as a way to control treatment side-effects. Burish and colleagues (1991) randomized participants into two groups: (a) Receipt of one to three sessions of progressive muscle relaxation and guided imagery, with additional sessions during chemotherapy infusions; or (b) a no-treatment control. Participants who received relaxation training reported less anticipatory nausea and less post-treatment emotional distress. Similar results were reported by others (Lerman et al., 1990; Walker, Nail, & Croyle, 1999). Jacobsen and colleagues (2002) compared one session of a professionally-administered relaxation training prior to chemotherapy with a self-administered relaxation training and a no-treatment control. Compared with participants receiving no treatment, participants who received the self-administered relaxation training reported greater quality of life and well-being. The professionally-administered relaxation training had no impact on quality of life and well-being.

One novel intervention approach that has recently received more empirical attention is a meaning-making intervention. These interventions are designed to assist individuals diagnosed with serious illness find purpose and meaning in life. Meaning-making coping includes attempts to reconcile priorities and assumptions about the world and one's life, which are typically challenged by the diagnosis of a life-threatening disease. Lee and colleagues (2006) conducted one of the only RCTs evaluating a meaning–making intervention. Individuals diagnosed with either colorectal or breast cancer were offered up to four sessions of meaning-making therapy or usual care. Individual sessions focused on: (a) Their responses to cancer, (b) the way they are coping with the cancer, (c) how they reflect on life priorities that have been challenged by the cancer diagnosis, and (d) their understanding of how life priorities have changed since the diagnosis. Results from the relatively small sample of participants ($n < 50$ in each group) indicated that participants in the meaning-making therapy reported significant increases in self-esteem, optimism, and self-efficacy, compared with the usual-care group.

Empirical Issues and Challenges for the Field

Before drawing conclusions about the role of coping in adaptation to cancer, it is important to review the widely-cited critiques of the general descriptive literature that examines the association between coping and psychological outcomes. Over the last three decades, there have been literally hundreds of studies published using standardized self-report coping checklists. Coyne and colleagues published two critiques of this literature, which summarized the key problems with this approach to measuring coping (Coyne and Gottlieb, 1996; Coyne & Racioppo, 2000). Rather than providing an exhaustive review of issues in the general coping literature, key issues that are relevant to the study of coping with cancer will be discussed.

One important issue is the mismatch of the approach used to measure coping strategies with the underlying theory. Although Lazarus and Folkman's theory proposes a process, which entails making judgments about the controllability and threat of a specific situation, and consequently selecting specific coping strategies to deal with the situation, followed by an evaluation of the effectiveness of the strategy and making adjustments if necessary, coping checklists do not approach the assessment in this manner. Rather, individuals are asked how often they used a particular strategy when dealing with a stressor, but they are only infrequently asked what appraisals they made regarding the stressor. Further, they are never asked whether they evaluated the strategy's effectiveness and made adjustments, or whether the coping strategy was effective.

Second, the instructional set of coping measures is typically vague, asking individuals to rate how they coped with the stress of "cancer." Thus, we do not know whether the individual is reporting that he or she *typically* uses a strategy, or if he or she used this strategy in a specific situation. Cancer is a complex condition with a number of controllable stressors (e.g., treatment options, selection of hospital and physician, how interpersonal stressors are handled, amount of self-disclosure) and uncontrollable stressors (e.g., disease stage and course, waiting for medical appointments, reactions of family and friends). The general nature of the instructional set in coping measures results in participants reporting coping strategies that they use with a variety of stressors. This complicates measurement, in addition to the factor of individual differences in the controllability and threat of the types of stressors selected.

A third issue is that there is often circularity with regard to the constructs of coping and distress. For example, if individuals are not experiencing negative emotion, they typically will not engage in attempts to delve into and understand emotions. It is unclear whether the attempts to understand negative emotions actually predict distress, or whether distress prompts attempts to comprehend one's emotions. A fourth problem is that most coping checklists do not ask participants whether they *consciously* selected a particular coping strategy, or whether the behavior was more a habit or routine. For example, it is unlikely that individuals consciously select self-criticism or wishful thinking as a way of coping with cancer. These behaviors most likely reflect less conscious, automatic responses to stressful situations that are based upon past history. Definitions of coping specify that the individual appraise a situation and select a way of dealing with the situation, rather than automatically responding to a stressor.

Finally, and perhaps most importantly, Coyne and Gottlieb (1996) point out that distress may not be an appropriate way of determining the coping outcomes. A person may judge a coping strategy to be effective, even though it causes more distress. For example, talking to a friend about an interpersonal conflict may be upsetting, but the coping strategy would be appraised as effective and successful, because the person was able to discuss the conflict with the friend and the friend altered his or her behavior. Thus, it is not always clear that distress is the most appropriate way of evaluating the effectiveness of coping efforts, at least in the short run.

Each of these criticisms is relevant to the literature on coping with cancer that was reviewed in this chapter. These perspectives influence the strength of the conclusions that can be made, regarding associations between coping and psychological adaptation to cancer. There are three additional weaknesses to the coping with cancer literature, which should also be acknowledged. First, many studies ask participants to rate coping "styles" (e.g., the Mental Adjustment to Cancer Scale), which reflect *dispositional* coping styles, rather than actual coping choices made by participants. Second, the way that coping strategies are grouped together to form constructs varies widely from study to study. Although the labels for the coping constructs are similar across studies, it is clear that coping strategies included in each construct differ. A lack of consistency, about which coping strategies are included in larger constructs, poses a problem in drawing conclusions about the effects of coping on adaptation.

Third, relatively few studies use longitudinal methodology. Among those studies employing longitudinal methods, analyses do not always use appropriate statistical methods, such as evaluating both changes in psychological outcome over time and changes in coping over time. More sophisticated methods such as growth curve modeling, which take into account trajectories of change in both coping and adaptation, have not typically been used.

Implications of Research

Despite the aforementioned weaknesses and criticisms of published research, there are consistent results across studies. Among women diagnosed with early stage breast cancer, observational studies suggest that avoidant coping strategies, which include both cognitive efforts to avoid thinking about the problem (e.g., wishful thinking) or behavioral efforts to avoid thinking about the problem (e.g., drinking or eating) have been found to be associated with poorer adaptation (Brain, Williams, Iredale, France, & Gray, 2006; Carver et al., 1993; Hack & Degner, 2004; List et al., 2002; McCaul et al., 1999; Stanton & Snider, 1993), although one study did not find such a relationship (Epping-Jordan et al., 1999;). Unfortunately, there is little evidence from intervention studies to bolster the conclusions about avoidance, because interventions have not focused solely on reducing avoidant coping. An implied focus on reducing avoidance is made in many cognitive-behavioral interventions. For example, both Antoni et al.'s CBSM (2001) and Andersen et al.'s group interventions (2005) teach assertiveness skills, and Nezu and colleagues (2003) focuses on active problem-solving. The focus on active coping with cancer implies that avoidance is not encouraged. However, there is no direct content targeted towards reducing avoidant coping; avoidant coping also is not assessed as a mediating mechanism for intervention effects.

There is less consistent evidence to support a beneficial role for practical and cognitive, active coping strategies, such as information-seeking, problem-solving, and cognitive restructuring in observational studies (Epping-Jordan et al., 1999; Ransom et al., 2005). However, it can be implied from intervention studies that target problem-solving (Nezu et al., 2003), stress management (Antoni et al., 2001), and relaxation and mindful meditation skills (Carlson & Garland, 2005), which actively attempt to manage symptoms and stress, are effective. A similar issue arises with evaluating what the mechanisms of change are for these interventions. The field has not progressed to the point in which mechanisms of change have been identified. The few studies that have examined mechanisms of change (Penedo et al., 2004) have not used coping measures that measure constructs from the coping literature. Penedo and colleagues (2004) found that stress-management skills mediated improvements in quality of life for participants in CBSM. Yet, stress-management skills do not comprise a coping strategy that is included in coping schemas. Therefore, it would be helpful if future intervention studies more clearly mapped intervention content to the coping strategies that are targeted by the intervention. If an intervention proved effective, then these coping strategies would be evaluated as mechanisms responsible for changes in quality of life.

Over the course of the last decade, there has been an increased interest in coping with cancer by emotional expression. Stanton and colleagues (2005) have reported that women, who are diagnosed with early stage breast cancer and who engage in emotional expression, reported lower levels of distress. However, there is other work suggesting that expressing emotions is not associated with distress (Walker et al., 1999). In addition, interventions focusing on assisting individuals express their emotional reactions (e.g., expressive writing) has either not supported the efficacy of these interventions on psychological outcomes (e.g., de Moor et al., 2002; Rosenberg et al., 2002), or suggested that expressive writing may reduce distress among subgroups of individuals, who use avoidant coping (Stanton et al., 2005), or who have unsupportive social networks (Zakowski, Ramati, Morton, Johnson, & Flanigan, 2004).

Overall, there has been a failure to link the content of psychological interventions with measures that evaluate coping and with the findings from the observational literature. While avoidance has consistently been found to be a strong correlate of poorer adaptation, reducing cognitive and behavioral avoidance is not explicitly targeted in the intervention, nor is it measured as an outcome or mediating mechanism. Similarly, although active problem-solving and cognitive restructuring are incorporated into many cognitive-behavioral interventions, these constructs are not measured in studies as either outcomes or mediators. Even in view of Coyne's position that scientists can learn more about coping's effects by focusing on the outcomes of clinical interventions (Coyne & Racioppo, 2000), the fact remains that the goals and targets of the vast majority of psychological interventions for individuals diagnosed with cancer are typically broader than simply instilling coping skills. Most interventions are multi-component interventions that incorporate other elements such as medical information, emotional support from peers with cancer, and non-specific components of most psychotherapies (e.g., bonding with therapists).

Finally, as can be easily seen from this literature review, most of the attention has been given to women diagnosed with breast cancer. Less is known about coping and adaptation to other types of cancer. Although it is probable that coping serves a similar function among individuals diagnosed with other types of cancer, it is likely that effective coping with more advanced stages of disease differs from earlier stages. It is also likely that different types of interventions, such as meaning-making or existential approaches, may prove more effective among individuals facing terminal illness.

Summary

In summary, there has been a great deal of observational and interventional research on individuals diagnosed with cancer, which has shed some light on the role of coping in adaptation to cancer. However, this literature suffers from many of the same flaws that characterize the general literature on coping. Although the field of coping research should probably not choose to "raze the slum before further building," as was suggested by Coyne & Racioppo (2000, p. 658), psycho-oncology researchers should attempt to assess coping using a more dynamic approach that includes appraisals of coping effectiveness, evaluations of the degree of choice in the usage of coping strategies, and an examination of changes in the use of coping strategies over the course of dealing with different stressors. There also should be some consensus with regard to measurement and categories of coping across studies. Research evaluating coping-skills interventions should include specific—not general—measures of coping, in order to evaluate whether coping strategies are indeed the mechanisms of change. Finally, future studies of coping strategies and future intervention studies would benefit from evaluating the impact of interventions upon participants' social and vocational functioning. As rates of cancer survivorship increase, long-term social and vocational functioning will become an important area of quality of life to evaluate.

References

Akechi, T., Kugaya, A., Okamura, H., Nishiwaki, Y., Yamawaki, S., & Uchitomi, Y. (1998). Predictive factors for psychological distress in ambulatory lung cancer patients. *Support Care Cancer, 6*, 281–286.

American Cancer Society. (2005). *Cancer Facts and Figures.* Retrieved July 6, 2006, from http://www.cancer.org/docroot/STT/content/STT_1x_Cancer_Facts__Figures_2005.asp

Andersen, B., Farrar, W., Golden-Kreutz, D., Glaser, R., Emery, C., Crespin, T., et al. (2005). Psychological, behavioral, and immune changes after a psychological intervention: A clinical trial. *Journal of Clinical Oncology, 22*, 3570–3580.

Antoni, M., Lehman, J., Kilbourn, K., Boyers, A., Culver, J. Alferi, S., et al. (2001). Cognitive behavioral stress management intervention decreases the prevalence of depression and enhances benefit-finding among women under treatment for early stage breast cancer. *Health Psychology, 20*, 20–32.

Barsevick, A. M., Swenney, C., Haney, E., & Chung, E. (2002). A systematic qualitative analysis of psychoeducational interventions for depression in patients with cancer. *Oncology Nursing Forum, 29*, 73–84.

Ben-Zur, H., Gilbur, O., & Lev, S. (2001). Coping with breast cancer: Patient, spouse, and dyad models. *Psychosomatic Medicine, 63*, 32–39.

Bjorck, J. P., Hopp, D. P., & Jones, L. W. (1999). Prostate cancer and emotional functioning: Effects of mental adjustment, optimism, and appraisal. *Journal of Psychosocial Oncology, 17*(1), 71–85.

Boesen, E., Ross, L., Frederickson, K., Thomsen, B., Dahlstrom, K., Schmidt, G., et al. (2005). Psychological intervention for patients with cutaneous malignant melanoma. *Journal of Clinical Oncology, 23*, 1270–1277.

Brain, K., Williams, B., Iredale, R., France, L., & Gray, J. (2006). Psychological distress in men with breast cancer. *Journal of Clinical Oncology, 24*(1), 95–101.

Burish, T., Snyder, S., & Jenkins, R. (1991). Preparing patients for cancer chemotherapy: Effect of coping preparation and relaxation interventions. *Journal of Consulting and Clinical Psychology, 59*, 518–525.

Carlson, L., & Garland, S. (2005). Impact of mindfulness based stress reduction on sleep, mood, stress and fatigue symptoms in cancer outpatients. *International Journal of Behavioral Medicine, 12*, 278–285.

Carlson, L., Ursuliak, Z., Goodey, E., Angen, M., & Speca, M. (2001). The effects of a mindfulness meditation-based stress reduction program on mood and symptoms of stress in cancer outpatients: 6 month follow up *Supportive Care in Cancer, 9*, 112–123.

Carver, C. S., Pozo, C., Harris, S. D., Noriega, V., Scheier, M. F., Robinson, D., et al. (1993). How coping mediates the effect of optimism on distress:A study of women with early stage breast cancer. *Journal of Personality and Social Psychology, 65*(2), 375–390.

Chan, D., Lee, P., Fong, D., Fung, A., Wu, L., Choi, A., et al. (2005). Effect of individual psychological intervention in chinese women with gynecologic malignancy: A randomized clinical trial. *Journal of Clinical Oncology, 23*, 4913–4924.

Compas, B. E., Stoll, M., Thomsen, A., Oppendisano, G., Epping-Jordan, J., & Krag, D. N. (1999). Adjustment to breast cancer: Age-related differences in coping and emotional distress. *Breast Cancer Research and Treatment, 54*, 195–203.

Constanzo, E. S., Lutgendorf, S. K., Rothrock, N. R., & Anderson, B. (2006). Coping and quality of life among women extensively treated for gynecologic cancer. *Psycho-Oncology, 15*, 132–142.

Coyne, J., & Gottlieb, G. (1996). The mismeasure of coping by checklist. *Journal of Personality, 54*, 959–991.

Coyne, J., & Racioppo, M. (2000). Never the twain shall meet? Closing the gap between coping research and clinical intervention research. *American Psychologist, 55*, 655–664.

Culver, J., Arena, P., Antoni, M., & Carver, C. (2002). Coping and distress among women under treatment for early stage breast cancer: Comparing African Americans, Hispanics, and non-Hispanic Whites. *Psychooncology, 11*, 495–504.

de Moor, C., Sterner, J., Hall, M., Warneke, C., Gilani, Z., Amato, R., et al. (2002). A pilot study of the effects of expressive writing on psychological and behavioral adjustment in patients enrolled in a Phase II trial of vaccine therapy for metastatic renal cell carcinoma. *Health Psychology, 21*(6), 615–619.

Devine, E. C., & Westlake, S. K. (1995). The effects of psychoeducational care provided to adults with cancer: Meta-analysis of 116 studies. *Oncology Nursing Forum, 22*, 1369–1381.

Dropkin, M. (2001). Anxiety, coping strategies, and coping behaviors in patients undergoing head and neck cancer surgery. *Cancer Nursing, 24*(2), 143–148.

Edwards, B. K., Brown, M. L., Wingo, P. A., Howe, H. L., Ward, E., Ries, L. A., et al. (2005). Annual report to the nation on the status of cancer, 1975–2002, featuring population-based trends in cancer treatment. *Journal of the National Cancer Institute, 97*(19), 1407–1427.

Engstrom, P. F., Benson, A., Chen, Y., Choti, M., Dilawari, R., Enke, C. et al. (2005). Colon cancer clinical practice guidelines in oncology. *Journal of the National Comprehensive Cancer Network, 3*, 468–491.

Epping-Jordan, J. E., Compas, B. E., Osowiecki, D. M., Oppedisano, G., Gerhardt, C., Primo, K., et al. (1999). Psychological adjustment in breast cancer: Process of emotional distress. *Health Psychology, 18*(4), 315–326.

Fisher, A., Anderson, S., Redmond, C., Wolmark, N., Wickerham, L., Cronin, W. M. (1995). Reanalysis and results after 12 years of follow up in a randomized clinical trial comparing total mastectomy and lumpectomy with or without irradiation in the treatment of breast cancer. *New England Journal of Medicine, 333*, 1456–1461.

Gaston-Johansson, F., Fall-Dickson, J., Nanda, J., Ohly, K., Stillman, S., Krumm, S., et al. (2000). The effectiveness of the Comprehensive Coping Strategy Program on clinical outcomes in breast cancer autologous bone marrow transplantation. *Cancer Nursing, 23*, 277–285.

Green, H. J., Pakenham, K. I., Headley, B. C., & Gardiner, R. A. (2002). Coping and health-related quality of life in men with prostate cancer randomly assisgned to hormonal medication or close monitoring. *Psycho-Oncology, 11*, 401–414.

Hack, T. F., & Degner, L. F. (2004). Coping responses following breast cancer diagnosis predict psychological adjustment three years later. *Psycho-Oncology, 13*(4), 235–247.

Holahan, C., & Moos, R. (1987). Personal and contextual determinants of coping strategies. *Journal of Personality and Social Psychology, 52*, 946–955.

Jacobsen, P., Meade, C., Stein, K., Chirikos, T., Small, B., & Ruckdeschel, J. (2002). Efficacy and costs of two forms of stress management training for cancer patients undergoing chemotherapy. *Journal of Clinical Oncology, 20*, 2851–2862.

Kuo, T., & Ma, F. (2002). Symptom distresses and coping strategies in patients with non-small cell lung cancer. *Cancer Nursing, 25*(4), 309–317.

Lazarus, R. T., & Folkman, S. (1984). *Stress, appraisal, and coping.* New York: Springer.

Lee, C., Cohen, S., Edgar, L., Laizner, A., & Gagnon, A. (2006). Meaning making intervention during breast or colorectal cancer treatment improves self-esteem, optimism and self-efficacy. *Social Science and Medicine, 62*, 3133–3145.

Lepore, S. J., Helgeson, V., Eton, D., & Schulz, R. (2003). Improving quality of life in men with prostate cancer: A randomized controlled trial of group education interventions. *Health Psychology, 22*, 443–452.

Lerman, C., Rimer, B., Blumberg, B., Cristinzio, S., Engstrom P., MacElwee, N., et al. (1990). Effects of coping style and relaxation on cancer chemotherapy side effects and emotional responses. *Cancer Nursing, 13*, 308–315.

List, M., Lee Rutherford, J., Stracks, J., Haraf, D., Kies, M., & Vokes, E. (2002). An exploration of the pretreatment coping strategies of patients with carcinoma of the head and neck. *Cancer, 95*(1), 98–104.

Manne, S., Ostroff, J., Winkel, G., Fox, K., Grana, G., Miller, E., et al. (2005). Couple-focused group intervention for women with early stage breast cancer. *Journal of Consulting and Clinical Psychology, 73*, 634–646.

Matsushita, T., Matsushima, E., & Maruyama, M. (2005). Psychological state, quality of life, and coping style in patients with digestive cancer. *General Hospital Psychiatry, 27*, 125–132.

McCaul, K., Sandgren, A., King, B., O'Donnell, S., Branstetter, A., & Foreman, G. (1999). Coping and adjustment to breast cancer. *Psychooncology, 8*(3), 230–236.

Newell, S., Sanson-Fisher, R., & Savolainen, N. (2002). Systematic review of psychological therapies for cancer patients: Overview and recommendations for future research. *Journal of the National Cancer Institute, 94*, 558–584.

Nezu, A., Nezu, C., Felgoise, S., McClure, K., & Houts, P. (2003). Project Genesis: Assessing the efficacy of problem-solving therapy for distressed adult cancer patients. *Journal of Consulting and Clinical Psychology, 71*, 1036–1048.

Nosarti, C., Roberts, J. V., Crayford, T., McKenzie, K., & David, A. S. (2002). Early psychological adjustment in breast cancer patients. *Journal of Psychosomatic Research, 53*, 1123–1130.

Osowiecki, D. M., & Compas, B. E. (1999). A prospective study of coping, perceived control, and psychological adaptation to breast cancer. *Cognitive Therapy and Research, 23*(2), 169–180.

Penedo, F., Dahn, J., Molton, I., Gonzalez, J., Kinsinger, D., Roos, B., et al. (2004). Cognitive behavioral stress management improves stress-management skills and quality of life in men recovering from treatment of prostate cancer. *Cancer, 100*, 192–200.

Perczek, R. E., Burke, M. A., Carver, C. S., Krongrad, A., & Terris, M. K. (2002). Facing a prostate cancer diagnosis: who is at risk for increased distress? *Cancer, 94*(11), 2923–2999.

Ransom, S., Jacobsen, P. B., Schmidt, J. E., & Andrykowski, M. A. (2005). Relationship of Problem-focused coping strategies to changes in quality of life following treatment for early stage breast cancer. *Journal of Pain and Symptom Management, 30*(3), 243–252.

Rosenberg, H., Rosenberg, S., Ernstoff, M., Wolford, G., Amdur, R., Elshamy, M., et al. (2002). Expressive disclosure and health outcomes in a prostate cancer population. *International Journal of Psychiatry in Medicine, 32*, 37–53.

Roth, S., & Cohen, L. J. (1986). Approach, avoidance, and coping with stress. *American Psychologist, 41*, 813–819.

Scardino, P. (2005). Update: NCCN prostate cancer clinical practice guidelines. *Journal of the National Comprehensive Cancer Network, 3*(Suppl.), S29–S33.

Scheier, M. F., Helgeson, V. S., Schulz, R., Colvin, S., Berga, S., Bridges, M. W., et al. (2005). Interventions to enhance physical and psychological functioning among younger women who are ending nonhormonal adjuvant treatment for early-stage breast cancer. *Journal of Clinical Oncology, 19*, 4298–4311.

Scott, J., Halford, K., & Ward, B. (2004). United we stand? The effects of a couple-coping intervention on adjustment to early stage breast or gynecological cancer. *Journal of Consulting and Clinical Psychology, 72*, 1122–1135.

Shapiro, C. E., Boggs, S. R., Rodrigue, J. R., Urry, H. L., Algina, J. J., Hellman, R., et al. (1997). Stage II breast cancer: Differences between four coping patterns in side effects during adjuvant chemotherapy. *Journal of Psychosomatic Research, 43*(2), 143–157.

Sheard, T., & Maguire, P. (1999). The effect of psychological interventions on anxiety and depression in cancer patients: results of two meta-analyses. *British Journal of Cancer, 80*, 1770–1780.

Sherman, A. C., Simonton, S., Adams, D. C., Vural, E., & Hanna, E. (2000). Coping with head and neck cancer during different phases of treatment. *Head & Neck, 22*(8), 787–793.

Speca, M., Carlson, L., Goodey, E., & Angen, M. (2000). A randomized, wait-list controlled clinical trial: the effect of mindfulness mediation-based stress reduction program on mood and symptoms of stress in cancer outpatients. *Psychosomatic Medicine, 62*, 613.

Stanton, A., Danoff-Burg, S., & Huggins, M. (2002). The first year after breast cancer diagnosis: Hope and coping strategies as predictors of adjustment. *Psychooncology, 11*(2), 93–102.

Stanton, A., Ganz, P, Kwan, P., Meyerowitz, B., Bower, J., Krupnick, J., et al. (2005). Outcomes from the Moving Beyond Cancer psychoeducational, randomized, controlled trial with breast cancer patients. *Journal of Clinical Oncology, 23*, 6009–6018.

Stanton, A., & Snider, P. (1993). Coping with a Breast Cancer Diagnosis: A prospective study. *Health Psychology, 12*, 16–23.

Trask, P., Paterson, A., Griffith, K., Riba, M., & Schwartz, J., (2003). Cognitive-behavioral intervention for distress in patients with melanoma. *Cancer, 98*, 854–864.

Walker, B., Nail, L., & Croyle, R. (1999). Does emotional expression make a different in reactions to breast cancer? *Oncology Nursing Forum, 25*, 1025–1032.

Walker, M. S., Zona, D. M., & Fisher, E. B. (2006). Depressive symptoms after lung cancer surgery: Their relation to coping style and social support. *Psycho-Oncology, 15*(8), 684–693.

Wasteson, E., Nordin, K., Hoffman, K., Glimelius, B., & Sjoden, P. (2002). Daily assessment of coping in patients with gastrointestinal cancer. *Psycho-Oncology, 11*, 1–11.

Zakowski, S., Ramati, A., Morton, C., Johnson, P., & Flanigan, R. (2004). Written emotional disclosure buffers the effects of social constraints on distress among cancer patients. *Health Psychology, 23*, 555–563.

11
Coping with Diabetes: Psychological Determinants of Diabetes Outcomes

Julie Wagner and Howard Tennen

Introduction

Diabetes is a stressful chronic disease. The goals of this chapter are to provide a primer on diabetes for the social scientist, and to review the literature on psychological determinants of diabetes outcomes, including temporally-primary, behavioral outcomes of adherence to the medical regimen, and temporally-secondary, physiological outcomes of disease control. This chapter is limited in its scope. It includes only research that examined psychological variables in established diabetes (as opposed to psychological variables as risk factors for incident diabetes). Additionally, this chapter is limited to the most common forms of diabetes: type 1 and type 2.

Medical Aspects of Diabetes

The Epidemiology and Burden of Diabetes

In 2005, 20.8 million people, or 7% of the US population had diabetes. Of them, 14.6 million were diagnosed and 6.2 million were undiagnosed (Centers for Disease Control [CDC], 2005). It is estimated that 41 million Americans also have pre-diabetes, a potent risk factor for type 2 diabetes and a serious health problem in it own right. Prevalence of type 2 diabetes is high and incidence is rising, with a 33% increase nationwide in the 1990s (Mokdad et al., 2000). Rising incidence can be attributed to national changes in risk-factor patterns, including rising rates of obesity and overweight people, an aging population, a larger proportion of racial and ethnic minorities in the general population, as well as lower thresholds for diabetes diagnosis.

Diabetes also incurs tremendous economic costs. In 2002, direct costs for diabetes (e.g., medication and medical professional services) were estimated to be $92 billion, and indirect costs (e.g., lost income and disability) were estimated to be $40 billion (CDC, 2005). Approximately half of this cost is spent on treatment of the metabolic condition per se, while the other half is spent on treatment of the long-term complications of diabetes. Thus, prevention of long-term complications is a primary goal of diabetes treatment.

Diabetes Etiology and Prevention

Diabetes is a heterogeneous group of glucose-dysregulation disorders, including type 1 diabetes, type 2 diabetes, gestational diabetes, pre-diabetes, and latent autoimmune diabetes in adults (LADA). An important related problem common to type 2 diabetes is the metabolic syndrome, which is the constellation of hypertension, dyslipidemia, hypercoagulability, glucose dysregulation, and adiposity. The two major subtypes of diabetes – type 1 and type 2 – will be the focus of this chapter.

Type 1

Type 1 diabetes is an autoimmune disorder characterized by an absolute insulin deficiency. In a healthy pancreas, beta cells produce insulin, a hormone that aids in the metabolism of glucose. In type 1 diabetes, these beta cells are destroyed by a malfunction of the body's own immune system. The result is an acute and permanent loss of insulin production, and as a consequence, elevated blood glucose, or hyperglycemia. Persons with type 1 diabetes must receive exogenous insulin for survival, which accounts for the previously-used term "insulin-dependent diabetes." The risk for type 1 diabetes involves genetic vulnerability, and persons of western European heritage are at increased risk for this type of diabetes. Onset is usually in childhood, with highest incidence during adolescence, which is why it was also previously referred to as "juvenile-onset" diabetes. Approximately 5% of individuals with diabetes have type 1 diabetes.

There is currently no cure for type 1 diabetes, but promising experimental protocols include beta-cell replacement. There is also no current prevention for type 1 diabetes. Two recent trials, which treated genetically at-risk relatives of individuals with type 1 diabetes with exogenous insulin, were not successful in preventing the onset of type 1 diabetes (Diabetes Prevention Trial-Type 1 Diabetes Study Group, 2002; Skyler et al., 2005). Work is underway to develop a vaccine to protect the beta cells from the autoimmune malfunction.

Type 2

Type 2 diabetes mellitus is a disorder characterized by a relative lack of insulin, due to progressive insulin resistance and gradual beta-cell failure, with individual variation in the contribution of each. Insulin resistance is the body's inability to properly use available insulin. In a process that is not fully understood, but is strongly related to adiposity, insulin resistance is the beginning of a cascade that can eventually lead to type 2 diabetes. Beta cells may compensate for insulin resistance by producing more insulin, a state referred to as hyperin-sulinemia. In many cases hyperinsulinemia successfully compensates for the insulin resistance. If, however, beta cells begin to fail, transient hyperglycemia results, 'impaired glucose tolerance' (IGT) or 'impaired fasting glucose' (IFG) can result. The presence of either IGT or IFG is referred to as 'pre-diabetes'. If beta-cell failure and/or insulin resistance progress further still, the result is overt type 2 diabetes. Because hyperglycemia develops gradually in type 2 diabetes, this form of diabetes frequently goes undiagnosed for many years. Delineating this cascade has proven to be important, because research suggests that the under-lying insulin resistance, not just overt hyperglycemia, is a strong independent risk factor for cardiovascular disease. It is estimated that over 20 million people have insulin resistance in the absence of pre-diabetes or diabetes (CDC, 2005).

Risk factors for type 2 diabetes include genetic vulnerability, obesity/overweight, physical inactivity, and race/ethnicity, with Native Americans, Hispanics, and African Americans at increased risk relative to non-Hispanic Whites. Increasing age is also a risk factor. While the majority of new cases are in adults, the incidence among children is rising, with most new cases coinciding with puberty. This is likely related to sedentary lifestyle, poor nutrition, and obesity in children.

Importantly, it is well demonstrated that type 2 diabetes can be prevented or delayed. The Diabetes Prevention Program showed that lifestyle modification (defined as 7% weight loss/management and 150 minutes of physical activity per week) decreased the incidence of type 2 diabetes by 58% (Knowler et al., 2002), and oral medication decreased incidence by 31%. International studies in Finland and China have shown similarly striking benefits for lifestyle interventions. Effectiveness trials are underway to translate these research protocols into practical interventions applicable to natural settings.

Long-Term Complications of Diabetes

Long-term complications of diabetes can be categorized as those affecting the macrovascular, microvascular, and neurological systems. Macrovascular compli-cations involve the arteries and large vessels that affect the heart and brain. The majority of morbidity and mortality in diabetes is due to cardiovascular disease. In fact, individuals with diabetes have risk of a myocardial infarction equal to individuals without diabetes who have already experienced an infarction (Haffner, Letho, Ronnemaa, Pyorala & Laakso, 1998). People with diabetes are more likely to develop cardiovascular disease, compared to individuals without diabetes (Jarrett, McCartney, & Keen, 1982), even after controlling for other risk factors (Kannel & McGee, 1979). Women with Type 2 are at particular risk. In fact, type 2 diabetes is the only disorder in which women have higher risk of coronary artery disease than men. Cerebrovascular disease, or stroke, is also a serious macrovascular complication. People with diabetes are two to four times more likely to have an ischemic stroke, and more likely to die once they have a stroke, than individuals without diabetes. Relative to Whites, African Americans are more likely to suffer strokes, secondary to diabetes (ADA, 2001).

Microvascular complications involve the small blood vessels, and primarily affect the eyes and kidneys. Diabetic eye disease, or retinopathy, is a common complication that involves changes in the retina, which can lead to vision impairment and blindness. Women, Hispanics, and African Americans are at increased risk for this complication, relative to men and non-Hispanic Whites (ADA, 2001). Kidney disease, or nephropathy, can lead to end-stage renal disease requiring dialysis or transplant. Rates of diabetic nephropathy are highest among Native Americans. Microvascular changes can occur in the sexual system, resulting in sexual dysfunction in men. Data show that individuals with diabetes are more aware of their risk for the disability associated with microvascular complications, than their risk for death by macrovascular complications (American Diabetes Association and the American College of Cardiology, 2002). Moreover, minorities are less aware of their risk for macrovascular disease than Whites (Wagner, Lacey, Abbott, de Groot, & Chyun, 2006).

Neurological complications affect the nervous system. Peripheral sensory neuropathy can be experienced as pain or as lack of sensation, particularly in the feet, and is present in 45–54% of individuals with diabetes (ADA, 2001). Peripheral neuropathy increases risk for puncture and laceration, which, in combination with impaired wound-healing, is a major contributor to lower limb amputation. Autonomic neuropathy can occur in the gastrointestinal system, resulting in gastroparesis, a disorder of gastric emptying. Most gravely, autonomic neuropathy can occur in the cardiac system, leading to silent myocardial ischemia, silent infarction, and sudden death.

Treatment of Diabetes and Prevention of its Complications

Several well-controlled trials with decades of follow-up show that the risk of some long-term complications can be reduced with proper diabetes treatment. The Diabetes Control and Complications Trial (Diabetes Control and Complications Trial Research Group, 1993) showed that intensive glycemic control significantly reduced risk of retinopathy, nephropathy, and neuropathy in individuals with type 1 diabetes. The United Kingdom Prospective Diabetes Study (UKPDS) showed similar results for individuals with type 2 (UKPDS Study Group, 1998). The gold standard indicator of glycemic control is a blood test of glycosylated hemoglobin A1c, also called 'A1c', which is routinely given in clinical practice. The A1c reflects average blood-glucose levels during the preceding six to ten weeks, with lower levels indicating tighter (better) glycemic control. Blood-pressure control and lipid management are also important treatment targets.

Diabetes Self-Management

The promise of the DCCT and UKPDS has not been translated into clinical practice for the majority of individuals with diabetes; tight glycemic control continues to be elusive for many. This is largely due to the numerous cognitive, psychological, social, and environmental barriers to diabetes self-care. Diabetes regimens contain all the aspects that make any regimen difficult to comply with. That is, lowest adherence rates occur: (a) Among individuals with have chronic disorders; (b) when lifestyle changes are required; (c) when treatment is complex, intrusive, and inconvenient; (d) when behaviors are not directly supervised; and (e) when prevention, instead of symptom reduction or cure, is the goal (Rodin & Salovey, 1989). Ruggiero et al. (1997) found that of 2056 respondents, 21.3% did not usually self-monitor blood glucose as prescribed, 58.5% did not usually exercise as prescribed, and 36.4% did not eat according to their prescribed meal plan. Adherence to medical components of the regimen (e.g., blood-glucose monitoring and medication administration) is typically higher than adherence to lifestyle components (e.g., exercise and nutrition).

Individuals with type 1 diabetes are usually prescribed a regimen of multiple daily insulin injections, or they may wear a 24-hour continuous subcutaneous insulin-infusion device (insulin pump). Although individuals with type 2 diabetes do not depend on insulin for survival, many require insulin for adequate glycemic control. Approximately 57% of individuals control their diabetes with oral agents only, and the remainder of individuals are fairly evenly split between insulin only, insulin plus oral agents, or diet only (CDC, 2005).

Diet is a cornerstone of diabetes care, and the typical diabetic food-plan emphasizes low-fat and high-fiber foods, avoidance of concentrated carbohydrates, and consumption of complex carbohydrates evenly across the course of the day. Regular physical activity is important for weight management, for the promotion of insulin sensitivity, and for the regulation of glucose levels. Interventions to improve self-management have shown varying success, with some also demonstrating improved glycemic control. For example, the Diabetes Stages of Change study used a theoretically-based intervention to improve smoking cessation, self-monitoring of blood glucose, and healthy eating among 1029 adults with diabetes. Results showed that relative to controls, the intervention group showed both improved self-care in the targeted areas, as well as improved glycemic control (Jones et al., 2003).

Short-Term Complications

The diabetes regimen is a balancing act, coordinating medication, carbohydrate intake, and physical activity. When this delicate balance is disrupted, as is often the case, short-term complications occur, which include episodes of hypo- and hyperglycemia. Furthermore, tightening glycemic control increases the likelihood of hypoglycemic episodes. Frequent and severe hypoglycemic episodes can lead to hypoglycemia unawareness, a dangerous condition in which the symptoms of hypoglycemia are not experienced.

*Hyper*glycemia results in idiosyncratic symptoms that may include thirst, nausea, fatigue, and vision changes. Hyperglycemia in type 1 diabetes can lead to diabetic ketoacidosis, an acute, life-threatening condition. Symptoms of *hypo*glycemia may include hunger, weakness, tremulousness, irritability, sweating, and impaired cognitive functioning. Hypoglycemia can be unpleasant, embarrassing, and dangerous. Untreated hypoglycemia can result in a range of problems, from unconsciousness, seizure, and death to accidents that can include driving mishaps (Cox et al., 2003).

Because individuals with diabetes are unreliable in their estimations of the treatment blood-glucose levels, and overconfident in their ability to make such estimations, the effectiveness of the treatment regimen must be continuously evaluated with multiple daily blood-glucose monitoring. Guidelines for insulin-users are typically four blood glucose checks per day, but many more are usually necessary to actually achieve tight glycemic control. Interventions to improve blood-glucose estimation accuracy have been shown to have long-term benefits for occurrence of, detection of, fear of, and response to hypoglycemia (Cox et al., 2001).

Stress and Coping in Diabetes

Sources of Diabetes-Related Stress

Diabetes-related stress is common; concern about long-term complications (Hendricks & Hendricks, 1998) and feeling deprived of food (Welch, Jacobson, & Polonsky, 1997) are some of the more common complaints. Risk factors for high levels of diabetes-related stress include diagnosis of type 1 (Polonsky et al., 1995), insulin use (Polonsky et al., 2005), female sex, significant psychiatric history, recent short-term complications (Snoek, Pouwer, Welch, & Polonsky, 2000), poor general health (CDC, 2004), and younger age (Polonsky et al., 2005).

The diabetes regimen is often viewed as a burden that interrupts normal daily activities. It can be financially costly, especially for the un- or under-insured. Treatment often increases in intensity over time: individuals with type 2 may progress from diet control to oral agents to insulin injections. Those with type 1 may be required to increase the number of daily injections or to transition to an insulin pump. Many individuals find this to be a difficult transition, and a phenomenon coined 'psychological insulin resistance' has been reported, wherein individuals are resistant to initiating insulin therapy (Polonsky et al., 2005; Snoek, 2002).

If and when the treatment regimen is mastered, there is often the frustration of not achieving treatment goals. A phenomenon called 'diabetes burnout' has been described, in which the chronic demands of the disease and its treatment, combined with the failure to achieve daily treatment goals, result in severe demoralization (Polonsky, 1999). Individuals with diabetes walk a fine line between the short-term complications of hypoglycemia and the fear of long-term complications, due to hyperglycemia. Fear of hypoglycemia can develop (Irvine, Cox, & Gonder-Frederick, 1992), especially after severe and frequent hypoglycemia, leading individuals to either become preoccupied with their blood glucose levels, or to deliberately allow their blood glucose to run high, in order to avoid hypoglycemia.

Social interactions can be made complicated by diabetes. Family members, health-care providers, co-workers, and friends may all pose social difficulties for persons with diabetes. Ineffective social problem-solving has been shown to be adversely associated with glycemic control (Hill-Briggs et al., 2006). Interventions, which include social skills-training, social problem-solving, and conflict resolution, have shown improvements for self-care and glycemic control (Grey et al., 1998).

Stress and Glycemic Control

Two hypothesized mechanisms link stress and blood glucose among individuals with diabetes. One mechanism is through the direct physiological effects of stress on the secretion of counter-regulatory hormones, which in turn increase blood glucose (Surwit & Feinglos, 1983). The other mechanism is indirect, through the disruption of an individual's adherence to the diabetes regimen.

While there is some evidence for a relationship between stress and blood glucose in animals, studies of the relationship in humans have provided less consistent support (Goetsch, 1989). Unfortunately, the human literature suffers from the same methodological limitations that permeate the broader stress and coping literature (Tennen, Affleck, & Armeli, 2003; Tennen, Affleck, Armeli, & Carney, 2000). Although it is beyond the scope of this chapter to provide a detailed critique of this literature, interested readers are encouraged to examine the literature demonstrating the limited reliability of retrospective measures of coping (Todd, Tennen, Carney, Armeli, & Affleck, 2004), and the mismatch between coping theory and research that is engendered by reliance on between-person coping phenomena (Tennen et al., 2003).

Field studies of the relationship between stress and glycemic control have focused either on everyday tribulations or major life events as stress indictors. For example, Aikens and Mayes (1997) asked individuals with type 2 diabetes to report the number and intensity of daily hassles that they experienced during the previous week. They concurrently completed a glucose check. Daily hassles and glucose showed a positive association even after controlling for long-term glycemic control (as measured by A1C), suggesting that the association is not the result of chronically compromised metabolic control. But as Aikens and Mayes (1997) noted, elevated glucose may lead to distress or a sense of helplessness that interferes with regimen adherence. In their study of major life stress and metabolic control among individuals with type 1 diabetes, Stenström, Wikby, Hörnqvist, and Andersson (1993) found gender differences in the relationship between recent major life events and glycemic control. Only women showed a positive relationship between the previous year's positive life events and a change for the better in A1c, whereas the relationship between negative life events and compromised metabolic control emerged only for men.

Gender and other between-person factors may well modify the relationship between stress and glycemic control; these effect modifiers may contribute to the inconsistent findings in this area of research.

Although most studies linking stress and metabolic control have failed to consider theoretically-derived effect modifiers/moderators, some investigations have demonstrated the promise of examining moderators of the stress-glycemic control relationship. For example, Griffith, Field, and Lustman (1990) found support for the buffering effect of social support. When life stress was high, individuals reporting greater perceived social support showed tighter glycemic control than their counterparts with lower levels of perceived support. When stress was low, social support was unrelated to glucose regulation.

Similarly, Peyrot and McMurry (1992) provided evidence consistent with their prediction that perceived stress was positively associated with blood glucose among individuals who reported using less effective coping strategies, and that stress and glucose were unrelated among participants who endorsed the use of more effective strategies. The moderated effects reported in these studies underscore the potential complexity of the association between stress and metabolic control in diabetes. They also highlight that such studies rely on retrospective reports of stress and the purported moderator, and that the operationalization of stress varies dramatically across studies, from major life events (Griffith et al. 1990; Stenström et al., 1993), to daily hassles (Aikens & Mayes, 1997), to perceived stress (Peyrot & McMurry, 1992).

Two studies in the area of stress, coping, and glycemic control stand out for their over-time designs and close to real-time assessment of stress and (in one study) regimen adherence. Aikens, Wallander, Bell, and Cole (1992) provided their type 1 diabetes participants with daily stress and regimen adherence questionnaires, which were completed in response to investigator-initiated telephone prompts on three consecutive days, during two different weeks, over the span of two months. These daily indicators were returned by mail. Aikens et al. found that *variability* in daily stress, but not the mean daily stress-level, was positively related to subsequent poor metabolic control. There was no evidence that regimen adherence mediated this relationship.

In a refreshing departure from the standard, between-person study design, Riazi, Pickup, and Bradley (2004) recently examined the relationship between daily stress and glycemic control among individuals with type 1 diabetes by having study participants report their stress each day for three weeks and take their blood-glucose measurements four times a day (see also Halford, Cuddihy, & Mortimer, 1990). Using time-series analysis, Riazi et al. found considerable variation in the magnitude and direction of blood-glucose response to daily stress. About one-third of their participants showed 'stress reactivity,' i.e., changes in stress were associated with same-day or next-day changes in blood-glucose levels. By relying on close to real-time assessments, this study suggests that although the glucose levels of a majority of individuals with type 1 diabetes may be unaffected by life's everyday slings and arrows, a sizeable minority of people with diabetes manifest stress-reactive changes in glycemic control.[1] This suggests that for these individuals, but not for others, targeted stress-management interventions might be particularly effective.

Overall, field studies examining the relationship between stress and glycemic control have produced inconsistent findings. Notable individual differences in the stress-glycemia relationship seem to exist, yet by and large studies have not been designed to examine theory-relevant moderators of the stress-glycemia association. Moreover, the operationalization of stress has spanned major life events, daily hassles, and perceived stress. Theoretical models linking stress, regimen adherence, and glycemic control have not explicated the temporal window during which stress should influence control directly or the hypothesized mediator of regimen adherence. If the imputed effects of stress on regimen adherence and glycemic control unfold within relatively brief periods of time, study designs will need to capture this brief temporal cycle.

Coping with Diabetes

Measurement Challenges

The promise of the coping construct in the broader literature has yet to be fulfilled by consistent empirical evidence that coping affects health outcomes, or that it modifies the relationship between stress and health or well-being (but see Peyrot & McMurry, 1992). Almost without exception, the literature on coping with diabetes has relied a retrospective coping reports and has determined *a priori* whether a coping strategy is adaptive or non-adaptive, despite converging evidence that the effectiveness of a coping strategy depends on the circumstances in which it is used (Conway & Terry, 1992; Felton & Revenson, 1984; Park, Armeli, & Tennen, 2004).

Retrospective reports of coping are the norm in the diabetes literature, and based on these reports, several investigators (e.g., Enzlin, Mathieu, & Demyttenaere, 2002) have concluded that men with diabetes use more active coping, less avoidant coping, and less support-seeking than women with diabetes. But as Porter and Stone (1995) demonstrated, gender differences such as the aforementioned emerge only when coping is assessed retrospectively. Real-time indicators of coping, free from retrospection decay and bias, do not support these coping differences between men and women.

Echoing the broader coping literature, emotion-focused coping (efforts to regulate emotions during stressful encounters) has been linked to poorer psychological and health outcomes, whereas problem-focused coping has been linked to better outcomes. However, a close examination of coping-scale items suggests

---

[1] See Goetsch, Abel, & Pope (1994) for a similar study of individuals with non-insulin-dependent diabetes, and Tennen, Affleck, Coune, Larsen & Delongis for a discussion of real-time and close to real-time measurement approaches.

that many of these items are not coping efforts at all, but rather catastrophic illness-related appraisals (e.g., *'diabetes is the worst thing that has ever happened to* me'), illness related self-appraisals (e.g., *'diabetes makes me feel different from everyone else'*), hopeless responses to the illness (e.g., *'I feel like just giving in to my diabetes'*), illness-related beliefs (e.g., *'I believe that research will discover a cure for diabetes before long'*), and distress-related self-appraisals (e.g., *'I blame myself'*).

Although the aforementioned coping items were derived from the recent reports of Karlsen and Bru (2002) and Gåfvels and Wändell (2006), they capture the coping indicators used in the vast majority of studies examining diabetes coping. These appraisals, beliefs, and responses are something quite different from the intentional efforts that define coping (Lazarus & Folkman, 1984). Furthermore, the consistent empirical association between these items on the one hand, and depression or global distress as 'outcomes' on the other hand, seems little more than the result of predictor-criterion content overlap.

Put simply, it should not be surprising that individuals who endorse negative views of themselves and their illness also report symptoms consistent with relatively poor psychosocial adjustment (e.g., White, Richter, & Fry, 1992; Willoughby, Kee, Demi, & Parker, 2000). Because the vast majority of diabetes coping research has relied on cross-sectional designs, any association between these so-called coping strategies and regimen adherence or glycemic control may reflect the fact that poor control prompts negative appraisals of the self, the illness, and the future. It can be concluded that even well-replicated associations between coping (as currently measured) and well-being or glycemic control in diabetes, and empirical confirmation of elegant models, in which the relationship between stress or coping and glycemic control is mediated through regimen adherence (e.g., Peyrot, McMurry, & Kruger, 1999), must be interpreted with caution.

Two emotion-related constructs have been by and large excluded from the diabetes coping literature: positive emotions and emotional-approach coping. Despite considerable evidence that positive emotions help in the regulation of negative emotions, foster resilience in response to health crises, and help people discover novel approaches to the problems they encounter (Frederickson, 1998), relatively few studies in the diabetes literature have incorporated positive emotions or positive well-being into their methods (see Karlsen, Idsoe, Hanestad, Murberg, & Bru, 2004 for an exception). Similarly, no study of diabetes related coping was found that included an indicator of coping through an emotional approach. Stanton and colleagues' program of research among individuals with cancer (Austenfeld & Stanton, 2004) demonstrates the adaptive potential of coping through acknowledging, understanding, and expressing emotion. Stanton's work also makes clear that the generally accepted conclusion in the diabetes literature – that emotion-focused coping is dysfunctional – is due to confounding of emotion-focused strategies with distress and self-deprecation. Thus, diabetes investigators and clinicians should consider positive emotions and emotional-approach coping in their research.

Additional Psychological Determinants of Diabetes Outcomes: Personality, Illness Appraisals, and Psychiatric Disorders

Numerous studies have examined personal characteristics of individuals with diabetes, which are associated with well-being, life quality, emotional distress, disease-management, regimen-adherence, glycemic control, and long-term complications. These characteristics can be categorized as: (a) Personality factors; (b) personal appraisal tendencies, most prominently self-efficacy expectations; and (c) psychiatric disorders. Because the literature is most advanced in the area of depression, that literature will be described in some detail.

Personality

Early studies of personality and diabetes unsuccessfully attempted to identify personality styles that increased risk for new-onset diabetes. The next generation of personality studies in diabetes was more successful in linking personality traits in individuals with diabetes with health outcomes. For example, Lustman, Frank, and McGill (1991) found that participants with higher levels of opportunism (i.e., individuals with high novelty-seeking, a low capacity to delay gratification, and a low harm-avoidance) showed poorer glucose control. Likewise, individuals who endorsed higher levels of alienated personality characteristics were also less likely to have adequate glycemic control.

Rose, Fliege, Hilderbrandt, Schirop, and Klapp (2002) reported a positive association between dispositional optimism and diabetes quality of life. Fournier, de Ridder, and Bensing (2002a, 2002b) found that among individuals with type 1 diabetes, optimism was related to lower levels of depression and anxiety. This inverse association between optimism and distress has been well documented in the broader health psychology literature (Scheier & Carver, 1992). The cross-sectional nature of these studies limits causal inferences.

Diabetes outcomes have also been investigated from the perspective of attachment theory. There is some evidence that patients with a dismissing attachment style can have greater difficulty engaging in a sustained, collaborative approach to their diabetes management, than patients with other attachment styles (Ciechanowski, Katon, Russo, & Walker, 2001). These patients may exhibit a 'self-reliant' approach to diabetes management which, in the absence of optimal provider-patient communication, is associated with worsened self-care (Ciechanowski et al., 2004) and glycemic control (Ciechanowski, Hirsch, & Katon, 2002).

Self-Efficacy

An individual's confidence that she or he can engage in a particular behavior (i.e., self-efficacy) is a potent predictor of subsequent behavior and has been linked to a wide range of health outcomes, particularly behaviors requiring persistence toward long-range goals (Bandura, 1997). Rose et al. (2002) found an association between self-efficacy for diabetes self-management and better self-reported life quality among individuals with diabetes. Similarly, Fournier et al. (2002b) found that self-efficacy expectations were related to lower levels of depression and anxiety. McCaul, Glasgow, and Schaefer (1987) found that among individuals with type 1 diabetes, self-efficacy beliefs were associated with adherence to treatment regimens both concurrently and prospectively.

Kavanaugh, Gooley, and Wilson (1993) pitted self-efficacy and previous adherence in predicting subsequent regimen adherence and glycemic control in a sample composed primarily of individuals with type 2 diabetes. Self-efficacy predicted subsequent adherence to the treatment regimen and was not accounted for by previous adherence. Adherence, in turn, predicted A1c, even after controlling for illness severity. The strengths of this study are its prospective design and its ability to demonstrate the predictive value of self-efficacy to regimen adherence, beyond the contribution of previous adherence.

Psychiatric Disorders

The prevalence of psychiatric disorders in diabetes has been examined. The most reliable evidence is for generalized anxiety disorder and panic disorder. Current and lifetime rates were generalized anxiety disorder: 13.5% and 20.5%; and panic disorder 1.3% and 1.9%, respectively (Grigsby, Anderson, Freedland, Clouse, & Lustman, 2002). Evidence is mixed as to whether rates are higher than in controls without diabetes. Rates of sub-clinical symptoms average 39%. Sperry (2006) used diabetes as a case study to depict how the existence of several types of personality disorders can interfere with health-related dynamics and, sometimes, with the ability to cope with diabetes.

When present, eating disorders are particularly problematic in diabetes. While rates of anorexia do not differ by diabetes status, rates of bulimia among individuals with diabetes are more than twice as high as non-diabetic controls (Mannucci et al., 2005). Intentional insulin-omission for weight control is sometimes seen in diabetes, and can be considered a compensatory behavior for the purposes of a bulimia diagnosis. Herpertz et al. (1998) found that 4.1% of people with diabetes report intentional and inappropriate insulin omission for the purposes of weight loss.

Depression, assessed as a continuous dimension and as a diagnostic entity, is the most extensively examined psychiatric problem in relation to diabetes. In the psychology literature, depression is often treated as an outcome. However, in the medical literature, depression is usually treated as an independent variable that affects diabetes self-management behaviors and diabetes outcomes. To the extent that the largely cross-sectional nature of the literature allows, this latter approach is taken in this review.

One area of considerable interest has been the prevalence of depression among adults with diabetes. Anderson, Freedland, Clouse, and Lustman (2001) reported the results of a meta-analysis of 39 studies (with over 20,000 partici-pants), including 20 that utilized a comparison group without diabetes. Anderson et al. concluded that diabetes doubles the odds of depression. Major depression (assessed primarily through structured diagnostic interviews) was present in 11% of individuals with diabetes, whereas elevated depressive symptoms (measured with standard depression scales) was present in 31% of the study participants across type 1 and type 2 diabetes. The latter figure is stunning, in view of evidence that even modest elevations in depressive symptoms are associated with impaired functioning and life-quality limitations (Jacobson, de Groot, & Samson, 1997).

Further, as summarized below, depressive symptoms have been linked to compromised treatment adherence, poorer glycemic control, and more long-term complications. Although depression may result from living with diabetes, or from neurobiological abnormalities associated with diabetes, Anderson et al. underscore that in prospective studies, depression doubles the risk of subsequent type 2 diabetes (e.g., Eaton, Armenian, Gallo, Pratt, & Ford, 1996). It may well be that the relationship is bi-directional, with depression increasing the risk for the onset of type 2 diabetes, and diabetes increasing the risk for subsequent depression.

The fact that nearly one in three individuals with diabetes report elevated depressive symptoms, combined with an 11% prevalence of depressive disorder, suggests that depression may play a significant role in predicting glycemic control. Lustman et al. (2000) examined the depression-glycemic control association. The meta-analysis included 24 studies and revealed that depression is associated with hyperglycemia. Lustman et al. note that although the effect size (0.17) is modest, it is clinically meaningful. Specifically, they calculated that the treatment of depression could increase the proportion of individuals with diabetes in adequate glucose control from 41% to 58%.

Two studies (de Groot, Jacobson, Samson, & Welch, 1999; Van Tilburg et al., 2001) suggest that the association between depression and glycemic control may be more reliable among individuals with type 1 diabetes, perhaps because the absolute insulin deficiency that characterizes type 1 diabetes is more vulnerable to disrupted self-care. When combined, these two studies point to a link between depression and control in type 1 diabetes, both when depression is treated as a clinical disorder (de Groot et al., 1999), or as a dimensional indicator (i.e., across the entire range of scores on a standard depression scale; Van Tilburg et al., 2001).

The documented association between depression and glycemic control does not, of course, imply that depression plays a causal role in glycemic control, nor does it suggest mechanisms that might link depression and disease control. It is quite plausible that maintaining good glucose control is more difficult for individuals with type 1 diabetes than it is for their type 2 counterparts. The repeated thwarting of efforts to attain glycemic control could lead to a sense of helplessness (Kuttner, Delamater, Santiago, 1990), and helpless pessimism, which are potential precursors to depression (Peterson, Maier, & Seligman, 1995). In a subsequent section of this chapter, several treatment studies are reviewed, which suggest a reciprocal relationship between depression and glycemic control. As de Groot et al. (1999) note, there are several plausible physiological and behavioral mechanisms that might underlie the association. These researchers summarize the potential hormonal and neurological links, but concluded that behavioral mechanisms, most notably regimen adherence, probably play a more prominent role in the relationship between depression and hyperglycemia.

Several studies have examined self-management as a mediator of the relationship between depression and glycemic control. Van Tilburg et al. (2001) found that diabetes self-management partially mediated the relationship between depressive symptoms and glycemic control. Similarly, in a longitudinal analysis, McKellar, Humphreys, and Piette (2004) found that depressive symptoms at baseline predicted a one-year change in symptoms of glucose dysreg-ulation, as measured through self-reported diabetes-related symptoms. But consistent with a mediational process, when self-care adherence was entered into the regression equation, the relationship between depressive symptoms and glucose dysregulation was no longer statistically significant. More recently, however, Lustman, Clouse, Ciechanowski, Hirsch, and Freedland (2005) found no evidence for a mediated relationship between depression and hyper-glycemia measured by A1c. Overall, the physiological and behavioral mecha-nisms linking depression and glucose dysregulation are only beginning to be understood.

Depression's prevalence among individuals with diabetes, and its association with poor glycemic control, suggest that depression might be associated with diabetes complications. Based on their meta-analytic review of 27 cross-sectional studies, de Groot, Anderson, Freedland, Clouse, and Lustman (2001) reported that for individuals with type 1 or type 2 diabetes, depression is consistently associated with diabetes complications, including retinopathy, neuropathy, sexual dysfunction, and macrovascular disease. De Groot and associates caution that depression may precede or follow the onset of diabetes complications.

It is tempting to speculate that depression manifests in motivational deficits which diminish diabetes self-management, thus worsening glycemic control and eventually leading to diabetes complications. However, Wing, Phelan and Tate (2002) have asserted that 'there is no evidence to support the hypothesis that adherence mediates the relationship between depression and [health] outcome' (p. 879). They, propose an alternative model in which adherence precedes and influences both mood states and health outcomes. Similarly, Sacco et al. (2005) found some cross-sectional support for a trajectory in which poor regimen adherence lowers self-efficacy, which in turn increases depressive symptoms. Thus the relationships among depression, adherence, and diabetes outcomes are complex and not fully understood.

This investigation is further complicated by any long-lasting effects of remitted depression. Evidence from cardiovascular disease (Wagner, Tennen, Mansoor, & Abbott, 2006), chronic pain (Fifield, Tennen, Reisine, & McQuillan, 1998; Fifield et al., 2001), as well as diabetes (Wagner & Tennen, in press), indicates that depression may be associated with health problems that are temporally distant from the depressive episode. Evidence also suggests that mood is more affected by day-to-day disease control among individuals with remitted depression, than never-depressed controls (Tennen, Affleck, & Zautra, 2006). Researchers are a long way from understanding the reciprocal influences that depression and glucose dysregulation may have on one another, and from appreciating the probable individual differences in depression's relationship with diabetes.

In sum, personality characteristics have been linked to quality of life, distress, self-management, and glycemic control. Consistent with the broader health-psychology literature, self-efficacy predicts adherence and glycemic control. Depression, both at the symptom-level and as a clinical disorder, is highly prevalent among individuals with diabetes, and has been linked empirically to regimen adherence, glycemic control, and diabetes complications.

Interventions

During the past 15 years investigators have turned their attention to psychosocial and educational interventions. Meta-analysis shows that while diabetes education has positive short-term effects on glycemic control, education alone is not sufficient for maintaining self-care behaviors and glycemic control over time (Norris, Lau, Smith, Schmid, & Engelgau, 2002).

Steed, Cooke, and Newman (2003) conducted a systematic review of the psychosocial outcomes associated with these interventions as they were described in 36 published studies. Steed et al. concluded that overall, the findings were distinctly mixed. Educational and self-management interventions that evaluated quality of life revealed a consistent advantage for self-management interventions. Interventions directed toward emotional distress, especially in randomized controlled trials, appeared to be associated more frequently with improvements in depression, as compared to educational or self-management interventions. However, this apparent advantage for psychological interventions is confounded by the fact that participants in the studies were more distressed upon study entry, than were their educational and self-management intervention counterparts, thus leaving more room for improvement. Since the publication of Steed et al.'s review, cognitive behavioral therapy (CBT) interventions, focusing on diabetes-related distress, continue to demonstrate their effectiveness (Karlsen, Idsoe, Dirdal, Hanestad, & Bru, 2004).

Stress & Coping Interventions

Stress-management interventions have been evaluated for their effects on diabetes outcomes. In one study, 108 individuals with type 2 diabetes were randomized to a five-session, group, diabetes-education program with or without stress-management training (Surwit et al., 2002). At one year follow-up, stress-management training was associated with a small (0.5%) but significant and clinically meaningful reduction in A1c. Trait anxiety did not predict response to treatment, showing that highly anxious patients did not derive more benefit from training. Other stress-management interventions with smaller samples have shown benefits for mood, but not glycemic control.

Coping interventions have been tested for their effect in individuals with diabetes. Coping-skills training typically incorporates skills that assist individuals in dealing with potential stressors and with the stress reactions that may result from these situations. Skills may include social problem-solving, communication, cognitive-behavioral modification, and conflict resolution. Coping-skills training interventions have shown benefits for adults and adolescents alike (Grey et al., 1998; Karlsen et al., 2004). For example, a randomized controlled trial of coping-skills training for adolescents with type 1 showed short term benefits for A1c, self-efficacy, and distress (Davidson, Boland, & Grey, 1997). Girls, but not boys, also enjoyed long-term effects on weight and hypoglycemic episodes (Grey, Boland, Davidson, & Tamborlane, 2000).

However, as stated previously regarding basic scientific measurement, it is not clear that the coping indicators, which were used as outcomes in these interventions, actually capture coping (Lazarus & Folkman, 1984) . For example, Grey et al. (1998, 2000) used the 'Upset' subscale of the 'Issues in Coping with IDDM' (Kovacs, Brent, Feinberg, Paulauskas, & Reid, 1986), which assesses the degree to which certain activities and thoughts about diabetes are experienced as upsetting. Furthermore, some of these interventions define healthy coping *a priori* as a 'style,' rather than as a goodness-of-fit between the stressor and the coping response (Karlsen et al., 2004). These randomized trials clearly show glycemic and other benefits for participants, and thus represent important interventions for the clinical care of individuals with diabetes. However, they are limited in their contribution to the understanding of coping as a psychological construct of inquiry.

Self-Efficacy Interventions

Self-efficacy in diabetes has been conceptualized by some investigators as empowerment. Empowerment is the discovery and development of one's inherent capacity to be responsible for one's own life (Funnell & Anderson, 2003). In addition to self-efficacy for diabetes self-management behaviors, empowerment focuses on psychosocial self-efficacy. This includes psychosocial issues such as managing stress, obtaining family support, negotiating with health-care professionals and employers, and dealing with uncomfortable emotions (Anderson, Funnell, Fitzgerald, & Marrero, 2000).

A randomized, wait-listed control group trial tested the effects of an empowerment intervention (Anderson, et al., 1995). Relative to controls, the intervention group showed improvements in self-efficacy and A1c. Within groups, an analysis of data from all program participants showed sustained improvements in self-efficacy and a modest improvement in blood glucose.

Interventions for Psychiatric Disorders

There is evidence for the effectiveness of pharmacological (Gulseren, Gulseren, Hekimsoy, & Mete, 2005; Lustman et al., 1995) and non-pharmacological (Boyle, Allan, & Millar, 2004; Snoek et al., 2001) treatment of anxiety and fear in diabetes, with some of both types of interventions showing benefits for glycemic control. Little work has been done to treat eating disorders in diabetes, but Kenardy, Mensch, Bowen, Green, and Walton (2002) did find that psychotherapy is effective in improving binge-eating and A1c in people with type 2 diabetes.

The evidence of intervention efficacy is strongest for treating depression in diabetes. Lustman and colleagues conducted randomized, double-blind, placebo-controlled trials to evaluate the effects of nortriptyline (Lustman et al., 1997) and fluoxetine (Lustman, Freedland, Griffith, and Clouse, 2000) on depression and glycemic control. In the eight-week nortriptyline trial, individuals with diabetes with poor glycemic control served as participants, with almost half meeting criteria for a current major depression. Although the reduction in depression symptoms was greater among nortriptyline-treated participants compared to participants who received placebo, the active medication was not superior to placebo in reducing A1c among the depressed participants. Further, there was some indication that the direct effect of nortripyline was to *worsen* glycemic control. In the fluoxetine trial, individuals with type 1 or type 2 diabetes and major depressive disorder received daily doses of fluoxetine or placebo for eight weeks. Again, participants receiving the active treatment showed a greater reduction in depressive symptoms, compared with placebo group. Although not achieving statistical significance, the fluoxetine group showed a trend toward greater improvement in glycemic control, compared to placebo-treated participants.

In a third randomized, controlled trial, Lustman, Griffith, Freedland, Kissel, and Clouse (1998) compared diabetes education to diabetes education plus 10 weeks of CBT. A greater proportion of CBT-treated participants, compared to controls, achieved depression remission. At six-month follow-up, CBT-treated participants had better glycemic control.

Finally, the Pathways study randomized 329 patients with diabetes mellitus and major depression and/or dysthymia to either: (a) Case management, which consisted of education, antidepressant medication support, or problem-solving therapy by the physician, or to (b) usual care (Katon et al., 2004). Compared to usual care, the collaborative care model improved depression levels and outcomes, but improved depression alone did not result in improved glycemic control. Together, these studies suggest that depression in individuals with diabetes can be treated effectively. It remains to be determined if pharmacological or psychological depression treatments reliably produce and maintain positive changes in glycemic control.

Effective strategies for depression screening and provision of depression treatment for persons with diabetes must also be established. Persons with diabetes typically welcome mood screening from health care providers, and are generally satisfied with depression treatment when it is provided (de Groot, Pinkerman, Wagner, & Hockman, 2006). However, approximately half of depression cases in diabetes go undetected by health-care providers (Wagner, Tsimikas, Heapy, de Groot, & Abbott, 2006). Furthermore, when depression is detected, African Americans with diabetes are less likely to receive pharmacotherapy than their White counterparts (Wagner, Tsimikas, et al., 2006). Effective depression treatments can achieve potential benefits only if they are delivered.

Summary and Implications

The increasing prevalence of diabetes, and the severity of its long-term complications, are a serious public health-threat. Psychological factors, including stress and coping, personality, self-efficacy, and psychiatric disorders, are important determinants of diabetes outcomes. In order for behavioral diabetes research to progress, scientific inquiry must improve upon current limitations. These limitations include cross-sectional designs, recalled coping strategies and stressful experiences, between-person investigations of inherently within-person processes, predictor-criterion content overlap in studies of coping, the exclusive use of negative affective states as indicators of adjustment, the rare use of close to real-time assessment, and the exclusion of positive affect. Furthermore, there is a pervasive confusion regarding mediated and moderated effects. Readers are reminded that a moderator affects the relationship between two variables, whereas a mediator identifies the mechanism through which the independent variable affects the dependent variable (Baron & Kenny, 1986; Holmbeck, 1997).

While this review has emphasized threats to the internal validity of published research, it should be noted that recently there has been increased attention paid to issues of external validity (Glasgow et al., 2006). It has been suggested that an emphasis on generalizability is necessary for greater translation of research findings into clinical practice. This is certainly true in clinical care of diabetes, where there is evidence for the benefit of psychosocial intervention; yet, few individuals with diabetes actually receive psychosocial services as part of, or as a complement to, their routine medical care.

As a major public health-problem, diabetes offers a significant opportunity for behavioral investigators to examine how psychosocial factors contribute to disease-onset, disease-management, and disease outcomes, as well as to evaluate the effectiveness of psychosocial interventions in reducing symptoms and affecting disease course. With greater attention to the measurement, methodological, and analytic and generalizability issues that were raised in this chapter, this area of inquiry can begin to fulfill its considerable promise.

References

Aikens, J. E., & Mayes, R. (1997). Elevated glycosylated albumin in NIDDM is a function of recent everyday environmental stress. *Diabetes Care, 20*, 1111–1113.

Aikens, J. E., Wallender, J. L., Bell, D. S., & Cole, J. A. (1992). Daily stress variability, learned resourcefulness, regimen adherence, and metabolic control in type I diabetes mellitus: evaluation of a path model. *Journal of Consulting and Clinical Psychology, 60*, 113–118.

American Diabetes Association (2001). *Diabetes 2001 Vital Statistics*. Alexandria, VA American Diabetes Association.

American Diabetes Association and the American College of Cardiology (2002). The Diabetes-Heart Disease Link. A report on the attitudes toward and knowledge of heart disease risk among people with diabetes in the U.S.

Anderson, R. J., Freedland, K. E., Clouse, R. E., & Lustman, P. J. (2001). The prevalence of comorbid depression in adults with diabetes. *Diabetes Care, 24*, 1069–1078.

Anderson R. M., Funnell M. M., Butler P. M., Arnold M. S., Fitzgerald J. T., & Feste C. C. (1995). Patient empowerment. Results of a randomized controlled trial. *Diabetes Care, 18*, 943–949.

Anderson, R. M., Funnell, M. M., Fitzgerald, J. T., & Marrero, D. G. (2000). The diabetes empowerment scale: A measure of psychosocial self-efficacy. *Diabetes Care, 23*, 739–743.

Austenfeld, J. L., & Stanton, A. L. (2004). Coping through emotional approach: A new look at emotion, coping and health-related outcomes. *Journal of Personality, 72*, 1335–1363.

Bandura, A. (1997). *Self-efficacy: The exercise of control*. New York: W. H. Freeman and Company.

Baron, R. M., & Kenny, D. A. (1986). The moderator-mediator variable distinction in social psychological research: Conceptual, strategic, and statistical considerations. *Journal of Personality and Social Psychology, 51*, 1173–1182.

Boyle, S., Allan, C., & Millar, K. (2004). Cognitive-behavioural interventions in a patient with an anxiety disorder related to diabetes. *Behaviour Research and Therapy, 42*, 357–366.

Centers for Disease Control and Prevention. (2004). Serious psychological distress among persons with diabetes – New York City, 2003. *Morbidity and Mortality, Weekly Report, 53*, 1089–1092.

Centers for Disease Control and Prevention. (2005). *National diabetes fact sheet: general information and national estimates on diabetes in the United States, 2005*. Atlanta, GA: U.S. Department of Health and Human Services, Centers for Disease Control and Prevention, 2005.

Ciechanowski, P. S., Hirsch, I. B., & Katon, W. J. (2002). Interpersonal predictors of HbA(1c) in patients with type 1 diabetes. *Diabetes Care, 25*, 731–736.

Ciechanowski, P. S., Katon, W. J., Russo, J. E., & Walker, E. A. (2001). The patient-provider relationship: attachment theory and adherence to treatment in diabetes. *American Journal of Psychiatry, 158*(1), 29–35.

Ciechanowski, P. S., Russo, J., Katon, W., Von Korff, M., Ludman, E., Lin, E., et al. (2004). Influence of patient attachment style on self-care and outcomes in diabetes. *Psychosomatic Medicine, 66*(5), 720–728.

Conway, V. J., & Terry, D. J. (1992). Appraised controllability as a moderator of the effectiveness of different coping strategies: A test of the goodness of fit hypothesis. *Australian Journal of Psychology, 44*, 1–7.

Cox, D. J., Gonder-Frederick, L., Polonsky, W., Schlundt, D., Kovatchev, B., & Clarke, W. (2001). Blood glucose awareness training (BGAT-2): long-term benefits. *Diabetes Care, 24,* 637–642.

Cox, D. J., Penberthy, J. K., Zrebiec, J., Weinger, K., Aikens, J. E., Frier, B., et al. (2003). Diabetes and driving mishaps: frequency and correlations from a multinational survey. *Diabetes Care, 26,* 2329–2334.

Davidson, M., Boland, E. A., & Grey, M. (1997). Teaching teens to cope: coping skills training for adolescent with diabetes mellitus. *Journal of Social and Pediatric Nursing, 2,* 65–72.

Diabetes Control and Complications Trial Research Group (1993). The effect of intensive treatment of diabetes on the development and progression of long-term complications in insulin-dependent diabetes mellitus. *New England Journal of Medicine, 329,* 977–985.

Diabetes Prevention Trial-Type 1 Diabetes Study Group (2002). Effects of insulin in relatives of patients with type 1 diabetes mellitus. *New England Journal of Medicine, 346,* 1685–1691.

de Groot, M. Anderson, R., Freedland, K. E., Clouse, R. E., & Lustman, P. J. (2001). Association of depression and diabetes complications: A meta-analysis. *Psychosomatic Medicine, 63,* 619–630.

de Groot, M., Jacobson, A. M., Samson, J. A., & Welch, G. (1999). Glycemic control and major depression in patients with type 1 and type 2 diabetes. *Journal of Psychosomatic Research, 46,* 425–435.

de Groot M., Pinkerman, B., Wagner, J., & Hockman, E. (2006). Depression treatment and satisfaction in a multicultural sample of type 1 and type 2 diabetic patients. *Diabetes Care, 29*(3), 549–553.

Eaton, W. W., Armenian, H. A., Gallo, J., Pratt, L., & Ford, D. E. (1996). Depression and the risk for onset of type 2 diabetes: a prospective population-based study. *Diabetes Care, 19,* 1097–1102.

Enzlin, P., Mathieu, C., & Demyttenaere, K. (2002). Gender differences in psychological adjustment to Type 1 diabetes mellitus: an explorative study. *Patient Education and Counseling, 48,* 139–145.

Felton, B. J., & Revenson, T. A. (1984). Coping with chronic illness: A study of illness controllability and the influence of coping strategies on psychological adjustment. *Journal of Consulting and Clinical Psychology, 52,* 343–353.

Fifield, J., McQuillan, J., Tennen, H., Sheeha, T. J., Reisine, S., Hesselbrock, V., et al. (2001). History of affective disorder and the temporal trajectory of fatigue in rheumatoid arthritis. *Annals of Behavioral Medicine, 23,* 34–41.

Fifield, J., Tennen, H., Reisine, S., & McQuillan, J. (1998). Depression and the long-term risk of pain, fatigue, and disability in patients with rheumatoid arthritis. *Arthritis and Rheumatology, 41,* 1851–1857.

Fournier, M., de Ridder, D., & Bensing, J. (2002a). Optimism and adaptation to chronic disease: The role of optimism in relation to self-care options of type 1 diabetes mellitus, rheumatoid arthritis and multiple sclerosis. *British Journal of Health Psychology, 7,* 409–432.

Fournier, M., de Ridder, D., & Bensing, J. (2002b). How optimism contributes to the adaptation to chronic illness: A prospective study into the enduring effects of optimism on adaptation moderated by the controllability of chronic illness. *Personality and Individual Differences, 33,* 1163–1183.

Frederickson, B. L. (1998). What good are positive emotions? *Review of General Psychology, 2,* 300–319.

Funnell, M. M., & Anderson, R. M. (2003). Patient empowerment: a look back, a look ahead. *Diabetes Educator, 29*, 454–458.

Gåfvels, C., & Wändell, P. E. (2006). Coping strategies in men and women with type 2 diabetes in Swedish primary care. *Diabetes Research and Clinical Practice, 71*, 280–289.

Glasgow, R. E., Green, L. W., Klesges, L. M., Abrams, D. B., Fisher, E. B., Goldstein, M. G., et al. (2006). External validity: we need to do more. *Annals of Behavioral Medicine, 31*, 105–108.

Goetsch, V. L. (1989). Stress and blood glucose in diabetes mellitus: A review and methodological commentary. *Annals of Behavioral Medicine, 11*, 102–107.

Goetsch, V. L., Abel, J. L., & Pope, M. K. (1994). The effects of stress, mood and coping on blood glucose in NIDDM: A prospective pilot evaluation. *Behavior Research and Therapy, 32*, 503–510.

Grey, M., Boland, E. A., Davidson, M., & Tamborlane, W. V. (2000). Coping skills training for youth with diabetes mellitus has long-lasting effects on metabolic control and quality of life. *Journal of Pediatrics, 137*, 107–113.

Grey, M., Boland, E. A., Davidson, M., Yu, C., Sullivan-Bolyai, S., & Tamborlane, W. V. (1998). Short-term effects of coping skills training as an adjunct to intensive therapy in adolescents. *Diabetes Care, 21*, 902–908.

Griffith, L. S., Field, B. J., & Lustman, P. J. (1990). Life stress and social support in diabetes: Association with glycemic control. *International Journal of Psychiatry in Medicine, 20*, 365–372.

Grigsby, A. B., Anderson, R. J., Freedland, K. E., Clouse, R. E., & Lustman, P. J. (2002). Prevalence of anxiety in adults with diabetes: a systematic review. *Journal of Psychosomatic Research, 53*, 1053–1060.

Gulseren, L., Gulseren, S., Hekimsoy, Z., & Mete, L. (2005). Comparison of fluoxetine and paroxetine in type II diabetes mellitus patients. *Archives of Medical Research, 36*, 159–165.

Haffner, S. M., Letho, S., Ronnemaa, T., & Pyorala, K. (1998). Mortality from coronary heart disease in subjects with type 2 diabetes and in non-diabetic subjects with and without previous myocardial infarction. *New England Journal of Medicine, 339*, 229–234.

Halford, W. K., Cuddihy, S., & Mortimer, R. H. (1990). Psychological stress and blood glucose regulation in type 1 diabetic patients. *Health Psychology, 9*, 516–528.

Hendricks, L. E., & Hendricks, R. T. (1998). Greatest fears of type 1 and type 2 patients about having diabetes: Implications for diabetes educators. *Diabetes Educator, 24*, 168–173.

Herpertz, S., Wagener, R., Albus, C., Kocnar, M., Wagner, R., Best, F., et al. (1998). Diabetes mellitus and eating disorders: A multicenter study on the comorbidity of the two diseases. *Journal of Psychosomatic Research, 44*, 503–515.

Hill-Briggs, F., Gary, T. L., Yeh, H.C., Batts-Turner, M., Powe, N. R., Saudek, C. D., et al. (2006). Association of social problem solving with glycemic control in a sample of rrban African Americans with type 2 diabetes. *Journal of Behavioral Medicine, 6*, 1–10.

Holmbeck, G. N. (1997). Toward terminological, conceptual, and statistical clarity in the study of mediators and moderators: Examples from the child-clinical and pediatric literatures. *Journal of Consulting and Clinical Psychology, 65*, 599–610.

Irvine, A. A., Cox, D., & Gonder-Frederick, L. (1992). Fear of hypoglycemia: Relationship to physical and psychological symptoms in patients with insulin-dependent diabetes mellitus. *Health Psychology, 11*, 135–138.

Jacobson, A. M., de Groot, M., & Samson, J. A. (1997). The effects of psychiatric disorders and symptoms on quality of life in patients with type I and type II diabetes mellitus. *Quality of Life Research, 6*, 11–20.

Jarrett, R. J., McCartney, P., & Keen, H. (1982). The Bedford survey: Ten year mortality rates in newly diagnosed diabetics, borderline diabetics and normoglycaemic controls and risk indices for coronary heart disease in borderline diabetics. *Diabetologia, 22*(2), 79–84.

Jones, H., Edwards, L., Vallis, T. M., Ruggiero, L., Rossi, S. R., Rossi, J. S., et al. (2003). Changes in diabetes self-care behaviors make a difference in glycemic control: The Diabetes Stages of Change (DiSC) study. *Diabetes Care, 26*, 732–737.

Kannel, W. B., & McGee, D. L. (1979). Diabetes and glucose tolerance as risk factors for cardiovascular disease: The Framingham study. *Diabetes Care, 2*(2), 120–126.

Karlsen, B., & Bru, E. (2002). Coping styles among adults with type 1 and type 2 diabetes. *Psychology, Health and Medicine, 7*, 245–259.

Karlsen, B., Idsoe, T., Dirdal, I., Hanestad, B. R., & Bru, E. (2004). Effects of a group-based counseling programme on diabetes-related stress, coping, psychological well-being and metabolic control in adults with type 1 or type 2 diabetes. *Patient Education and Counseling, 53*, 299–308.

Katon, W. J., Von Korff, M., Lin, E. H., Simon, G., Ludman, E., Russo, J., et al. (2004). The Pathways Study: A randomized trial of collaborative care in patients with diabetes and depression. *Archives of General Psychiatry, 61*, 1042–1049.

Kavanaugh, D. J., Gooley, S., & Wilson, P. H. (1993). Prediction of adherence and control in diabetes. *Journal of Behavioral Medicine, 16*, 509–522.

Kenardy, J., Mensch, M., Bowen, K., Green, B., & Walton, J. (2002). Group therapy for binge eating in type 2 diabetes: a randomized trial. *Diabetes Medicine, 19*, 234–239.

Knowler, W. C., Barrett-Connor, E., Fowler, S. E., Hamman, R. F., Lachin, J. M., Walker, E. A., et al. (2002). Reduction in the incidence of type 2 diabetes with lifestyle intervention or metformin. *New England Journal of Medicine, 7*, 393–403.

Kovacs, M., Brent, D., Feinberg, T. F., Paulauskas, S., & Reid, J. (1986). Children's self-reports of psychologic adjustment and coping strategies during the first year of insulin-dependent diabetes mellitus. *Diabetes Care, 9*, 472–479.

Kuttner. M. J., Delamater, A. M., & Santiago, J. V. (1990). Learned helplessness in diabetic youths. *Journal of Pediatric Psychology, 15*, 581–594.

Lazarus, R. S., & Folkman, S. (1984). *Stress, appraisal, and coping.* New York: Springer.

Lustman, P. J., Anderson, R. J., Freedland, K. E., de Groot, M., Carney, R. M. & Clouse, R. E. (2000). Depression and poor glycemic control: A meta-analytic review of the literature. *Diabetes Care, 23*, 934–942.

Lustman, P. J., Clouse, R. E., Ciechanowski, P. S., Hirsch, I. B., & Freedland, K. E. (2005). Depression-related hyperglycemia in type 1 diabetes: A mediational approach. *Psychosomatic Medicine, 67*, 195–199.

Lustman, P. J., Frank, B. L., & McGill, J. B. (1991). Relationship of personality characteristics to glucose regulation in adults with diabetes. *Psychosomatic Medicine, 53*, 305–312.

Lustman, P. J., Freedland, K. E., Griffith, L. S., & Clouse, R. E. (2000). Fluoxetine for depression in diabetes: A randomized double blind placebo-controlled trial. *Diabetes Care, 23*, 618–623.

Lustman, P. J., Griffith, L. S., Clouse, R. E., Freedland, K. E., Eisen, S. A., Rubin, E. H., et al. (1995). Effects of alprazolam on glucose regulation in diabetes. Results of double-blind, placebo-controlled trial. *Diabetes Care, 18*, 1133–1139.

Lustman, P. J., Griffith, L. S., Clouse, R. E., Freedland, K. E., Eisen, S. A., Rubin, E. H., et al. (1997). Effects of nortryptyline on depression and glycemic control in diabetes: results of a double blind, placebo-controlled trial. *Psychosomatic Medicine, 59*, 241–250.

Lustman, P. J., Griffith, L. S., Freedland, K. E., Kissel, S. S., & Clouse, R. E. (1998). Cognitive behavior therapy for depression in type 2 diabetes mellitus: A randomized, controlled trial. *Annals of Internal Medicine, 129*, 613–621.

Mannucci, E., Rotella, F., Ricca, V., Moretti, S., Placid, G. F., & Rotella, C. M. (2005). Eating disorders in patient with type 1 diabetes: A meta-analysis. *Journal of Endocrinological Investigation, 28*, 417–419.

McCaul, K. D., Glasgow, R. E., & Schaefer, L. C. (1987). Diabetes regimen behaviors predicting adherence. *Medical Care, 25*, 868–881.

McKellar, J. D., Humphreys, K., & Piette, J. D. (2004). Depression increases diabetes symptoms by complicating patients' self-care adherence. *The Diabetes Educator, 30*, 485–492.

Mokdad, A. H., Ford, E. S., Bowman, B. A., Nelson, D. E., Engelgau, M. M., Vinicor, F., et al. (2000). The continuing increase of diabetes in the US. *Diabetes Care, 24*(2), 412.

Norris, S. L., Lau, J., Smith, S. J., Schmid, C. H., & Engelgau, M. M. (2002). Self-management education for adults with type 2 diabetes: a meta-analysis of the effect on glycemic control. *Diabetes Care, 25*, 1159–1171.

Park, C. L., Armeli, S., & Tennen, H. (2004). Appraisal-coping goodness of fit: A daily internet study. *Personality and Social Psychology Bulletin, 30*, 558–569.

Peterson, C., Maier, S. F., & Seligman, M. E. P. (1995). *Learned helplessness: A theory for the age of personal control.* New York: Oxford University Press.

Peyrot, M. F., & McMurry, J. F., Jr. (1992). Stress buffering and glycemic control: The role of coping styles. *Diabetes Care, 15*, 842–846.

Peyrot, M. F., McMurry, J. F., Jr., & Kruger, D. F. (1999). A biopsychosocial model of glycemic control in diabetes: Stress, coping and regimen adherence. *Journal of Health and Social Behavior, 40*, 141–158.

Polonsky, W. H. (1999). *Diabetes burnout: Preventing it, surviving it, finding inner peace.* American Diabetes Association Alexandria, VA.

Polonsky, W. H., Anderson, B. J., Lohrer, P. A., Welch, G., Jacobson, A. M., Aponte, J. E., et al. (1995). Assessment of diabetes-related distress. *Diabetes Care, 18*, 754–760.

Polonsky, W. H., Fisher, L., Earles, J., Dudl, R.J., Lees, J., Mullan, J., et al. (2005). Assessing psychosocial distress in diabetes: development of the diabetes distress scale. *Diabetes Care, 28*, 626–631.

Riazi, A., Pickup, J., & Bradley, C. (2004). Daily stress and glycemic control in type 1 diabetes: individual differences in magnitude, direction, and timing of stress-reactivity. *Diabetes Research and Clinical Practice, 66*, 237–244.

Rodin, J., & Salovey, P. (1989). Health Psychology. *Annual Review of Psychology, 40*, 533–579.

Rose, M., Fliege, H., Hilderbrandt, M., Schirop, T., & Klapp, B. F. (2002). The network of psychological variables in patients with diabetes and their importance for quality of life and metabolic control. *Diabetes Care, 25*, 35–42.

Ruggiero, L., Glasgow, R., Dryfoos, J. M., Rossi, J. S., Prochaska, J. O., Orleans, C. T., et al. (1997). Diabetes self-management: Self-reported recommendations and patterns in a large population. *Diabetes Care, 20*, 568–576.

Sacco, W. P., Wells, K. J., Vaughan, C. A., Friedman, A., Perez, S., & Matthew, R. (2005). Depression in adults with type 2 diabetes: The role of adherence, body mass index, and self-efficacy. *Health Psychology, 24*, 630–634.

Scheier, M. F., & Carver, C. S. (1992). Effects of optimism on psychological and physical well-being: Theoretical overview and empirical update. *Cognitive Therapy and Research, 16*, 201–228.

Skyler, J. S., Krischer, J. P., Wolfsdorf, J., Cowie, C., Palmer, J. P., Greenbaum, C., et al. (2005). Effects of oral insulin in relatives of patients with type 1 diabetes: The Diabetes Prevention Trial-Type 1. *Diabetes Care, 28*, 1068–1076.

Snoek, F.J. (2002). Breaking the barriers to optimal glycaemic control – what physicians need to know from patients' perspectives. *International Journal of Clinical Practice Supplement, 129*, 80–84.

Snoek, F. J., Pouwer, F., Welch, G. W., & Polonsky, W. H. (2000). Diabetes-related emotional distress in Dutch and U.S. diabetic patients: cross-cultural validity of the problem areas in diabetes scale. *Diabetes Care, 23*, 1305–1309.

Snoek, F. J., van der Ven, N. C., Lubach, C. H., Chatrou, M., Ader, H. J., Heine, R. J., et al. (2001). Effects of cognitive behavioural group training (CBGT) in adult patients with poorly controlled insulin-dependent (type 1) diabetes: A pilot study. *Patient Education and Counseling, 45*, 143–148.

Sperry, L. (2006). *Psychological treatment of chronic illness: The biopsychosocial therapy approach*. Washington, DC: American Psychological Association.

Steed, L., Cooke, D., & Newman, S. (2003). A systemic review of psychological outcomes following education, self-management and psychological interventions in diabetes mellitus. *Patient Education and Counseling, 51*, 5–15.

Stenström, U., Wikby, A., Hörnqvist, J.O., & Andersson, P. (1993). Recent life events, gender, and the control of diabetes mellitus. *General Hospital Psychiatry, 15*, 82–88.

Surwit, R. S., & Feinglos, M. N. (1983). The effects of relaxation on glucose tolerance in non-insulin- dependent diabetes. *Diabetes Care, 6*, 176–179.

Surwit, R.S., van Tilburg, M. A., Zucker, N., McCaskill, C. C., Parekh, P., Feinglos, M. N., et al. (2002). Stress management improves long-term glycemic control in type 2 diabetes. *Diabetes Care, 25*, 30–34.

Tennen, H., Affleck, G., & Armeli, S. (2003). Daily processes in health and illness. In J. Suls and K. Wallston (Eds.), *The social psychological foundations of health and illness* (pp. 495–529). Oxford: Blackwell Publishers.

Tennen, H., Affleck, G., Armeli, S., & Carney, M. A. (2000). A daily process approach to coping: Linking theory, research and practice. *American Psychologist, 55*, 626–636.

Tennen, H., Affleck, G., Coyne, J. C., Larsen, R. J., & DeLongis, A. (2006) Paper *and plastic in daily diary research: Comments on Green, Rafaeli, Balger, Shrout & Reis (2000). *Psychological Methods, 11*, 112–118.

Tennen, H., Affleck, G., & Zautra, A. (2006). Depression history and coping with chronic pain: A daily process analysis. *Health Psychology, 25*, 370–379.

Todd, M., Tennen, H., Carney, M. A., Armeli, S., & Affleck, G. (2004). Do we know how we cope? Relating daily coping reports to global and time-limited retrospective assessments. *Journal of Personality and Social Psychology, 86*, 310–319.

UKPDS Study Group (1998). Intensive blood-glucose control with sulphonylureas or insulin compared with conventional treatment and risk of complications in patients with type 2 diabetes. *Lancet, 12*, 837–853.

Van Tilburg, M. A. L., McCaskill, C. C., Lane, J. D., Edwards, C. L., Bethel, A., Feinglos, M. N., et al. (2001). Depressed mood is a factor in glycemic control in type 1 diabetes. *Psychosomatic Medicine, 63*, 551–555.

Wagner, J., Lacey, K., Abbott, G., de Groot, M., & Chyun, D. (2006). Knowledge of heart disease risk in a multicultural community sample of people with diabetes. *Annals of Behavioral Medicine, 31*, 224–230.

Wagner, J., & Tennen, H. (in press). History of major depressive disorder and diabetes outcomes among diet and tablet treated postmenopausal women: A case control study. *Diabetic Medicine*.

Wagner, J., Tennen, H., Mansoor, G., & Abbott, G. (2006). History of major depressive disorder and endothelial function in postmenopausal women. *Psychosomatic Medicine, 68*, 80–86.

Wagner, J., Tsimikas, J., Heapy, A., de Groot, M., & Abbott, G. (2006). Ethnic and racial differences in diabetic patients' depressive symptoms, diagnosis, and treatment. *Diabetes Research and Clinical Practice, 75*, 119–112.

Welch, G. W., Jacobson, A. M., & Polonsky, W. H. (1997). The problem areas in diabetes scale. An evaluation of its clinical utility. *Diabetes Care, 20*, 760–766.

White, N. E., Richter, J. M., & Fry. C. (1992). Coping, social support, and adaptation to chronic illness. *Western Journal of Nursing Research, 14*, 211–224.

Willoughby, D. F., Kee, C. C., Demi, A., & Parker, V. (2000). Coping and psychosocial adjustment of women with diabetes. *The Diabetes Educator, 26*, 105–112.

Wing, R. R., Phelan, S., & Tate, D. (2002). The role of adherence in mediating the relationship between depression and health outcomes. *Journal of Psychosomatic Research, 53*, 877–881.

12
Coping with Epilepsy: Research and Interventions

Malachy Bishop and Chase A. Allen

Epilepsy is an umbrella diagnosis covering a range of etiologies and presentations, with the unifying factor being recurrent seizures. Due in part to the unpredictable and intrusive nature of seizures, epilepsy has the potential to significantly impact personal experience and functioning across the wide range of physical, psychological, and social domains of living. Along with the potential physical and cognitive problems associated with seizures, epilepsy has been associated with psychological and emotional problems, social isolation, and problems in education, employment, family life, and leisure activities (Thompson & Oxley, 1993).

The frequently significant psychosocial impact and consequences of epilepsy cannot, however, be fully explained as resulting directly from the occurrence of seizures, but rather as the result of a complex interaction of neurological, psychological, physical and social factors, and the stigma historically associated with this condition. Indeed, Engel (2000) suggested that epilepsy, "perhaps more than any other disorder, is associated with profound deleterious psychological and sociological consequences that are not directly related to the actual disease process" (p. xiii–xiv).

"Coping is concerned with the thoughts and actions a person makes in response to a taxing situation" (Reeve & Lincoln, 2002, p. 33). Understanding the complex mechanisms through which epilepsy affects psychosocial function, and the processes that people employ to cope with this impact, are a critical focus of epilepsy research, for it is through such understanding that effective clinical interventions emerge. This chapter explores the topic of coping with epilepsy, beginning with an overview of epilepsy, including its etiology, prevalence, and treatment. The psychosocial impact of epilepsy and a review of research related to coping with epilepsy are then presented. Finally, various physical, psychosocial, behavioral and environmental interventions, which have been hypothesized to promote effective coping, are described.

Overview: Incidence, Prevalence, and Etiology

Epilepsy is one of the most common neurological disorders (Livneh & Antonak, 1997). The word epilepsy is a generic term, synonymous with convulsive disorder or seizure disorder. These terms refer to a wide variety of seizure conditions, rather than a single condition (Engel & Pedley, 1997; Fraser, Glazer, & Simcoe, 1992). For this reason, epilepsy is also referred to as *the epilepsies*, reflecting the fact that the condition results from a group of chronic neurological conditions characterized by recurrent epileptic seizures (Engel, Birbeck, Gallo Diop, Jain, & Palmini, 2005). Epilepsy may develop from a wide variety of causes and a definitive etiology is identified in only about one-third of all newly diagnosed cases (Epilepsy Foundation, 2006; Hauser, 1997).

Seizures are sudden, involuntary, time-limited alterations in behavior, which include a change in consciousness, motor activity, autonomic function, or sensation, and are accompanied by abnormal electrical discharge in the brain (Leppik, 1997). A seizure involves a disruption of the normal electrical activity of the brain, in which neurons become unstable and fire in an abnormally rapid manner. This excessive electrical discharge may be confined to one area of the brain (partial seizure), or may occur throughout the brain in entirety (generalized seizure). "Depending on the patient, seizures may occur frequently or infrequently, only at night or after awakening, in a cyclic pattern, suggesting hormonal influences, only with highly specific triggers, in many other permutations, and, most commonly, without any apparent predictability" (Engel & Pedley, 1997, p. 4).

Incidence and Prevalence of Epilepsy

Although incidence studies around the world have produced a wide variety in estimates, most studies in the developed world suggest an incidence of between 40 and 70 per 100,000 (Cockerell, 2003). In developing nations, the estimates are considerably higher, ranging from 120 to 190 per 100,000 (Cockerell, 2003). The incidence of epilepsy in the U.S. is generally agreed to be between 1% and 2% of the population (Livneh & Antonak, 1997). Males appear to be slightly more likely to develop epilepsy than females. The incidence of epilepsy is greater in African-American and socially disadvantaged populations (Epilepsy Foundation, 2006).

With regard to age, the incidence of epilepsy is bimodal, occurring most frequently among the very young and the elderly. Incidence is highest under the age of 2 and over 65 (Epilepsy Foundation, 2006). This pattern is explained to a great extent by the etiologies of epilepsy, which are discussed below. It is estimated that in the U.S., 45,000 children under the age of 15 develop epilepsy each year. Between 40% and 50% of seizures arise in persons aged 20-years and younger, with the highest incidence among those under the age of 10 (Cockerell, 2003; Epilepsy Foundation, 2006). Good evidence indicates that epilepsy is more common among the elderly now than in the past

(Cockerell, 2003). Thus, there appears to be a trend toward decreased incidence in children and increased incidence in the elderly (Epilepsy Foundation, 2006).

As with the incidence rates, the reported prevalence of epilepsy varies widely in different studies, due to both geographic variations and differences in methodology. Estimates of the prevalence of active epilepsy (i.e., ongoing epileptic seizures, as opposed to epilepsy in remission) in the U.S. typically range from 4 to 7 per 1000 persons (Cockerell, 2003; Engel et al., 2005) or approximately 2.7 million people. Prevalence rates are higher among racial minorities than among Caucasians (Epilepsy Foundation, 2006). The prevalence of epilepsy in the developing world varies widely by region, but in many regions is reported to be significantly higher than in developed nations (Engel et al., 2005).

Etiology

In considering the etiology of epilepsy, it is important to distinguish between the cause of isolated, provoked seizures and the cause of epilepsy, or recurrent and unprovoked seizures. Isolated seizures can be caused by nearly any condition that affects brain function (Bromfield, 1997). This may include, for example, toxic-metabolic disturbances, such as disturbances in glucose, electrolyte balance, renal failure, or drug intoxication or withdrawal. Although these metabolic conditions and drug or medication effects may be recurrent, they would not lead to a diagnosis of epilepsy, because they are at least potentially preventable (Bromfield, 1997).

Epilepsy, or recurrent, unprovoked seizures, can appear secondary to a known and enduring disturbance to the brain, or can be due to unknown causes (Engel et al., 2005). A number of potential causes and risk factors for epilepsy have been identified, and these vary depending on the age of the individual. For example, among the elderly, central nervous-system injury, due to stroke, dementia and neurodegenerative diseases, trauma, and vascular disease, are leading risk factors for epilepsy. Acute neurological conditions, such as stroke or trauma, even if functionally minor, may produce structural damage to the brain and permanently alter neuronal excitability and synchronization, resulting in a tendency toward recurrent unprovoked seizures (Bromfield, 1997). Most studies of epilepsy in the elderly have found some form of vascular disease to be responsible for the majority of those cases, for which a cause is identified (Bromfield, 1997).

In newborns, infants, and young children, risk factors for epilepsy include low weight for gestational age, having a seizure in the first month of life, fever-related (febrile) seizures that are unusually long, being born with abnormal brain structures, infection or metabolic imbalance, and lack of oxygen to the brain (Schachter, 2001). Other general risk factors for epilepsy include head injury, serious brain injury or lack of oxygen to the brain, brain tumors, infections of the brain, such as abscess, meningitis, or encephalitis, stroke, cerebral palsy, a family history of epilepsy or fever-related seizures, exposure to toxic substances, and use of illegal drugs such as cocaine (Engel et al., 2005; Epilepsy Foundation, 2006; Schachter, 2001).

Individuals with other existing conditions are at an increased risk for developing epilepsy. For example, it is estimated that epilepsy can be expected to develop in 10% of children with mental retardation or cerebral palsy, and 50% of children with both disabilities (Epilepsy Foundation, 2006). Persons with Alzheimer's disease have a 10% chance of developing epilepsy, as do 22% of stroke patients. Approximately 8.7% of children of mothers with epilepsy, and 2.4% of children of fathers with epilepsy can be expected to develop epilepsy. Further, whereas approximately 70% of people with epilepsy can be expected to experience remission, which is defined as five or more years seizure-free on medication, this will be the case for only 35% of people with mental retardation, cerebral palsy, or other neurological conditions (Epilepsy Foundation, 2006).

Seizure Classification and Treatment

Classification of Seizures and Syndromes

The classification of seizures is important for a number of reasons, including the identification of treatment approach and prognosis, enhancement of professional communication and collaborative research, and understanding of the functions of the central nervous system (Dreifuss, 1993; Engel et al., 2005). Although revised classification and diagnostic schemes have recently been proposed (Baykan et al., 2005; Engel et al., 2005), and their use will likely become more prevalent as limitations to the existing schemes are recognized and addressed, two systems of classification of epilepsies are in use today: the International League Against Epilepsy (ILAE) Classification of Epileptic Seizures (Commission on Classification and Terminology of the International League Against Epilepsy, 1981) and the ILAE Classification of Epilepsies and Epileptic Syndromes (Commission on Classification and Terminology of the International League Against Epilepsy, 1989).

The ILAE Classification of Epileptic Seizures divides seizures into three types: partial, generalized, and unclassifiable, and identifies subtypes of each. Partial seizures are seizures in which the initial activation of a system of neurons is limited to one part of a single cerebral hemisphere. A partial seizure is classified primarily according to whether consciousness is impaired or not. When consciousness is impaired, the seizure is classified as a complex partial seizure. If consciousness is not impaired, the seizure is classified as a simple partial seizure. Simple partial seizures may evolve into complex partial seizures; and a partial seizure may progress to a generalized seizure (involving both cerebral hemispheres).

Generalized seizures are those in which the seizures appear to begin simultaneously in both hemispheres. Consciousness is usually impaired and this impairment may be the first manifestation. Generalized seizures include absence seizures (formerly called petit mal seizures, characterized by brief episodes of staring with impairment of awareness and responsiveness), myoclonic seizures (characterized by muscular jerking, primarily around bedtime or waking hours), tonic seizures (more common during sleep, associated with sudden stiffening movements of the body, arms, and legs, generally lasting less than 20 seconds), clonic seizures (involving jerking movements on both sides of the body, without the stiffening tonic component), tonic-clonic seizures (formerly called grand mal seizures), and atonic seizures (or "drop attacks", characterized by sudden loss of muscle tone) (Devinsky, 1994).

This system has a number of limitations, including that an individual may have more than one type of seizure, either simultaneously or in sequence, and that many individuals' seizures change over the course of their illness (Loughlin, 2005). The ILAE Classification of Epilepsies and Epileptic Syndromes (1989) was designed in part to address these limitations, and is meant to supplement the previous classification, not to replace it (Loughlin, 2005). According to this system, epilepsies are divided into four broad syndromatic groups: (1) Localization-related, (2) generalized, (3) undetermined whether localized or generalized, and (4) special syndromes. Within the localized and generalized groups, there are further subdivisions into idiopathic (unknown cause), symptomatic (identifiable cause), or cryptogenic (hidden cause) (Engel et al., 2005; Loughlin, 2005).

Treatment of Epilepsy

Because epilepsy is a term for a seizure disorder with a multitude of potential causes, it is more appropriate to discuss seizure control than cure, the former of which is achieved for 60–70% of those with epilepsy (Epilepsy Foundation, 2006; Fraser et al., 1992). Although a number of recent advances have made surgical and other treatments more prevalent, the majority of persons with epilepsy are treated with anticonvulsant or anti-epilepsy drugs. The form of treatment prescribed depends on several factors, including the type, frequency, and severity of the seizures, as well as the person's age, health, and medical history. An accurate diagnosis of the epilepsy syndrome is also critical to choosing the treatment.

The duration of treatment with anti-epilepsy drugs depends on a number of variables, including the underlying cause, seizure and syndrome type, and other factors. Many individuals can be taken off treatment after a few years, while other types of epilepsy require life-long treatment (Epilepsy Foundation, 2006). Approximately 75% of people who are seizure-free on medication for two to five years can be successfully withdrawn from medication.

Anti-epilepsy medications are frequently associated with significant adverse side effects, which may include double vision, fatigue, nervousness or agitation, difficulty concentrating, nausea, dizziness, gum overgrowth, facial hair growth, sexual dysfunction, and, occasionally, more severe side effects (Baker, Jacoby, Buck, Stalgis, & Monnet, 1997; Epilepsy Foundation, 2006; Fraser & Clemmons, 1983). Generally, at least one side effect will be experienced (Baker et al., 1997). In a recent large community-based U.S. study, Fisher et al. (2000)

found that almost one out of five people reported that the side effects and the cost of anti-epilepsy medication were the "worst" things about having epilepsy.

Surgical removal of seizure-producing areas of the brain has been an accepted form of treatment for over 50 years. However, recent developments in imaging and surgical techniques have made surgery an increasingly effective and more frequently utilized treatment approach. Most individuals with epilepsy do not require epilepsy surgery. Furthermore, surgery is not appropriate for many people for a number of reasons. Yet, if seizures are not controlled after a trial of two or three medications, then the option of surgery is frequently considered. According to the Epilepsy Foundation (2006), out of the 30% of individuals whose seizures cannot be controlled with medications, approximately one-third may be candidates for surgery.

Two additional treatment approaches, the ketogenic diet and vagus-nerve stimulation, have also received increased attention and use in recent years. The ketogenic diet is a high-fat, low-carbohydrate, adequate-protein diet that has been used for more than eight decades for the treatment of refractory (i.e., non-responsive) epilepsy in children. The ketogenic diet is used most frequently in children with seizures that have not responded to medication therapy (Epilepsy Foundation, 2006). Despite the long history of this treatment, the mechanisms by which the diet exerts its anti-seizure action are not fully understood (Stafstrom & Bough, 2003).

Vagus nerve stimulation (VNS) therapy was approved by the FDA as a treatment for epilepsy in 1997. VNS therapy involves a minor surgery to implant a small stimulator, similar to a pacemaker, under the skin in the upper chest. Stimuli are delivered at a determined frequency from the device through the vagus nerve to relay nuclei in the pons and medulla, and interfere with cortical and subcortical excitability (Engel et al., 2005). The treatment appears to be effective for seizures that do not respond well to medications alone, decreasing seizure frequency by approximately one-half in 40–50% of individuals (Engel et al.). Although the majority of individuals continue taking medications after the stimulator has been placed, many people may take fewer medicines (Epilepsy Foundation, 2006).

The Psychosocial Impact of Epilepsy

Historically, research on the psychosocial impact of epilepsy has focused on exploring and explaining the high rate of psychological distress or psychiatric co-occurrence among persons with epilepsy. Research in this area has provided an important understanding of the well-established relationship between epilepsy, depression, and anxiety (Robertson, 1989). However, because the impact of epilepsy on a person's life is multidimensional, and can span a range of functional and psychosocial domains, the need for more comprehensive models of assessing and delineating epilepsy's impact has increasingly been recognized (e.g., Bishop & Allen, 2003; Engel, 2000).

In recent years, epilepsy researchers have increasingly applied a multidimensional quality of life (QOL) perspective to exploring and understanding the psychosocial impact of epilepsy. The resulting research has underscored the complexity of epilepsy's impact and the importance of understanding and assessing epilepsy's impact beyond measures of psychological distress. The following discussion reviews the extant research on the psychosocial impact of epilepsy from both perspectives, and provides a framework for the ensuing discussion of coping responses.

Epilepsy, Depression, and Anxiety

Although the association between epilepsy, depression, and anxiety has been well established (Hermann, Seidenberg, & Bell, 2000; Robertson, 1989), the relationship is a complex one. The research concerning this relationship has been characterized by methodological differences with regard to patient groups (i.e., community versus clinical populations), diagnostic criteria, and methods of assessment. However, recent reviews in which these differences were controlled for (e.g., Hermann et al., 2000; Swinkels, Kuyk, van Dyck, & Spinhoven, 2005) suggest that the following general conclusions with regard to epilepsy and psychiatric diagnoses can be made:

1. The risk of experiencing an Axis I disorder (i.e., a clinical disorder) is elevated in people with chronic epilepsy, with mood disorders (e.g., anxiety and depression) being the most prevalent.
2. Major depression is the most prevalent mood disorder and it occurs more frequently than in the general population.
3. Major depression is more prevalent in clinical populations (where epilepsy is more severe and intractable) than in community samples.

In the search for causality in the complex relationship between epilepsy and depression, it has been consistently found that factors directly related to the disease process rarely are the sole factors accounting for depression and other psychiatric diagnoses. Interestingly, however, features of the disease process (i.e., seizure-related variables) have been the almost-exclusive focus of research attention. For example, across the 36 studies reviewed by Hermann et al. (2000), 60 different variables were examined for their relationship to depression in epilepsy. Potential predictor variables fell into four categories: (a) Neuroepilepsy (e.g., age of onset, laterality, duration of disorder, etiology, and seizure type); (b) psychological and social (e.g., adjustment to epilepsy, perceived stigma or discrimination, and stressful life events); (c) medication (e.g., monotherapy vs. polytherapy, use of barbiturate medications, and blood levels); and (d) sociodemographic factors (e.g., age, gender, education).

Although neuroepilepsy variables were the most frequently investigated predictors of depression, they resulted in the fewest positive findings. Psychological and social variables and medication variables were evaluated less commonly (representing 15% and 12% of the analyses respectively), but were associated *more frequently* with depression than the neuroepilepsy variables. This finding is essentially typical of the extant research concerning this relationship, in that level of depression is not usually well-accounted for by seizure variables (type, frequency, severity), suggesting that other factors play a significant part in this relationship. In the last decade, the relationship has been further complicated by evidence that people with major depression are at a higher risk for the development of epilepsy (e.g., Kanner & Nieto, 1999).

It has been suggested that protracted anxiety, as may result from living with a chronic and unpredictable seizure disorder, may be a precursor of depression (Robertson, 1989). Certainly, being in a situation of always wondering when one might have a seizure may be expected to lead to significant anxiety. This dynamic of epilepsy has led some researchers to represent the experience of living with epilepsy in the context of learned helplessness (e.g., DeVellis, DeVellis, Wallston, & Wallston, 1980; Hermann, Trenerry, & Colligan, 1996). However, generalized anxiety and depression are likely also to be the result of factors not directly related to seizure activity, such as social stigma, iatrogenic interactions, and various social, practical, and vocational limitations and restrictions.

Epilepsy and Quality of Life

In the last two decades, QOL has become an important and frequently utilized outcome measure in epilepsy clinical care. A multidimensional QOL framework has been identified as appropriate and useful for understanding the psychosocial impact of epilepsy, and for discussing coping responses (e.g., Bishop & Allen, 2003; Bishop, Berven, Hermann, & Chan, 2002; Chaplin, Yepez, Shorvon, & Floyd, 1990; Collings, 1995; Jacoby, 1992; Jacoby, Baker, Smith, Dewey, & Chadwick, 1993; O'Donoghue, Duncan, & Sander, 1998). A number of interesting and important observations can be made about this body of research. First, comparative studies found, with some consistency across a relatively small number of studies (e.g., Chubon, 1995; Hermann et al., 1996; Schiffer & Babigan, 1984; Scott, Lhatoo, & Sander, 2001; Wiebe, Bellhouse, Fallahay, & Eliasziw, 1999), that people with epilepsy report lower QOL, compared both to persons without chronic illnesses or disabilities (CID) and persons with other CIDs. Second, as with the question of depression, the relationship between epilepsy and QOL has been found to be far more complex than can be accounted for by seizure variables alone (e.g., Bishop et al., 2002; Jacoby et al., 1993; O'Donoghue et al., 1998). Rather, a number of psychosocial variables, which are associated with living with epilepsy, appear to play an important role in this relationship.

Some researchers, who use a QOL perspective to explore the impact of epilepsy, have defined QOL more narrowly, such as from a health-related QOL perspective in which social, mental, and physical health are the foci. Others have used a more comprehensive approach, defining QOL as including a broader range of domains, such as family function, financial situation, self-esteem and identity, employment status, and social function (Bishop et al., 2002). In the following discussion, findings are incorporated from research that are inclusive of both approaches.

Chronicity

As with any chronic illness, a diagnosis with epilepsy typically means the beginning of a long-term, sometimes life-long relationship with seizures, medications and treatments, medical care, and the coloring of one's experience by epilepsy (Coping with Epilepsy, 2003; Murray, 1993). People are generally uncomfortable with the sense of immutable permanence, and find stressful the lack of control, the lack of the ability to change, and the lack of flexibility associated with the concept of chronicity (Bishop, 2001). The post-diagnosis realization of the chronic nature of epilepsy and of the absence of a "cure" as commonly conceived represents a significant issue to cope with for those who are recently diagnosed.

Stigma and Identity

"Epilepsy has often been regarded as one of the most stigmatizing medical impairments" (Livneh, Wilson, Duchesneau, & Antonak, 2001, p. 535). Although data reveal regional and national differences, stigmatizing perceptions, negative attitudes, and misperceptions about persons with epilepsy have been found to exist in samples across the world (Livneh & Antonak, 1997). The stigma of epilepsy consists of deeply discrediting attributes (e.g., a propensity to crime and violence, sexual deviance, inheritability, and mental illness); restrictions or denials of common benefits (e.g., a drivers' license or life insurance); and limitations on opportunities that lead to independence (e.g., housing or employment discrimination) (Livneh & Antonak, 1997, Livneh et al., 2001).

The limitations and restrictions associated with the diagnosis of epilepsy can have a significant impact on one's sense of identity. In a number of complex ways, epilepsy has the potential to change the way individuals do things, the way others see them, and the way they see themselves. By limiting access to or otherwise affecting the roles engaged in, by the nature of participation in valued by activities, and the ensuing loss of confidence, epilepsy has the potential both to alter one's identity and to reduce perceptions of control.

Fear and Uncertainty

Fear is the factor most frequently identified as being the worst thing about having epilepsy (Fisher et al., 2000). Seizures are, of course, the hallmark symptom of epilepsy, and although seizures cannot solely account for the psychosocial problems experienced by persons with epilepsy, they certainly represent a fundamental element in this relationship. Although generally relatively brief, seizures nevertheless have the potential to be tremendously disruptive, and fear of, or concern about seizures has consistently been found to affect social, psychological, and vocational function (Baker et al., 1997) and QOL (Bishop & Allen, 2003). Specific fears frequently identified by adults with epilepsy include fear of dying, fear that their children will witness a seizure and be upset, fear of having a seizure in public, fear of losing employment, and fear of having a seizure while driving (Fisher et al., 2000).

Social Function and Isolation

Epilepsy is, for many, an isolating condition. This isolation frequently occurs as a bi-directional process, in which people around the individual with epilepsy withdraw due to discomfort, stigma, and so on, and the individual simultaneously engages in active withdrawal of opportunities for social engagement. Although many people with epilepsy may have few, if any, disruptions of social interaction and functioning, others have severe problems that prevent them from engaging in fully productive lives; adults with epilepsy have been found to have a higher prevalence of social problems and social isolation than people in the general population (Austin & deBoer, 1997).

In their survey of 92 adults examining the psychosocial effects of poorly controlled epilepsy, Thompson and Oxley (1988) found that social function was the area of greatest dissatisfaction. Sixty-eight percent of the participants reported having no personal friends, and 34% stated that they never formed true friendships. Only 8% were married or cohabiting, 8% were involved in a steady relationship, and 57% had never had such a relationship. Collings (1990) found similar experiences of social isolation in his research with people with epilepsy. Among the proposed explanations for problems in social functioning are: (a) The development of a dependency role (e.g., due to parental overprotectiveness), (b) severe and frequent seizures and embarrassment or concerns about participating in activities involving social interaction, because of fear of having a seizure, (c) low self-esteem from having a chronic disease that carries a stigma, (d) concomitant conditions or deficits, and (e) academic underachievement (Austin & deBoer, 1997; Fisher et al., 2000).

Employment

Employment is a highly valued personal and social role, and an important means of accessing both financial security and, for many, medical insurance. For many people with epilepsy, access to employment is a significant concern. The problematic employment situation for people with epilepsy has been well-researched, and an extensive body of literature exists on this topic (see for example, Bishop, 2002, 2004; Bishop & Allen, 2001; Fraser & Clemmons, 1983; Thorbecke & Fraser, 1997). In the U.S., over 50% of individuals with moderately severe epilepsy listed employment as a concern, and over 20% considered it to be the most important concern in relation to living with recurrent seizures (Gilliam, Kuzniecky, Faught, Black, Carpenter, & Schrodt, 1996).

The unemployment rate among individuals with epilepsy, who are eligible workers or who are maintaining an active job search in the U.S., ranges from 13% to 25% (Fisher et al., 2000; Thorbecke & Fraser, 1997). Employment status has been found to be associated with seizure type (i.e., individuals who had seizures classified as tonic-clonic were less likely to be employed; Jacoby, Baker, Steen, Potts, & Chadwick, 1996). Numerous psychosocial factors have been implicated in the high unemployment rate among individuals with epilepsy, including: (a) Social isolation, (b) lack of information, (c) social skills deficits, (d) lack of family support, and (e) fears about and experiences with negative attitudes on the part of employers (Devinsky, 1994; Thorbecke & Fraser, 1997).

Family Functioning

Family functioning and family support have been found to be important determinants of adjustment, coping, and quality of life among persons with epilepsy (Loring, Meador, & Lee, 2004; Mirnics, Bekes, Rózsa, & Halász, 2001). Unfortunately, however, epilepsy has frequently been found to have a significant negative impact on family, both for adults (i.e., marriage and family life), and for children with epilepsy and their siblings. There is evidence that people with epilepsy are less likely to marry and have children. This is particularly true if the epilepsy is severe, or if it exists in the presence of additional illnesses or disabilities (Dansky, Andermann, & Andermann, 1980; Jacoby, 1992). Higher rates of divorce than the general population have also been found among parents of children with epilepsy (Sillanpaa, 1973). In addition, siblings of children with epilepsy appear to be at a greater risk for psychiatric disturbance (Hoare & Kerley, 1991). Families of children with epilepsy have been found to be less cohesive, have lower levels of self-esteem and communication, and have lower levels of social support than families of children with other chronic conditions (Austin, 1988; Ferrari, Matthews, & Barabas, 1983).

Coping with Epilepsy: Overview and Research

Unfortunately, despite a growing body of research concerning the psychosocial impact of epilepsy, there is relatively little research specifically addressing either the mechanisms of coping with epilepsy or the interventions that promote effective coping. This is particularly true when compared with the extensive research of this type that has been conducted among persons with other chronic illnesses, such as AIDS, arthritis, cancer, and diabetes. Further, in evaluating the coping research in the field of epilepsy, a number of important limitations are evident. These include a narrow focus, in many studies, on specific subgroups of persons with epilepsy, particularly children and adolescents; an over-reliance on cross-sectional, rather than longitudinal research; and lack of a consistent approach to defining coping outcomes. [See Livneh et al. (2001, p. 541) for a comprehensive discussion of methodological and conceptual limitations in this literature.] Although further attention to coping with epilepsy is clearly necessary, the following discussion summarizes the research on coping to date.

Research has demonstrated that the use of specific coping styles and strategies has an influential effect on the psychosocial adjustment of individuals with epilepsy (Snyder, 1990; Upton & Thompson, (1992). In their comprehensive review of the extant literature on coping with epilepsy, Livneh et al. (2001) considered both general and more specific coping styles and their relationship to psychosocial adaptation in people with epilepsy. Their overview suggested that personal resourcefulness (Rosenbaum & Palmon, 1984), a general propensity for problem-solving (Snyder, 1990), and higher self-efficacy (Tedman, Thorton, & Baker, 1995) were associated with better psychosocial outcomes (generally characterized by lower anxiety and depression), as well as better subjective perceptions of health, higher self-esteem, and reduced feelings of stigma. In terms of more specific coping strategies, planful problem-solving and cognitive restructuring were identified as strategies that appear to be associated with lower levels of anxiety, depression, and other measures of psychosocial well-being. Alternately, the use of what have been termed "disengaging" coping strategies (such as avoidance, wishful thinking, and self-blame) have been associated with higher anxiety and depression scores.

It should be noted that although there is a tendency among coping researchers to consider some coping strategies as inherently more likely to promote successful psychosocial outcomes, while associating other strategies with negative outcomes, "the majority of coping strategies fail to be accounted for in such a simplistic dichotomy" (Livneh et al., 2001, p. 534). For example, in the relationship between specific coping strategies and various psychosocial outcomes, some strategies (e.g., denial) appear to be beneficial for some people, and less so for others. One explanation for such inconsistencies is that coping strategies emerge and shift over time and experience (e.g., Folkman & Moskowitz, 2004). This perspective suggests that coping strategies and adaptive coping mechanisms are developed, engaged in, and revised or discarded as the source of stress, and one's experience with it, change.

Some strategies may effectively promote coping at one specific stage of the disease process (e.g., at and immediately post-diagnosis) and other strategies may be more effective at others (e.g., after several years of living with the condition). Such a dynamic has been suggested, for example, in the work of Leventhal (e.g., Leventhal & Diefenbach, 1991). Longitudinal research, which has been almost nonexistent in the epilepsy coping literature to date, would help to explore this dynamic process among persons with epilepsy.

Interventions that Promote Effective Coping

A number of psychotherapeutic and psychoeducational approaches have been evaluated and found to be associated with various positive outcomes in the epilepsy research. Several forms of psychological intervention, which are aimed at promoting effective coping with epilepsy, are described below, including psychotherapeutic approaches and psychoeducational programs and interventions. Following this, assistive and rehabilitation-technology interventions, and other environmentally-focused approaches, which can be used to enhance coping, are described.

Psychotherapeutic Approaches

Psychotherapeutic approaches include counseling or psychotherapy interventions that promote effective coping, acceptance, or psychosocial adaptation. Cognitive-behavioral approaches, progressive relaxation therapy, and family therapy have each been explored and shown to have beneficial effects for coping with epilepsy, as described below.

Cognitive-Behavioral Approaches

There have been relatively few studies in which specific therapies have been developed or evaluated for their ability to assist individuals with epilepsy to engage in effective coping strategies, or to modify less effective strategies. There is, however, evidence that some cognitive-behavioral approaches do promote such an effect. For example, Rösche, Uhlmann, and Weber (2004) recently reported a study in which the use of a "holistic therapeutic approach" resulted in an increase in the use of problem-focused coping and a decrease in emotion-focused coping or avoidance-oriented coping among 65 individuals with therapy-refractory epilepsy. This effect was independent of seizure control or antidepressant medication. Similarly, Goldstein, McAlpine, Deale, Toone, and Mellers (2003) reported that cognitive-behavior therapy with a small sample of adults with chronic, poorly controlled seizures and co-existing psychiatric and/or psychosocial difficulties reduced the deleterious impact of epilepsy on participants' daily lives. It also resulted in significant improvements in their self-rated work and social adjustment, and a decreased use of escape-avoidance coping strategies. These findings occurred despite the absence of a significant decrease in seizure frequency.

A number of specific cognitive-behavioral techniques have been evaluated for their ability to enhance coping. For example, Upton and Thompson (1992) found that the use of the coping strategy, "cognitive restructuring," described as efforts at finding positive aspects of the experience of epilepsy, was associated with better acceptance of disability and lower levels of depression, anxiety, and social avoidance. Additionally, the "information-seeking" coping strategy, while found to be associated with higher levels of anxiety, was also found to be associated with lower levels of social avoidance. Alternately, Krakow, Bühler, and Haltenhof (1999) found that high seizure frequency and the use of coping strategies deemed ineffective, such as denial and wishful thinking, were associated with high levels of depression and poor psychosocial adjustment.

Progressive Relaxation Training

Progressive relaxation training (PRT) for seizure reduction entails the method described by Wolpe (1969), in which the individual with epilepsy initially learns deep muscular relaxation, and is then encouraged to reproduce those feelings of relaxation when the individual thinks a seizure is forthcoming (Fenwick, 1991). In a study that examined the use of this method in individuals with poorly controlled epilepsy, Rousseau, Hermann, and Whitman (1985) found that implementing PRT resulted in a 30% reduction in median seizure frequency. In another study investigating the use of PRT, Whitman, Dell, Legion, Eibhlyn, and Statsinger (1990) found that median seizure frequency decreased 21% after two months, 41% after four months, and 54% after six months. Puskarich, Whitman, Dell, Hughes, Rosen, and Hermann (1992) found that PRT was more effective than placebo (sitting quietly) in reducing seizures, and reported that the PRT group showed a significant 29% decrease in mean seizure frequency and a 54% decrease in median seizure frequency.

Although these three investigations used varying follow-up intervals, different relaxation training protocols, and different therapists, the consistent evidence of seizure reduction is noteworthy. Nonetheless, while these studies appear to provide support for the use of PRT to reduce seizures, the mechanism by which PRT seems to reduce seizure frequency is unclear (Puskarich et al., 1992). Because daily stress has been found to be a significant predictor of seizure activity (Temkin & Davis, 1984), PRT may decrease the frequency of seizures by reducing stress. Williams and Koocher (1998) observed that relaxation techniques involve a paradox, noting that "in order to gain control, an individual must be able to 'let go' and relax" (p. 334). For those who cannot relinquish control, training in relaxation techniques has the potential of increasing anxiety.

Other behavioral approaches have also been reported to control seizures. For example, Kobau and DiLorio (2003) reported that a substantial number of participants indicated using their own behavioral approaches to controlling seizures, either by avoiding their seizure triggers or by trying to stop a seizure in their own way. This finding is consistent with other studies (e.g., Reiter & Andrews, 2000; Spector, Cull, & Goldstein, 2001), in which some individuals with epilepsy were able to successfully implement behavioral approaches to control seizures.

Family Therapy

Family therapy often becomes an essential component of the management of epilepsy, especially when a disruptive family pattern is a source of chronic stress for an individual with epilepsy (Miller, 1994). For families of a person with epilepsy, a fundamental element of successful family therapy is the family's acceptance of the diagnosis and the treatment, as well as the family's willingness to collaborate (Miller, 1994). Miller suggested that whereas a family's support may help the family member with epilepsy to overcome any hesitations about accepting the diagnosis, a family's rejection of the diagnosis may undermine the family member's acceptance of his or her own epilepsy.

Numerous issues (e.g., dependency, communication patterns, family structure) may be appropriately and effectively addressed within family therapy. "Family sessions should help families make the necessary changes in their concept of the patient's condition, to avoid blaming the patient for the illness, and to hopefully achieve a new family homeostasis" (Miller, 1994, p. 741).

Psychoeducational Programs and Interventions

The foremost aims of psychoeducational interventions for people with epilepsy are the improvement of knowledge, medication compliance, and coping with epilepsy, as well as the enhancement of QOL (May & Pfäfflin, 2005). May and Pfäfflin propose that any psychoeducational program designed for individuals with epilepsy should address the following domains: (a) Understanding epilepsy (e.g., prevalence, etiology, the various forms of epilepsies and types of seizures); (b) managing seizures (e.g., comprehending what seizures are, identifying potential seizure precipitants, the usefulness of documenting the details of seizures, anti-epilepsy drug therapy); (c) understanding treatment options (e.g., improving of compliance, advantages and disadvantages of various options); (d) self-control of seizures (e.g., self-control strategies, lifestyle options); and (e) social consequences and restrictions due to ever-present seizures (e.g., driving). May and Pfäfflin also suggest that group discussions and exchanges between group members about their own personal experiences are indispensable components of psychoeducational programs, especially in terms of improving the ability to cope with epilepsy.

The need for psychoeducational interventions has been solidly established in research, showing that many people with epilepsy have deficits concerning their knowledge of their diagnosis (e.g., Schneider & Conrad, 1986), seizure precipitants or triggers (Dawkins, Crawford, & Stammers, 1993; Mittan, 1986; Unsworth, 1999), seizure type (Goldstein, Minchin, Stubbs, & Fenwick, 1997; Unsworth, 1999), the purpose and potential side effects of anti-epilepsy drugs (Goldstein et al., 1997; Thompson & Oxley, 1993), safety (Goldstein et al., 1997; Long, Reeves, Moore, Roach, & Pickering, 2000), and the potential consequences of seizures (Mittan, 1986).

Noncompliance with anti-epilepsy drug therapy is also a frequent problem among individuals with epilepsy (Cramer, Glassman, & Rienzi, 2002; Leppik, 1990; Specht, Elsner, May, Schimichowski, & Thorbecke, 2003). Self-efficacy, or confidence in one's capabilities to initiate and successfully perform particular tasks at designated levels, has been demonstrated to be a significant predictor of successful medication management for individuals with epilepsy (DiLorio, Faherty, & Manteuffel, 1992; DiLorio, Faherty, & Manteuffel, 1994). "It is likely that the sense of one's ability to cope with the disease encourages actual coping, such as taking medication and performing other actions known to increase self-management" (Amir, Roziner, Knoll, & Neufeld, 1999, p. 221).

Tedman et al. (1995) found that individuals with epilepsy who had higher perceptions of self-efficacy also reported reduced perceptions of epilepsy impact and stigma.

Only a few comprehensive psychoeducational programs have been evaluated for their ability to promote effective coping with epilepsy. Two such programs are described below: the Seizures and Epilepsy Education Program (SEE), and the Modular Service Package Epilepsy (MOSES).

Seizures and Epilepsy Education (SEE)

The Seizures and Epilepsy Education (SEE; formerly known as Sepulveda Epilepsy Education) program (Helgeson, Mittan, Tan, & Chayasirisobhon, 1990) is a two-day psychoeducational treatment intervention for adults with epilepsy, which places a heavy emphasis on medication compliance in order to achieve the best possible seizure control. The underlying belief of SEE is that an adequate understanding of epilepsy is essential to effective coping with epilepsy. This program uses a psychoeducational approach to deliver health education, psychosocial help, and to enable individuals with epilepsy to better cope with their disability. While there is only one published investigation of the SEE program and its effectiveness with adults with epilepsy (Helgeson et al., 1990), a recent poster session (Shore, Perkins, & Austin, 2005) presented findings on the efficacy of the SEE program for adolescents with epilepsy and their parents.

Helgeson and colleagues' (1990) study found that, in comparison to the waiting-list control group ($n = 18$), the treatment group ($n = 20$) demonstrated a significant decrease in their level of fear of death and brain damage resulting from seizures, and a significant decrease in overall level of misinformation and misconceptions about epilepsy. In addition to the self-report measures concerning anti-epilepsy drug (AED) compliance, this study used an objective measure of AED serum levels, and the results indicated that the SEE program was effective at improving medication compliance. The authors noted that, "It was particularly significant that the blood level increase was maintained for months after the program. Moreover, none of the increased blood levels were in generally accepted toxic ranges, nor were there any reports of increase in toxic symptoms" (Helgeson et al., 1990, p. 81).

Thus, the SEE program demonstrated that a psychoeducational program can improve medication compliance in adults with epilepsy. Further, although statistically significant differences were lacking between the treatment group and the waiting-list control group on the scales of the Washington Psychosocial Seizure Inventory (WPSI; Dodrill, Batzel, Queisser, & Temkin, 1980), which is an instrument that assesses the social and emotional concerns of individuals with epilepsy, Helgeson and colleagues found that the treatment group displayed continued trends of improvement in numerous domains of adjustment (e.g., emotional, interpersonal, vocational, and seizure-related) from the immediate post-assessment to the four-month follow-up.[1]

Modular Service Package Epilepsy (MOSES)

The Modular Service Package Epilepsy (MOSES; Ried, Specht, Thorbecke, Goecke, & Wohlfarth, 2001) is designed to support individuals with epilepsy in becoming experts in managing their own disability by attempting to change their attitudes and behavior, rather than merely conveying theoretical knowledge. As an interactive program, MOSES was specifically developed to be used in a small-group learning environment (ideally between seven and 10 participants; Ried et al., 2001). Ried and colleagues noted that training in small groups offers numerous advantages, such as: (a) Opportunities for sharing experiences with other participants, (b) other participants acting as models from which to learn, and (c) motivating one another.

The structure of MOSES, as the name implies, is modular, and consists of nine modules, or units, which involve the following topics: Living with epilepsy, epidemiology, basic knowledge, diagnostics, therapy, self-control, prognosis, psychosocial aspects, and network epilepsy (Ried et al., 2001). May and Pfäfflin (2002) report that the program typically involves approximately 14 lessons (each lasting one-hour). Spreading the course out over many sessions allows participants the opportunity to interact with one another, practice what they have learned, and get feedback.

The educational aims of MOSES are to improve participants' knowledge about epilepsy, its consequences, and common diagnostic tests (e.g., electroencephalography, magnetic resonance imaging); to improve participants' understanding of psychosocial and vocational issues; and to learn effective coping strategies (Ried et al., 2001). May and Pfäfflin (2002) note that the program focuses on enhancing the participants' self-help abilities and on encouraging the participants to become experts of their own lives in dealing with epilepsy.

In a controlled, randomized study, May and Pfäfflin (2002) investigated the efficacy of MOSES for adults with epilepsy. While MOSES was developed so that the various modules would be offered to a small group over a span of several weeks, this study modified the program and presented MOSES as a two-day course. Even so, the results are rather impressive. Compared to the waiting-list control group ($n = 129$), the MOSES group ($n = 113$) reported significantly fewer seizures. As the researchers stated, this finding was particularly noteworthy

---

[1] The SEE program has been revised since the publication of Helgeson and colleagues' (1990) study, and information may be found on the World Wide Web (http://www.theseeprogram.com/index.html). Information from this website contains details about the SEE topics, which include medical aspects of epilepsy (e.g., explanation of epilepsy, diagnosis, anti-epilepsy drug therapy, first-aid) and social and emotional aspects of epilepsy.

because most of the participants had had long-standing seizures and had previously received specialized treatment. They assumed that the MOSES program led to an improved compliance with anti-epilepsy drugs and to a lifestyle adjustment.

More recently, May and Pfäfflin (2005) explained that the MOSES program emphasizes the identification and avoidance of seizure precipitants and the use of seizure-control methods; when taken together with improved anti-epilepsy drug compliance, a reduction in seizure frequency may indeed result (May & Pfäfflin, 2005). Concerning the study's claim that the MOSES program improved participants' coping with epilepsy, May and Pfäfflin (2002) suggested that the MOSES program was successful in providing information, self-management strategies, and possibilities for participants to gather and locate information independently. The researchers viewed this as supporting the active role of the individual with epilepsy in dealing with his or her disability. Although the MOSES program was developed for German-speaking countries, a translation into the English language is in progress (May & Pfäfflin, 2005).

Assistive and Rehabilitation Technology and Environmental Interventions that Promote Coping

Seizures that result in the temporary loss of consciousness and function are accompanied by risks for a variety of injuries, such as fractures, dislocations, concussions, burns, and even death (Breningstall, 2001; Spitz, 1998). Assistive and rehabilitation technology can help individuals with epilepsy maintain their independence while maximizing their safety, thereby promoting their integration into society. These interventions range in sophistication from grab bars or safety rails to monitoring and tracking systems that are designed to locate an individual, who may have wandered away from home during a seizure (Schuch, 1998).

Within an individual's place of residence, several types of assistive technology may be used to maintain independence. For example, for individuals with epilepsy who experience nocturnal seizures, Applied Health-care Ltd., a company based in the United Kingdom, manufactures an anti-suffocation pillow, which is made of ripple foam inside a netting cover, which is designed to prevent suffocation due to vomiting during a seizure.

Showers have proven to be safer than baths in terms of the risk of drowning (e.g., Ryan and Dowling, 1993). In a retrospective review of the medical examiner's investigations into deaths from drowning in Alberta, Canada between 1981 and 1990, Ryan and Dowling (1993) identified 25 people whose death by drowning was considered to be directly related to seizures. Of these, 15 (60%) occurred while the individual was taking an unsupervised bath, and only one occurred while the person was taking a shower. The other deaths by drowning occurred in rivers, lakes, public and private pools, and a Jacuzzi.

Nonetheless, several studies (e.g., Buck, Baker, Jacoby, Smith, & Chadwick, 1997; Spitz, Towbin, Shantz, & Adler, 1994), investigating injuries as a consequence of seizures in individuals with epilepsy, have found that a subset of individuals with epilepsy are at increased risk for burns received while showering. Investigating risk factors and circumstances for burns, Spitz and colleagues (1994) surveyed 244 consecutive individuals with epilepsy attending the University of Colorado Health Sciences Center Seizure Clinic and found that 16% of injuries occurred while showering; showering was the second most common activity associated with a burn, with cooking on a stove the primary cause of burn injuries.

Yet, most shower-related burns are avoidable, as modern water heaters have thermostats that can be set to limit the maximum temperature of the water (Spitz et al., 1994). Another precaution that individuals with epilepsy may consider is to install an anti-scald safety device (Spitz, 1998). These devices limit the flow of water to a mere trickle when the temperature reaches a predetermined temperature (e.g., 120 degrees F). It is also recommended that individuals with epilepsy use showers equipped with pirouetting taps which, even when accidentally struck, are less likely to lead to dangerous increases in water temperature (Unglaub, Woodruff, Ulrich, & Pallua, 2005). According to Unglaub (2005), pirouetting tap systems, better known in the U.S. as a "single lever handle," meet requirements of the Americans with Disabilities Act. Other common recommendations for the shower area include grab bars, bathtub rails, shower seats, and the removal of existing glass shower-doors (Vogtle, 2003). Another example of assistive or rehabilitation technology that may benefit individuals with uncontrolled seizures is a shower that uses infrared technology to shut off the water supply when an individual falls (Schuch, 1998).

Seizure-Response Dogs

Several recent studies conducted in the United Kingdom have investigated the use of specially trained assistance dogs to provide a warning of an impending seizure to individuals with epilepsy (e.g., Brown & Strong, 2001; Strong, Brown, Huyton, & Coyle, 2002; Strong, Brown, & Walker, 1999). Anecdotal evidence has suggested that many individuals with epilepsy who have trained assistance dogs experience a reduction in seizure frequency (e.g., Brown & Strong, 2001; Strong et al., 1999). A pilot study by Strong et al. (2002) provides empirical support for this finding.

Strong and colleagues (2002) described the findings of 10 consecutive referrals of individuals with tonic-clonic seizures, none of which experienced any type of aura, to the Seizure Alert Dogs® program. Seizure frequency was monitored over a span of 48 weeks, which included a 12-week baseline period, a 12-week training period, and a 24-week follow up. Results indicated a significant drop in seizure frequency during the first four weeks of training and a further drop during the last four weeks of training. This final reduction in seizure frequency was maintained through the 24-week follow-up. While more evidence is needed, one major benefit that such specially trained dogs offer is the potential to reduce the stress that is related to not knowing when a seizure will occur (Strong & Brown, 2000). Specially trained dogs may also be trained to help during a seizure by pushing life-alert buttons, helping and/or comforting a person during a seizure, and getting help or the phone for the person experiencing a seizure. Within the U.S., there are several organizations that train and place various types of assistance dogs with individuals with epilepsy and other disabilities.

Conclusion

The complexity and individually unique experience of epilepsy undoubtedly contributes to the limitations in the scope and extent of coping research that are noted in this chapter. However, some final conclusions can be made when considering the state of this pursuit. First, there simply has not been sufficient empirical research attention conducted on coping in the area of psychosocial aspects of epilepsy. This is underscored by the comparison of the number of articles on the topic of coping with epilepsy with that of other chronic conditions. More longitudinal research, such as has been highlighted in this chapter (Livneh et al., 2001), is particularly needed.

Second, there is a need for further theory-development in the area of coping with epilepsy. It is likely that general coping theories, such as those described in the first section of this text, can be fruitfully applied in the context of epilepsy. Given the unique features of the condition, however, the further development and evaluation of epilepsy-specific models of coping, and interventions to aid in coping (e.g., the psychoeducational programs described in this chapter) are necessary. Finally, as is the case for all the conditions discussed in this text, understanding and promoting the process of effectively coping with epilepsy requires a focus not only on the individual, but on the interrelationships between the individual and the social, legal, medical, and physical contexts in which he or she lives.

References

Amir, M., Roziner, I., Knoll, A., & Neufeld, M. Y. (1999). Self-efficacy and social support as mediators in the relation between disease severity and quality of life in patients with epilepsy. *Epilepsia, 40*(2), 216–224.

Austin, J. K. (1988). Childhood epilepsy: Child adaptation and family resources. *Journal of Child and Adolescent Psychiatric Mental Health Nursing, 1*(1), 18–24.

Austin, J. K., & deBoer, H. M. (1997). Disruptions in social functioning and services facilitating adjustment for the child and adult. In J. Engel Jr. & T. A. Pedley (Eds.), *Epilepsy: A comprehensive textbook* (pp. 2191–2201). Philadelphia: Lippincott-Raven.

Baker, G. A., Jacoby, A., Buck, D., Stalgis, C., & Monnet, D. (1997). Quality of life of people with epilepsy: A European study. *Epilepsia, 38*(3), 353–362.

Baykan, B., Ertas, N. K., Ertas, M., Aktekin, B., Saygi, S., & Gokyigit, A. (2005). Comparison of classifications of seizures: A preliminary study with 28 participants and 48 seizures. *Epilepsy & Behavior, 6*, 607–612.

Bishop, M. (2001). The recovery process and chronic illness and disability: Applications and implications. *Journal of Vocational Rehabilitation, 16*(1), 47–52.

Bishop, M. (2002). Barriers to employment among people with epilepsy: Report of a focus group. *Journal of Vocational Rehabilitation, 17,* 281–286.

Bishop, M. (2004). Determinants of employment status among a community-based sample of people with epilepsy: Implications for rehabilitation interventions. *Rehabilitation Counseling Bulletin, 47,* 112–120.

Bishop, M., & Allen, C. (2001). Employment concerns of people with epilepsy and the question of disclosure: Report of a survey of the epilepsy foundation. *Epilepsy & Behavior, 2*(5), 490–495.

Bishop, M., & Allen, C. A. (2003). The impact of epilepsy on quality of life: A qualitative analysis. *Epilepsy & Behavior, 4,*226–233.

Bishop, M., Berven, N. L., Hermann, B., & Chan, F. (2002). Quality of life in epilepsy: An exploratory model. *Rehabilitation Counseling Bulletin, 45,* 41–70.

Bromfield, E. B. (1997). Epilepsy and the elderly. In S. C. Schachter & D. L. Schomer (Eds.), *The comprehensive evaluation and treatment of epilepsy* (pp. 233–254). San Diego, CA: Academic Press.

Breningstall, G. N. (2001). Mortality in pediatric epilepsy. *Pediatric Neurology, 25,* 9–16.

Brown, S. W., & Strong, V. (2001). The use of seizure-alert dogs. *Seizure, 10,* 39–41.

Buck, D., Baker, G. A., Jacoby, A., Smith, D. F., & Chadwick, D. W. (1997). Patients' experiences of injury as a result of epilepsy. *Epilepsia, 38*(4), 439–444.

Chaplin, J. E., Yepez, R., Shorvon, S., & Floyd, M. (1990). A quantitative approach to measuring the social effects of epilepsy. *Neuroepidemiology, 9,* 151–158.

Chubon, R. A. (1995). *Manual for the life situation survey.* Columbia, SC: University of South Carolina Rehabilitation Counseling Program.

Cockerell, O. C. (2003). *Epilepsy: Current concepts* (2nd ed.). London: Current Medical Literature Ltd.

Collings, J. A. (1990). Epilepsy and well-being. *Social Science and Medicine, 31,* 165–170.

Collings, J. A. (1995). Life fulfillment in an epilepsy sample from the United States. *Social Science and Medicine, 40,* 1579–1584.

Commission on Classification and Terminology of the International League Against Epilepsy. (1981). Proposal for revised clinical and electroencephalographic classification of epileptic seizures. *Epilepsia, 22,* 489–501.

Commission on Classification and Terminology of the International League Against Epilepsy. (1989). Proposal for revised classification of epilepsies and epileptic syndromes. *Epilepsia, 30,* 389–399.

Coping with Epilepsy (2003). *Epilepsia, 44*(Suppl. 6), 43–44.

Cramer, J. A., Glassman, M., & Rienzi, V. (2002). The relationship between poor medication compliance and seizures. *Epilepsy & Behavior, 3,* 338–342.

Dansky, L.V., Andermann, E., & Andermann, F. (1980). Marriage and fertility in epileptic patients. *Epilepsia, 21,* 261–271.

Dawkins, J. L., Crawford, P. M., & Stammers, T. G. (1993). Epilepsy: A general practice study of knowledge and attitudes among sufferers and non-sufferers. *British Journal of General Practice, 43,* 453–457.

DeVellis, R. F., DeVellis, B. M., Wallston, B. S., & Wallston, K. A. (1980). Epilepsy and learned helplessness. *Basic and Applied Social Psychology, 1,* 241–253.

Devinsky, O. (1994). *A guide to understanding and living with epilepsy.* Philadelphia: F. A. Davis Co.

DiLorio, C., Faherty, B., & Manteuffel, B. (1992). Self-efficacy and social support in self-management of epilepsy. *Western Journal of Nursing Research, 14,* 292–303.

DiLorio, C., Faherty, B., & Manteuffel, B. (1994). Epilepsy self-management: Partial replication and extension. *Research in Nursing & Health, 17*, 167–174.

Dodrill, C. B., Batzel, L. W., Queisser, H. R., & Temkin, N. R. (1980). An objective method for the assessment of psychological and social problems among epileptics. *Epilepsia, 21*, 123–135.

Dreifuss, F. E. (1993). Classification of epilepsies in childhood. In W. E. Dodson & J. M. Pellock (Eds.), *Pediatric epilepsy: Diagnosis and therapy* (pp. 45–56). New York: Demos.

Engel, J., Jr. (2000). Foreward. In G. A. Baker & A. Jacoby (Eds.), *Quality of life in epilepsy: Beyond seizure counts in assessment and treatment* (pp. xiii–xiv). London: Harwood Academic Publishers.

Engel, J., Jr., Birbeck, G. L., Gallo Diop, A., Jain, S., & Palmini, A. (2005). What is epilepsy? In T. L. Munsat (Series Ed.) and J. Engel, G. L. Birbeck, A. Gallo Diop, S. Jain, & A. Palmini (Volume Eds.) *World Federation of Neurology Seminars in Clinical Neurology: Vol. 2. Epilepsy: Global issues for the practicing neurologist* (pp. 1–11). New York: Deimos Medical Publishing.

Engel, J., Jr., & Pedley, T. A. (1997). Introduction: What is epilepsy? In J. Engel Jr. & T. A. Pedley (Eds.), *Epilepsy: A comprehensive textbook* (pp. 1–10). Philadelphia: Lippincott-Raven.

Epilepsy Foundation (2006). Retrieved January 3, 2006, from http://www.epilepsyfoundation.org/

Fenwick, P. (1991). Evocation and inhibition of seizures: Behavioral treatment. *Advances in Neurology, 55*, 163–183.

Ferrari, M., Matthews, W. S., & Barabas, G. (1983). The family and the child with epilepsy. *Family Process, 22*(1), 53–59.

Fisher, R. S., Vickrey, B. G., Gibson, P., Hermann, B., Penovich, P., Scherer, A., et al. (2000). The impact of epilepsy from the patient's perspective I: Descriptions and subjective perceptions. *Epilepsy Research, 41*, 39–51.

Folkman, S., & Moskowitz, J. T. (2004). Coping: Pitfalls and promise. *Annual Review of Psychology, 55*, 745–774.

Fraser, R. T., & Clemmons, D. (1983). Epilepsy rehabilitation: Assessment and counseling concerns. *Journal of Applied Rehabilitation Counseling, 14*(3), 26–31.

Fraser, R. T., Glazer, E., & Simcoe, B. J. (1992) Epilepsy. In M. G. Brodwin, F. Telez, & S. K. Brodwin (Eds.), *Medical, psychosocial and vocational aspects of disability* (pp. 439–454). Athens, GA: Elliott & Fitzpatrick.

Gilliam, F., Kuzniecky, R., Faught, E., Black, L., Carpenter, G., & Schrodt, R. (1996). Patient-validated content of epilepsy-specific quality of life measurement. *Epilepsia, 36*, 233–236.

Goldstein, L. H., McAlpine, M., Deale, A. Toone, B. K., & Mellers, J. D. C. (2003). Cognitive behaviour therapy with adults with intractable *epilepsy* and psychiatric co-morbidity: Preliminary observations on changes in psychological state and seizure frequency. *Behaviour Research & Therapy, 41*, 447–461.

Goldstein, L. H., Minchin, L., Stubbs, P., & Fenwick, P. B. (1997). Are what people know about their epilepsy and what they want from an epilepsy service related? *Seizure, 6*, 435–442.

Hauser, W. A. (1997). Incidence and prevalence. In J. Engel Jr. & T. A. Pedley (Eds.), *Epilepsy: A comprehensive textbook* (pp. 47–57). Philadelphia: Lippincott-Raven.

Helgeson, D. C., Mittan, R., Tan, S. Y., & Chayasirisobhon, S. (1990). Sepulveda epilepsy education: The efficacy of a psychoeducational treatment program in treating medical and psychosocial aspects of epilepsy. *Epilepsia, 31*, 75–82.

Hermann, B. P., Seidenberg, M., & Bell, B. (2000). Psychiatric co-morbidity in chronic epilepsy: Identification, consequences and treatment of major depression. *Epilepsia, 41*(Suppl. 2), 31–41.

Hermann, B. P., Trenerry, M. R., & Colligan, R. C. (1996). Learned helplessness, attributional style, and depression in epilepsy. *Epilepsia, 37*, 680–686.

Hermann, B. P., Vickrey, B., Hays, R. D., Cramer, J., Devinsky, O., Meador, K., et al. (1996). A comparison of health-related quality of life in patients with epilepsy, diabetes, and multiple sclerosis. *Epilepsy Research, 25*, 113–118.

Hoare, P., & Kerley, S. (1991). Psychosocial adjustment of children with chronic epilepsy and their families. *Developmental Medicine & Child Neurology, 33*(3), 201–215.

Jacoby, A. (1992). Epilepsy and the quality of everyday life: Findings from a study of people with well-controlled epilepsy. *Social Science and Medicine, 34*, 657–666.

Jacoby, A., Baker, G. A., Smith, A., Dewey, N., & Chadwick, D. W. (1993). Measuring the impact of epilepsy: The development of a novel scale. *Epilepsy Research, 16*, 83–88.

Jacoby, A., Baker, G., Steen, N., Potts, P., & Chadwick, D. (1996). The clinical course of epilepsy and its psychosocial correlates. *Epilepsia, 37*, 148–161.

Kanner, A. M., & Nieto, J. C. R. (1999). Depressive disorders in epilepsy. *Neurology, 53*(Suppl. 2), s26–s32.

Kobau, R., & DiLorio, C. (2003). Epilepsy self-management: A comparison of self-efficacy and outcome expectancy for medication adherence and lifestyle behaviors among people with epilepsy. *Epilepsy & Behavior, 4*, 217–226.

Krakow, K., Bühler, K. E., & Haltenhof, H. (1999). Coping with refractory epilepsy. *Seizure, 8*, 111–115.

Leppik, I. E. (1990). How to get patients with epilepsy to take their medication. The problem of noncompliance. *Postgraduate Medicine, 88*, 253–256.

Leppik, I. E. (1997). *Contemporary diagnosis and management of the patient with epilepsy*, (3rd ed.). Newtown, PA: Handbooks in Health Care.

Leventhal, H., & Diefenbach, M. (1991). The active side of illness cognition. In J. A. Skelton & R. T. Croyle (Eds.), *Mental representation in health and illness* (pp. 247–272). New York: Springer Verlag.

Livneh, H., & Antonak, R. (1997). *Psychosocial adaptation to chronic illness and disability*. Gaithersburg, MD: Aspen Publishers Inc.

Livneh, H., Wilson, L. M., Duchesneau, A., & Antonak, R. F. (2001). Psychosocial adaptation to epilepsy: The role of coping strategies. *Epilepsy and Behavior, 2*, 533–544.

Long, L., Reeves, A. L., Moore, J. L., Roach, J., & Pickering, C. T. (2000). An assessment of epilepsy patients' knowledge of their disorder. *Epilepsia, 41*, 727–731.

Loring, D. W., Meador, K. J., & Lee, G. P. (2004). Determinants of quality of life in epilepsy. *Epilepsy & Behavior, 5*, 976–980.

Loughlin, J. (2005). *Classification of epilepsies and epileptic syndromes*. Retrieved December 27, 2005, from http://www.epilepsy.com/articles/ar_1063752242.html

May, T. W., & Pfäfflin, M. (2002). The efficacy of an educational treatment program for patients with epilepsy (MOSES): Results of a controlled, randomized study. *Epilepsia, 43*(5), 539–549.

May, T. W., & Pfäfflin, M. (2005). Psychoeducational programs for patients with epilepsy. *Disability Manage Health Outcomes, 13*(3), 185–199.

Miller, L. (1994). The epilepsy patient: Personality, psychodynamics, and psychotherapy. *Psychotherapy, 31,* 735–743.

Mirnics, Z., Békés , J., Rózsa, S., & Halász, P. (2001). Adjustment and coping in epilepsy. *Seizure, 10,* 181–187.

Mittan, R. (1986). Fear of seizures. In S. Whitman & B. P. Hermann (Eds.), *Psychopathology in epilepsy: Social dimensions* (pp. 90–121). New York: Oxford University Press.

Murray, J. (1993). Coping with the uncertainty of uncontrolled epilepsy. *Seizure, 2,* 167–178.

O'Donoghue, M. F., Duncan, J. S., & Sander, J. W. A. S. (1998). The subjective handicap of epilepsy: A new approach to measuring treatment outcome. *Brain, 121,* 317–343.

Puskarich, C. A., Whitman, S., Dell, J., Hughes, J. R., Rosen, A. J., & Hermann, B. P. (1992). Controlled examination of effects of progressive relaxation training on seizure reduction. *Epilepsia, 33,* 675–680.

Reeve, D. K., & Lincoln, N. B. (2002). Coping with the challenge of transition in older adolescents with epilepsy. *Seizure, 11,* 33–39.

Reiter, J. M., & Andrews, D. J. (2000). A neurobehavioral approach for treatment of complex partial epilepsy: Efficacy. *Seizure, 9,* 198–203.

Ried, S., Specht, U., Thorbecke, R., Goecke, K., & Wohlfarth, R. (2001). MOSES: An educational program for patients with epilepsy and their relatives. *Epilepsia, 42*(Suppl. 3), 76–80.

Robertson, N. M. (1989). The organic contribution to depressive illness in patients with epilepsy. *Journal of Epilepsy, 2,* 189–230.

Rösche, J., Uhlmann, C., & Weber, R. (2004). Changes of coping strategies in patients with therapy refractory epilepsy in the course of a ward based treatment with a holistic therapeutic approach. *Psychotherapie, Psychosomatik, Medizinisch Psychologie, 54,* 4–8.

Rosenbaum, M., & Palmon, N. (1984). Helplessness and resourcefulness in coping with epilepsy. *Journal of Consulting and Clinical Psychology, 52,* 244–253.

Rousseau, A., Hermann, B., & Whitman, S. (1985). Effects of progressive relaxation on epilepsy: Analysis of a series of cases. *Psychological Reports, 57,* 1203–1212.

Ryan, C. A., & Dowling, G. (1993). Drowning deaths in people with epilepsy. *Canadian Medical Association Journal, 148,* 781–784.

Schachter, S. C. (2001). Epilepsy. *Neurologic Clinics, 19*(1), 57–78.

Schiffer, R. B., & Babigan, H. M. (1984). Behavioral disorders in multiple sclerosis, temporal lobe epilepsy, and amyotrophic lateral sclerosis: An epidemiological study. *Archives of Neurology, 41,* 1066–1070.

Schneider, J. W., & Conrad, P. (1986). Doctors, information and the control of epilepsy. In S. Whitman & B. P. Hermann (Eds.), *Psychopathology in epilepsy: Social dimensions* (pp. 69–89). New York: Oxford University Press.

Schuch, J. Z. (1998). Living safely with seizures: Assistive technology, rehabilitation technology, and resources. *Clinical Nursing Practice in Epilepsy, 5*(1), 13.

Scott, R. A., Lhatoo, S. D., & Sander, J. W. (2001). The treatment of epilepsy in developing countries: Where do we go from here? *Bulletin of the World Health Organization, 79*(4), 344–351.

Shore, C. P., Perkins, S. M., & Austin, J. K. (2005). Efficacy of the S.E.E. program on quality of life, seizure management and cost of savings for adolescents with epilepsy and their parents [Abstract]. *Epilepsia, 46*(Suppl. 8), 21.

Sillanpaa, M. (1973). Medico-social prognosis of children with epilepsy: Epidemiological study and analysis of 245 patients. *Acta Paediatrica Scandinaica Suppl., 237*, 3–104.

Snyder, M. (1990). Stressors, coping mechanisms, and perceived health in persons with epilepsy. *International Disability Studies, 12*, 100–103.

Specht, U., Elsner, H., May, T. W., Schimichowski, B., & Thorbecke, R. (2003). Postictal serum levels of antiepileptic drugs for detection of noncompliance. *Epilepsy & Behavior, 4*, 487–495.

Spector, S., Cull, C., & Goldstein, L. H. (2001). High and low perceived self-control of epileptic seizures. *Epilepsia, 42*, 556–564.

Spitz, M. C. (1998). Injuries and death as a consequence of seizures in people with epilepsy. *Epilepsia, 39*, 904–907.

Spitz, M. C., Towbin, J. A., Shantz, D., & Adler, L. E. (1994). Risk factors for burns as a consequence of seizures in persons with epilepsy. *Epilepsia, 35*, 764–767.

Stafstrom, C. E., & Bough, K. J. (2003). The ketogenic diet for the treatment of epilepsy: A challenge for nutritional neuroscientists. *Nutritional Neuroscience, 6*(2), 67–79.

Strong, V., & Brown, S. W. (2000). Should people with epilepsy have untrained dogs as pets? *Seizure, 9*, 427–430.

Strong, V., Brown, S., Huyton, M., & Coyle, H. (2002). Effect of trained Seizure Alert Dogs® on frequency of tonic-clonic seizures. *Seizures, 11*, 402–405.

Strong, V., Brown, S. W., & Walker, R. (1999). Seizure-alert dogs – fact or fiction? *Seizure, 8*, 62–65.

Swinkels, W. A. M., Kuyk, J., van Dyck, R., & Spinhoven, P. (2005). Psychiatric comorbidity in epilepsy. *Epilepsy & Behavior, 7*, 37–50.

Tedman, S., Thorton, E., & Baker, G. (1995). Development of a scale to measure core beliefs and perceived self-efficacy in adults with epilepsy. *Seizure, 4*, 221–231.

Temkin, N. R., & Davis, G. R. (1984). Stress as a risk factor for seizures among adults with epilepsy. *Epilepsia, 25*, 450–456.

Thompson, P. J., & Oxley, J. (1988). Socioeconomic accompaniments of severe epilepsy. *Epilepsia, 29*(Suppl. 1), s9–s18.

Thompson, P., & Oxley, J. (1993). Social aspects of epilepsy. In J. Laidlaw, A. Richens, & D. Chadwick (Eds.), *A textbook of epilepsy* (4th ed., pp. 661–704). London: Churchill Livingstone.

Thorbecke, R., & Fraser, R. T. (1997). The range of needs and services in vocational rehabilitation. In J. Engel Jr. & T. A. Pedley (Eds.), *Epilepsy: A comprehensive textbook* (pp. 2211–2225). Philadelphia: Lippincott-Raven Publishers.

Unglaub, F. (2005). Response: Pirouetting tap. *Epilepsia, 46*, 1153.

Unglaub, F., Woodruff, S., Ulrich, D., & Pallua, N. (2005). Severe burns as a consequence of seizure while showering: Risk factors and implications for prevention. *Epilepsia, 46*, 332–333.

Unsworth, C. (1999). Living with epilepsy: Safety during home, leisure and work activities. *Australian Occupational Therapy Journal, 46*, 89–98.

Upton, D., & Thompson, P. J. (1992). Effectiveness of coping strategies employed by people with chronic epilepsy. *Journal of Epilepsy, 5*(2), 119–127.

Vogtle, L. K. (2003). Assistive technology applications for older persons with epilepsy. *Technology Special Interest Section Quarterly, 13*(1), 1–3.

Whitman, S., Dell, J., Legion, V., Eibhlyn, A., & Statsinger, J. (1990). Progressive relaxation for seizure reduction. *Journal of Epilepsy, 3*, 17–22.

Wiebe, S., Bellhouse, D. R., Fallahay, C., & Eliasziw, M. (1999). Burden of epilepsy: The Ontario Health Survey. *Canadian Journal of Neurological Science, 26*(4), 263–270.

Williams, J., & Koocher, G. P. (1998). Addressing loss of control in chronic illness: Theory and practice. *Psychotherapy, 32*, 325–335.

Wolpe, J. (1969). *The practice of behavior therapy.* Elmsford, NY: Pergamon Press.

13
Coping and Heart Disease: Implications for Prevention and Treatment

Kymberley K. Bennett and Jennifer L. Boothby

What Is Cardiovascular Disease?

Cardiovascular diseases include stroke, congenital heart defects, heart failure, and other cardio-circulatory ailments. Yet, the most common form of cardiovascular disease is coronary heart disease (CHD). CHD is usually marked by one of three symptoms: *angina, myocardial infarction, or sudden cardiac death* (Walker & Lorimer, 2004). Each of these symptoms typically stems from partial or complete blockages of the vessels that prevent normal blood flow to and from the heart; the degree of severity, or damage to the heart, runs along a continuum from angina to sudden cardiac death.

At one end of the severity spectrum, angina is severe chest pain usually experienced due to insufficient blood flow supplied to the heart (Walker & Lorimer, 2004). Although painful and frightening, angina represents the least serious of the symptoms of CHD, often signaling to the individual that drastic lifestyle changes are necessary. Myocardial infarction (MI), or heart attack, involves damage or death to part of the heart muscle on account of a lack of oxygenated blood to that area. Unlike angina, however, MIs result in actual damage, or infarcts, to the heart muscle. Regardless of the size of the infarct, the area of muscle damage subsequently forms scar tissue, thereby disrupting normal heart activity. Pain from MIs is similar to that experienced in individuals with angina, but individuals with MI have the possibility of much more severe and long-lasting discomfort.

At the other end of the spectrum, some individuals' first symptoms of CHD culminate in sudden cardiac death. Sudden cardiac death is defined as a death that occurs instantaneously on account of CHD symptoms, or death that occurs up to 24 hours following the onset of symptoms. Ventricular fibrillation, a rapid and uncoordinated pumping of the blood through the heart, is often the cause of sudden cardiac death. The American Heart Association (AHA; 2006) estimates that approximately 7.2 million individuals suffer MIs annually. The AHA also estimates that approximately 6.5 million individuals, who are diagnosed with

CHD, experience some form of angina during the course of the disease. Further, it is estimated that 335,000 people die each year on account of sudden cardiac deaths.

The Incidence, Prevalence, and Impact of Cardiovascular Disease

Cardiovascular diseases are the number one cause of death in the U.S., with the AHA (2006) estimating that approximately 37% of deaths in this country are a result of one form of the disease. The most current data show that in 2003, over 910,000 individuals died as a result of cardiovascular diseases. Furthermore, the AHA estimates that one in three adults in the U.S. has one form of the disease—that is, approximately 71.3 million individuals are currently estimated to be afflicted with a cardiovascular disease.

The AHA (2006) reports that if all forms of cardiovascular disease were eliminated, the current projected lifespan of Americans would lengthen by seven years—from approximately 77 years to 84 years. The AHA also estimates that 13.2 million Americans are diagnosed with CHD, with approximately 650,000 deaths annually related to CHD. Furthermore, it is estimated that approximately every 30 seconds someone in the U.S. will experience a cardiac event and that nearly every minute someone will die from CHD in the U.S. In addition, the direct and indirect costs associated with CHD are staggering—the AHA estimates these costs to be $142.5 billion in 2006.

Risk Factors for Cardiovascular Disease

With the marked increase in the incidence of CHD in the United States over the past few decades, much research attention has been paid to better understanding the risk factors that contribute to the onset and progression of CHD. The three main risk factors, or what Daly-Nee, Brunt, and Jairath (1990) call the "classic triad" (p. 7), are elevated cholesterol, hypertension, and smoking. Other important (and related) risk factors are sedentary lifestyles, obesity, and diabetes. The AHA (2006) reports that only 30% of U.S. adults report regular leisure-time activity; that is, less than one-third of Americans report engaging in physical activity for at least 30 minutes per day for five or more times per week. In a related vein, the AHA reports that 136.5 million adults were overweight in 2003 and that an additional 64 million adults were obese. Additionally, risk for death as a result of CHD is two to four times higher among individuals with diabetes than their non-affected counterparts. Age and family history are also important risk factors for CHD. Research indicates that one's risk steadily increases with age and that having a first-degree relative with the disease sharply increases one's chances of being diagnosed with CHD (Walker & Lorimer, 2004).

In addition to these risk factors, social scientists are elucidating psychosocial constructs that play an important role in understanding the etiology (and recurrence) of CHD. First, there is a vast literature suggesting that economic deprivation, as measured by socioeconomic status (SES), is related to CHD (Lynch, Kaplan, & Salonen, 1997). That is, research has firmly established that individuals of relatively low SES are more likely to be diagnosed with CHD than their middle SES and high SES counterparts (Chesney, 1996). In a comprehensive review of SES and CHD, Kaplan and Keil (1993) concluded that low SES is an *independent* risk factor for the disease, even after controlling for behavioral risk factors. These authors suggest that the conditions of life, which are associated with poverty and economic deprivation (e.g., unsafe and unstable living conditions, onerous working conditions, family and marital conflict), are related to increased levels of chronic stress, which in turn negatively impact cardiovascular functioning (see Sapolsky, 2004, for a review of the linkages between chronic stressors, the body's stress response, and cardiovascular functioning).

In addition, there are data suggesting the importance of hostility as a risk factor for CHD. Although much media attention was paid to the "Type A" personality construct, as proposed by Friedman and Rosenman (1959), contemporary researchers have isolated the most toxic of the components comprising the constellation of "Type A" behaviors, namely, hostility. Research has shown that hostile individuals are at a higher risk for developing CHD than their non-hostile counterparts. Furthermore, once diagnosed, hostile individuals with CHD are at a heightened risk for subsequent cardiac complications, relative to non-hostile individuals (Miller, Smith, Turner, Guijarro, & Hallet, 1996). A recent study by Sher (2004) identified a new personality construct, "Type D," which may also function as a risk factor for CHD. "Type D," or the "distressed" personality, is characterized by a combination of negative affectivity and social inhibition. Even after controlling for other known risk factors, Sher found "Type D" personality to substantially increase the risk of cardiac-related death among a group of individuals undergoing cardiac rehabilitation. Future research on this personality variable will provide important information about CHD risk and prevention.

Depression is another psychosocial risk factor for CHD that has received a growing amount of attention within the field of behavioral medicine. The negative affectivity component of "Type D" personality likely reflects features of depression. Several studies have found that major depression and subclinical levels of depressive symptoms are related to the development of CHD, particularly with respect to first-time MIs (Barefoot & Schroll, 1996; Cohen, Madhavan, & Alderman, 2001; Kubzansky & Kawachi, 2000). Furthermore, major depression and symptoms of depression are linked to greater risk for recurrence among individuals with CHD (Frasure-Smith, Lesperance, & Talajic, 1995a, 1995b; Lesperance, Frasure-Smith, & Talajic, 1996).

With regard to psychosocial functioning, depressive symptoms following a cardiac event have been negatively linked to perceptions of quality of life (Shen, Myers, & McCreary, 2006). The importance of studies linking depression to cardiac-related morbidity and mortality is underscored by the prevalence of depressive disorders among individuals who have been diagnosed with CHD. It is estimated that between 16% and 22% of individuals with MI meet diagnostic criteria for major depression in the year following their MIs (Carney & Freedland, 2000), whereas less than 7% in the general population meet these criteria in any given year (Kessler, Berglund, Demler, Jin, & Walters, 2005). This is nearly a three-fold increase in the rates of depression among individuals with cardiac problems, relative to the general population.

Treatments for Cardiovascular Disease

Paralleling the advances in our understanding of risk factors for CHD, vast medical advances have been made in our treatment of CHD. For individuals with angina, several medications can be prescribed. Nitrates often represent the centerpiece of any anti-anginal medication therapy. Nitrate medications work to reduce required oxygen levels by dilating blood vessels, thereby decreasing the workload of the heart. Beta blockers are also commonly prescribed, because they dampen the body's automatic stress response via the sympathetic nervous system; these drugs slow heart rate and decrease blood pressure, again decreasing the overall workload of the heart. Calcium channel blockers also reduce blood pressure by reducing the rate at which calcium passes into the heart muscle and vessels, thereby allowing the vessels to relax, causing blood to flow more freely (McInnes, Curzio, & Kennedy, 2004).

For individuals who have MI and who have partial or complete blockages, other medical treatments are often necessary. Blockages are commonly treated through percutaneous coronary intervention (PCI; formerly known as percutaneous transluminal coronary angioplasty, or PTCA) or through coronary artery bypass graft (CABG). PCI involves inserting a catheter with an un-inflated balloon at its tip into the groin area, and extending the catheter to the artery in the heart that has been identified as being blocked. The tiny balloon at the tip of the catheter is then inflated at the spot of this blockage, and this balloon compresses the plaque (or fatty deposits) that once occluded the artery.

It is estimated that approximately 90% of PCIs are successful in clearing blockages (Balachandran & Oldroyd, 2004). The AHA (2006) reports that approximately 664,000 PCI procedures were performed on individuals with cardiovascular disease in 2003. Furthermore, some PCI procedures also involve the placement of a stent, a tiny mesh tube that is placed at the spot of the blockage after the surrounding plaque has been compressed. The use of stents has increased sharply in the past decade (i.e., 147% in the latter half of the 1990s, AHA), due to their ability to protect against subsequent arterial collapse and restenosis, or narrowing of the artery.

For individuals with more severe or numerous blockages, CABG is often the preferred treatment. CABG involves using an artery from another part of the body (usually from the leg or chest) to "bypass" a blocked one in the heart;

the new (or "harvest") artery is attached to the aorta on one end, with the other end of the new artery attached beyond the spot of the blockage. CABG allows the blood to avoid the blocked area completely, redirecting the blood through the newly-attached artery (Scheidt, 1996). The AHA (2006) reports that over 465,000 CABG procedures were performed on individuals with cardiovascular disease in 2003.

Coping with Heart Disease

A wealth of research exists on how individuals with CHD cope with their illness and on how different coping styles influence medical and psychosocial outcomes for individuals with CHD. Studies have been mixed with respect to the kinds of coping strategies that are employed most often by individuals with CHD and the outcomes associated with those strategies (see Livneh, 1999 for a review). More definitive studies are urgently needed, especially because an understanding of coping with CHD can potentially elucidate additional areas for intervention.

Coping Strategies Used by Individuals with Cardiovascular Disease

Individuals with cardiovascular disease have been found to cope with their illness in a variety of ways. On average, it appears that these individuals tend to use healthy and adaptive coping strategies. For example, several studies have found that individuals with CHD report using optimistic coping, active coping, active problem solving, positive reappraisal, and seeking social support as their most frequently employed coping styles (Kinne, Droste, Fahrenberg, & Roskamm, 1999; Kristofferzon, Lofmark, & Carlsson, 2005a, 2005b; Stewart, Hirth, Klassen, Makrides, & Wolf, 1997; van Rijen et al., 2004). Research with both healthy and chronically ill populations consistently finds these types of coping strategies to be associated with positive outcomes. Even more striking is the finding that individuals awaiting heart transplantation, who are arguably the most severely ill of those with cardiovascular disease, also report using healthy coping strategies more than unhealthy coping. For example, Porter et al. (1994) found these individuals use positive thinking and humor most frequently in coping with their illness.

Although many studies find individuals with cardiovascular disease use adaptive coping styles, studies that have compared coping of those with CHD and with healthy matched controls do not always report similar findings. For example, one study compared types of coping and levels of burnout between a sample of women with CHD and a sample of healthy matched controls (Hallman, Thomsson, Burell, Lisspers, & Setterlind, 2003). Burnout in this study referred to "exhaustion that might be a consequence of long-term stress" (p. 434). Women with CHD used more emotion-focused coping, reported higher levels of burnout and, overall, indicated lesser coping abilities than matched controls. Examples of emotion-focused coping strategies include avoidance, escape, emotional distancing, and self-control. Although univariate analyses revealed that having CHD and using emotion-focused coping were each related to levels of burnout, emotion-focused coping was found to exert the greatest influence in predicting burnout in multivariate analyses.

Another study employing healthy, matched controls found few differences between controls and individuals with CHD in coping styles (van Rijen et al., 2004). However, when this study explored gender differences in coping, several differences emerged. Although there was no difference in the use of emotion-focused coping as found by Hallman et al. (2003), females with CHD engaged in less active problem-solving than their female peers. Adaptive coping is often associated with higher levels of active problem-focused coping and lower levels of emotion-focused coping. Males with CHD in this study demonstrated greater use of seeking social support and less use of passive reactions and expression of emotions, as compared to their male peers. Thus, males with CHD appeared to be using more constructive coping methods than male healthy controls. It is worth noting that the controls in this study were largely members of the general population, and were not necessarily experiencing any significant stressors at the time that they completed the measure of coping.

Coping and the Development of CHD

Longitudinal studies have attempted to explicate those medical and psychosocial factors predictive of the development of heart disease. A German study followed 416 middle-aged blue-collar workers for six years, tracking their work conditions, coping styles, coronary risk factors, and development of CHD (Siegrist, Peter, Junge, Cremer, & Seidel, 1990). Six percent of the sample had suffered an MI by the six-year follow-up. Psychosocial factors, such as high work pressure, low work-status control and a high need for control, were predictive of an MI. Those who developed CHD were shown to demonstrate a coping style characteristic of "exhaustive coping," whereby they continuously attempted to gain a sense of control at work and experienced negative emotions during the process. Interestingly, psychosocial variables, including coping style, were more predictive of CHD than demographic factors, such as age and body mass index.

A cross-sectional study with correctional officers explored the association of coping styles and signs of CHD on electrocardiogram recordings (Harenstam, Theorell, & Kaijser, 2000). Men, who reported high levels of covert coping, and women, who reported low levels of open coping, displayed the most signs of CHD. Covert coping was defined as not displaying any emotional reactions in difficult situations at work, whereas open coping was defined as dealing openly and directly with problems in the workplace. The associations between coping and signs of CHD were more robust than conventional risk factors, such as body mass index, cholesterol level, blood pressure, and smoking.

Coping and Psychosocial Outcomes

In terms of emotional adaptation to CHD, many studies have reported that denial (also called avoidance or repression in some studies) is associated with positive emotional outcomes in the short-term following a cardiac event (Havik & Maeland, 1988; Levenson, Mishra, Hamer, & Hastillo, 1989; Soloff, 1980; Soloff & Bartel, 1979; van Elderen, Maes, & Dusseldorp, 1999). The impact of denial on longer-term emotional functioning or psychosocial adaptation is unclear. For example, some studies found that denial is not associated with psychosocial adaptation in the longer-term (van Elderen et al., 1999), whereas other studies report that denial can be emotionally damaging when used on a longer-term basis (Doering et al., 2004; Levine et al., 1987). Cross-sectional research among individuals with CHD has found avoidant coping to be associated with higher levels of anxiety, depressive, and anger symptoms (Maes & Bruggemans, 1990). The more global coping style of emotion-focused coping has also been associated with greater psychological distress among individuals with CHD (Terry, 1992).

Hughes et al. (2004) examined social support and religiosity as they relate to anxiety among individuals with cardiac disease. Given that anxiety is associated with increased risk for CHD and increased mortality due to cardiovascular disease (Sirois & Burg, 2003), the authors suggest that understanding those variables associated with anxiety is important for cardiac health. The study examined 228 individuals hospitalized due to CHD. It was found that higher levels of social support and religiosity were associated with lower levels of anxiety. However, after controlling for social support in further analyses, religiosity was no longer a significant predictor of anxiety. Thus, social support may impact cardiac health in both direct and indirect ways. Religious coping is increasingly being examined as a predictor of health outcomes (Pargament, Ano, & Wachholtz, 2005), and it is likely that the area of cardiac health will see a similar increase in focus on religious coping.

Coping and Health-Related Outcomes

The impact of coping on health-related outcomes is clearly an important area of research, and one that has been explored in several studies. Stewart et al. (1997) examined 100 individuals with CHD, who were just released from the hospital. Among individuals who had just experienced their first CHD-related hospitalization, the use of seeking social support was predictive of readmission within four months. In contrast, for individuals with a history of prior hospitalization, less use of the coping strategy of accepting responsibility was associated with readmission during the four-month follow-up period. The authors suggested that these findings may reflect the use of more active coping strategies by individuals with less severe or less advanced stages of CHD, and more passive coping strategies by individuals with multiple hospitalizations. As chronic illness progresses or persists, many individuals develop a sense of helplessness and feelings of a lack of control. Passive coping strategies would be consistent with the belief that one has no control over illness. Similarly, Kinne et al. (1999) found that symptomatic individuals reported higher levels of helplessness and lower scores on a measure of active coping, as compared to asymptomatic individuals.

Shen, McCreary, and Myers (2004) examined the relationhips between active coping (e.g., planning, taking actions, and seeking emotional support), negative coping (e.g., self-blame, denial, and behavioral disengagement), social support, dispositional optimism, hostility, depression, and physical health. Greater optimism and social support were the only variables to demonstrate significant direct relations with physical functioning. Negative coping impacted physical health indirectly as a mediator. For example, more optimistic individuals used fewer negative coping strategies, which led to improved physical functioning at a six-week follow-up. Similarly, individuals with greater social support adopted fewer negative coping strategies, which also led to better physical health at the follow-up. Although some studies have found active coping to be associated with improved long-term physical outcomes (Suls & Fletcher, 1985), Shen et al. (2004) did not find active coping to be associated with positive or negative physical health indicators.

Denial appears to affect adaptation to CHD in different ways. Its varied impact on psychosocial functioning has already been discussed. With respect to health-related outcomes, studies have found denial to be associated with less time in the hospital (Levine et al., 1987), lower mortality rates, and less interference with activities (Havik & Maeland, 1988).

Although treatment attendance is not a physical health outcome, per se, showing up for treatment certainly has implications for health outcomes. Whitmarsh, Koutantji, and Sidell (2003) explored whether attenders and non-attenders of cardiac rehabilitation differed in terms of psychological symptoms, illness beliefs, and coping. The authors found that individuals who used problem-focused and emotion-focused coping strategies more frequently were more likely to attend cardiac rehabilitation than individuals who used fewer of these coping strategies. Thus, individuals with larger coping repertoires more frequently attended treatment. There was no difference between attenders and non-attenders in their use of non-adaptive coping strategies (e.g., denial, behavioral and mental disengagement). It is also noteworthy that attenders had significantly higher scores on measures of anxiety and depression, as compared to non-attenders. It may be that psychological distress serves as a motivator for treatment in this population.

Gender and Cultural Differences in Coping

Several studies have explored differences in coping between men and women with CHD. Research has consistently found that women use more supportive coping and report having larger social support networks than men (Kristofferzon, Lofmark, & Carlsson, 2003, 2005b; van Rijen et al., 2004). However, women receive less informational and instrumental support than men (Young & Kahana, 1993). Men tend to perceive their spouses as more supportive and also rely on their spouses for more support than do women (Kristofferzon et al., 2005b). There is little support for gender-differentiated coping styles. Although previous research in other populations has found that men tend to use more active or problem-focused coping strategies and women tend to use more passive or emotion-focused strategies, there is no clear gender-role pattern in research on coping with CHD. Individuals tend to use both problem-focused and emotion-focused coping strategies, depending on their specific needs and situations (Kristofferzon et al., 2003, 2005b). However, several studies have found that women reported using more coping strategies overall than do men (Bogg, Thornton, & Bundred, 2000; Kristofferzon et al., 2005b). This may reflect that women experience CHD as more stressful than men, and thus, have a need for more extensive coping repertoires.

Research on cultural differences in coping with cardiovascular disease is somewhat limited. Many studies have documented differential treatment and outcomes for individuals with cardiac disease, based on race and ethnicity (Carlisle, Leake, & Shapiro, 1997; Giles, Anda, Casper, Escobedo, & Taylor, 1995; Vaccarino et al., 2005; Yarzebski, 2004), but few studies have examined differences in coping among various racial and ethnic groups (e.g., Saab, 1997; Taylor-Piliae, 2001). Given the potential impact of coping on cardiac outcomes, it follows that research should be extended into this area.

Interventions to Promote Coping Behavior

Coping with the stress of a cardiovascular disease represents a great challenge to many individuals. Pharmacological and surgical advances in the treatment of heart disease have allowed many individuals to survive diagnoses, which several years ago were tantamount to death sentences. With the increased medical technology available to individuals with heart disease (and concomitant survival rates), it becomes necessary to help individuals adjust to their new diagnosis—individuals must now adjust to new aspects of life, such as limited physical repertoires, acknowledgement of behavioral risk factors, changing social expectations from friends and family, and facing psychological burdens in the form of depression and anxiety. These new challenges faced by individuals with heart disease can be mitigated by programs aimed in assisting individuals to integrate their new-found realities into their day-to-day lives. Research has shown that intervention programs, whether strictly targeting exercise regimens or ones more holistic in nature, have the capacity to exert positive change within the lives of individuals with CHD (e.g., Lavie & Milani, 1999b; Maines et al., 1997; Ornish et al., 1990).

Cardiac Rehabilitation

As a starting point, exercise represents an important means of coping with CHD. Many individuals with heart disease participate in cardiac rehabilitation programs that encourage regular exercise and the modification of other lifestyle risk-factors (e.g., smoking). In fact, cardiac rehabilitation has grown substantially within the last 20 years in its focus and efficacy in treating individuals recovering from CHD (Donker, 2000). Cardiac rehabilitation programs typically follow a three-phase approach. Phase I involves the actual cardiac event and is usually marked by the period of hospitalization. Phase II is an outpatient program, in which individuals participate in exercise sessions and other lifestyle-change classes, such as stress-management training. Individuals who are referred to cardiac rehabilitation begin their Phase II activities at a time when their primary physicians or cardiologists believe it is safe for them to do so; it is common for individuals who experience a severe cardiac event, like PCI, to require more time between Phase I and Phase II than individuals experiencing a less severe cardiac event, such as angina. Individuals participating in Phase II exercise sessions are monitored while they exercise; heart monitoring is done as a precautionary measure to ensure that individuals' hearts are functioning properly and to ensure that individuals exercise at the optimal level for their stage of recovery. Phase III is a maintenance period, during which individuals participate in lifestyle-change classes and non-monitored exercise sessions. The overall aim of cardiac rehabilitation programs is to provide an environment which facilitates lifestyle changes in individuals that, in turn, will reduce their risk factors for subsequent cardiac complications.

Data collected on the efficacy of cardiac rehabilitation programs have shown a positive effect on physical health among individuals with cardiac diagnoses. Specifically, research shows significant improvements in a host of cardiopulmonary outcomes after participation in cardiac rehabilitation: peak oxygen consumption (Lavie & Milani, 1999a), exercise capacity (Fitchet et al., 2003), heart rate (Duru et al., 2000), cholesterol levels (Maines et al., 1997), blood pressure (Morrin, Black, & Reid, 2000), and body mass index (Lavie & Milani, 1999b). In addition, recent meta-analyses suggest that participation in rehabilitation can reduce risk for death by 20% among individuals who experienced MIs (Miller, Balady, & Fletcher, 1997), and that rehabilitation programs that utilize psycho-educational practices, in addition to exercise-based training, can reduce cardiac-related mortality by as much as 30% (Dusseldorp, van Elderen, Maes, Meulman, & Kraaij, 1999). Furthermore, the Dusseldorp et al. meta-analysis showed that program success on proximal cardiac markers (e.g., blood pressure and smoking cessation) moderated the programs' long-term impact on physical health. That is, rehabilitation programs that reported success on proximal outcomes had greater reductions in recurrence (36% versus 2%) and mortality (31% versus 14%) than programs that did not achieve significant progress on proximal outcomes.

Although exercise is still a key component to contemporary cardiac rehabilitation programs, they are, at present, much more comprehensive in their scope, targeting psychological adjustment (e.g., stress management) and the importance of social support. Some programs even include spouses (e.g., spousal support, dietary/cooking classes). This shift to comprehensive rehabilitation mirrors the emergence of the biopsychosocial model, replacing strictly biomedical orientations to treating illness and disease. McIntosh (2004) cites a quote from the

Scottish Intercollegiate Guideline Network (SIGN) that illustrates this shift in orientation in many cardiac rehabilitation programs: "Cardiac rehabilitation is the process by which individuals with cardiac disease, in partnership with a multidisciplinary team of health-care professions, are encouraged and supported to achieve and maintain optimal *physical and psychological health*" (p. 272, italics added). As cardiac rehabilitation programs move to a more holistic view of recovery, studies on the efficacy of psychosocial interventions are becoming more numerous.

Large-Scale Intervention Studies

The most famous large-scale cardiac intervention studies have been led by Dean Ornish. In their first comprehensive intervention, Ornish and colleagues (1983) randomly assigned individuals with heart disease to a usual-care control group or to a treatment group that received an intensive, away-from-home, 3½ week program. The intervention program consisted of: (a) Moderate exercise; (b) a strict vegetarian, low-fat diet; and (c) stress-management techniques, such as meditation and breathing exercises. Results of this initial intervention were positive; individuals in the treatment group showed significant improvements in exercise duration and cholesterol levels relative to their control group counterparts. With these intervention data in hand, Ornish and colleagues (1990) conducted a follow-up intervention study that included a measure of atherosclerosis (i.e., the extent to which coronary arteries are clogged). As in the first intervention, individuals in the second study were randomly assigned to a usual-care control group or to a treatment group, which was prescribed a low-fat and low-calorie diet, stress management techniques, and moderate exercise. Results from this intervention were similarly encouraging; one year later, individuals in the treatment group evidenced significant reductions in their degree of atherosclerosis, compared to individuals in the control group (Billings, Scherwitz, Sullivan, Sparler, & Ornish, 1996). Although these intervention data are promising, Linden (2000) noted that few individuals may be willing to comply with such an intensive rehabilitation program. Furthermore, even among those individuals who are motivated to make drastic changes, few may be able to afford (in time or money) such a comprehensive approach.

Another large-scale cardiac intervention program was the Recurrent Coronary Prevention Project (RCCP) led by Friedman and colleagues. The aim of the RCCP was to target and reduce "Type A" behaviors, thereby leading to improvements in cardiopulmonary indicators and psychological functioning (Friedman et al., 1984). Post-MI individuals in the RCCP were randomly assigned to cardiac counseling only (e.g., information about medications, risk-factor modification through diet and exercise, and psychological distress) or to cardiac counseling with an accompanying intervention for "Type A" behaviors (e.g., recognition of stress triggers, relaxation techniques, and cognitive restructuring of stress-related thoughts). Three years into the 4½ year study, results showed that the fatal and non-fatal recurrence rate was significantly lower in the counseling group with the "Type A" intervention, compared to the group that received cardiac counseling only. In addition, documented "Type A" behaviors were significantly lower among the treatment group with the "Type A" intervention component, as compared to those who received cardiac counseling alone. Follow-up results six years later showed similar trends: mortality, recurrence, and "Type A" behaviors were reduced among the "Type A" intervention group, in comparison to the group that received the standard, cardiac counseling (see Linden, 2000).

The Ischemic Heart Disease Life Stress Monitoring Program (IHDLSM) was an intervention conducted by Frasure-Smith & Prince (1989) that focused on distress screening and "stress monitoring" by nurses. Male, post-MI individuals were randomly assigned to a control condition, in which they received usual care or were assigned to a treatment condition that required them to be screened monthly for psychological distress. Within the treatment group, when distress levels were elevated, nursing professionals delivered home-based interventions comprised of education, social support, and referrals. Results were encouraging at the first-year mark: individuals in the treatment group had significantly lower mortality rates than individuals in the control group. However, by the four-year follow-up, improvements in the treatment group disappeared. In attempting to explain this decline in treatment effects, Frasure-Smith (1991) divided the sample into "high" baseline stress and "low" baseline stress groups. Results showed significant reductions in mortality rates among the treatment group with "high" stress levels, in comparison to their "high" stress counterparts in the control group. These results suggest that the intervention was most successful among individuals manifesting stress during the intervention (i.e., a moderating effect of baseline stress on treatment effectiveness). In an attempt to replicate the original IHDLSM study, Frasure-Smith et al. (1997) conducted a follow-up intervention with post-MI males and females. However, no significant differences between the treatment and control groups emerged in this study.

Most recently, the Enhancing Recovery in Coronary Heart Disease (ENRICHD) intervention study was conducted, in order to test the effects of a psychological intervention that was specifically designed to treat depression among individuals with CHD (ENRICHD Investigators, 2003). The ENRICHD study collected data from post-MI individuals who manifested depression and/or low perceived social support. Individuals were randomly assigned to a control group that received usual care or to a treatment group that received a cognitive-behavioral therapy (CBT)-based psychosocial intervention. Individuals in the treatment group participated in six months of individual CBT sessions and group-therapy sessions, and, in some cases, were prescribed antidepressant medications. Initial results from the study were positive: individuals in the treatment group evidenced significantly lower levels of depressive symptoms than their control group counterparts. At the three-year follow-up, however, no significant benefits to psychological functioning, due to the intervention, were evident. Furthermore, although the study results confirmed that major depressive disorder is an independent risk factor for cardiac-related mortality, there were no significant differences in mortality rates between the treatment and control groups

(Carney et al., 2004). Post-hoc analyses suggest that the intervention was most effective among Caucasian men (Schneiderman et al., 2004). When dividing their sample into groups based on gender and minority status, the ENRICHD researchers found that Caucasian men in the treatment group had lower rates of mortality and MI recurrence than ethnic minority men, and lower rates than women, regardless of their ethnic background.

Summary of Intervention Studies

Results summarized above from the major intervention studies provide mixed results on the efficacy of psychosocial treatments. In addition to the large studies discussed above, many other researchers have studied the impact of treatment interventions among individuals with CHD. Linden (2000) recently conducted a meta-analysis of 23 studies in order to quantify the effect of psychosocial interventions on physical health (i.e., cardiac endpoints, such as morbidity and mortality) and on psychological adjustment among individuals with cardiovascular disease. Results showed that the treatment group had a 46% reduction in recurrence, compared to their control-group counterparts, in short-term follow-ups (i.e., less than two years in length, with an average of 12 months). In long-term follow-ups (i.e., greater than two years, with an average of five years), the treatment group demonstrated a 39% reduction in recurrence, relative to the control group. For mortality as the outcome, results showed that the short-term treatment group had a significant reduction of 41%, and long-term reductions represented a non-significant trend of 26%. Results of the meta-analysis also showed significant improvements in distress, heart rate, cholesterol, and systolic blood pressure among individuals in treatment groups across the studies.

An increase can be noted in the number of intervention trials that target psychological adjustment, in addition to physical recovery, among individuals with heart disease, although much work is yet to be done. Whereas some large-scale interventions yielded promising findings (e.g., Ornish et al., 1983, 1990), others have failed to improve recovery among individuals (e.g., follow-up to IHDLSM). Linden (2000) suggests that the current state of knowledge in this area implies that intervention efforts must be carefully screened and tailored to the needs of individuals with CHD. As evidenced by the Frasure-Smith (1991) study, it is possible that individuals must be screened for distress before offering interventions. If individuals do not manifest distress, it may not be cost-effective to offer services to them. In addition, there may be ceiling effects in recovery and adjustment because "standard" cardiac care has improved. Therefore, being able to document significant improvements in recovery by psychosocial interventions above-and-beyond usual care becomes increasingly more difficult. Linden also notes that because many early intervention efforts targeted males, the accumulating data, to date, may reflect the intervention needs of males, more so than females (e.g., Frasure-Smith & Prince, 1989), and of Caucasian individuals, more so than individuals from ethnic minority backgrounds (e.g., Schneiderman et al., 2004). Even so, the emerging picture of psychosocial interventions for improving recovery among individuals with heart disease is very encouraging.

Vocational and Social Implications of Treating Heart Disease

Research has firmly established the effectiveness of cardiac rehabilitation programs in improving cardiopulmonary outcomes among individuals with cardiac problems. Although findings are mixed with regard to psychosocial interventions in improving psychological adjustment among individuals with cardiac problems, data are amassing that a key component to any successful intervention is its ability to tailor the program to the specific needs of individuals. Future intervention research that focuses on the match between individuals' needs and intervention strategies will improve the understanding of the mechanisms by which physical and psychological recovery processes can be maximized.

The risk of not furthering the understanding about the processes involved in recovery is large, given the staggering costs of heart disease to society. The AHA (2006) estimates that direct and indirect costs associated with all forms of cardiovascular disease in the United States will amount to $403.1 billion in 2006. With regard to CHD specifically, the AHA estimates that the total costs will be $142.5 billion in 2006. This figure breaks down as follows: $75.2 billion is estimated to be expended on direct costs such as hospital care, physician-related expenses, home-health-care, nursing-home professionals, and medications. Indirect costs, such as low productivity in the workforce as a result of morbidity and mortality are estimated to be $67.3 billion. By comparison, the AHA states that in 2004, all cancers combined were estimated to cost the United States $190 billion in direct and indirect expenses. Furthermore, in 1999 the cost of HIV infections was estimated to amount to $28.9 billion for the United States in direct and indirect costs.

The *indirect* costs associated with heart disease could be mitigated by programs aimed at enhancing individuals' return to work in a timely and safe manner. For employers, research suggests that providing paid leave during recovery from a cardiac event significantly increases the odds that a person will return to work (e.g., Earle, Ayanian, & Heymann, 2006). It is hypothesized that a paid leave period during recovery promotes returning to work because it increases feelings of commitment to one's employer. Paid leaves also allow employees to recuperate fully by caring for themselves, resulting in their ability to resume work at full productivity levels.

On the medical treatment side, research by Engblom, Korpilahti, Hamalainen, Ronnemaa, and Puukka (1997) suggests that traditional cardiac rehabilitation programs focused on exercise training may have a positive influence on whether individuals return to work. In their study of individuals with CABG, these researchers found a higher proportion of individuals in the treatment group that received cardiac rehabilitation had returned to their jobs at the three-year follow-up, compared to individuals in their control group. However, Engblom et al. failed to find a significant difference between the groups at the five-year follow-up period, suggesting that long-term occupational status may be the result of more complex rehabilitation processes.

Mital et al. (2000) tested the efficacy of a job-simulated cardiac rehabilitation program among individuals who underwent bypass and angioplasty. The job-simulated program was comprised of low-intensity, non-aerobic activities that mirror many tasks required of industrial and manufacturing workers. Participants were randomly assigned to a control condition of traditional cardiac rehabilitation or to a treatment condition that focused on improving functioning via simulated elements of industrial and manufacturing occupations. Examples of the simulated elements include carrying a wooden box up and down stairs, moving a wooden box onto a shelf at the participant's maximum reach, and turning the body while holding on to a wooden box. These activities were meant to enhance flexibility and dexterity. Results from the study showed that significantly more individuals in the job-simulated treatment condition returned to their professions at the end of Phase II than their control-group counterparts.

Even though the job-simulated training consisted of low-impact activities, results from the Mital et al. study showed that individuals in the treatment-group made significant improvements from the beginning of Phase II to the end of Phase II in aerobic capacity. In fact, improvements in aerobic capacity seen in the treatment group were statistically indistinguishable from the improvements made in the aerobic-focused, traditional Phase II rehabilitation control group. The findings suggest that cardiac rehabilitation centers can enhance individuals' return to work by incorporating job-related activities into their existing exercise programs. Shrey and Mital (2000) also suggest that including vocational rehabilitation specialists on cardiac rehabilitation teams will enhance recovery and ease individuals' transitions back to work.

In addition to adding occupation-focused activities to cardiac rehabilitation programs, research suggests that targeting the types of beliefs held about one's cardiac event can be a powerful predictor of returning to work. For example, Petrie, Weinman, Sharpe, and Buckley (1996) studied how beliefs about cardiac events shaped individuals' return to their pre-MI occupations. Questionnaire data were collected from individuals at the time of their hospitalization and again three and six months later. Results showed that individuals, who believed their MIs would have serious consequences in their lives and who believed that their MIs would last a long time, took significantly longer to return to their jobs than individuals, who considered their MIs to be less serious and last only a short time. These findings imply that encouraging people to view their cardiac events in realistic and optimistic ways may translate to more hopeful orientations about recovery, thereby impacting their willingness to return to work.

Given the staggering costs for treating heart disease, policy-makers are turning their attention to ways of more effectively promoting prevention efforts, in addition to treatment interventions, in the general public. The Centers for

Disease Control and Prevention (CDC, 2003) outlined two main requirements for prevention and control efforts in the future: first, we must communicate to the general public the "... urgent need and unprecedented opportunity to prevent heart disease and stroke in order to establish widespread awareness and concern about these conditions..." (p. 8). Second, the CDC states that we must target the nation's public-health system in order that leaders can coordinate partnerships and collaborations, which will be able to implement the education and behavior-change strategies needed. In order to achieve these two requirements, the report makes several summary recommendations including: (a) Policies for prevention must be made at the national, state, and local levels; (b) treatment and prevention interventions must be carried out in multiple settings, in order to reach all age groups—and especially those at highest risk for heart disease; (c) we must strengthen the capacities and training offered through public-health agencies; and, (d) innovative ways of monitoring and evaluating public-health efforts must be developed, in order to continually improve the services provided.

Conclusion

Cardiovascular diseases are the number one cause of death in the United States. Much is known regarding biological and psychosocial risk factors for CHD, but much remains to be learned about effective means of improving recovery and modifying risk factors among individuals with cardiac disorders. Research on coping suggests that the manner in which individuals with CHD cope with their illness is predictive of short and long-term recovery. Although cardiac rehabilitation programs have demonstrated some success, incorporating interventions that target coping skills may bolster outcomes. Furthermore, tailoring treatment to the specific psychosocial needs of individuals is likely to improve outcomes as well.

References

American Heart Association (2006). *Heart Disease and Stroke Statistics—2006 Update*. Dallas, TX: American Heart Association. Retrieved April 1, 2006, from http://www.americanheart.org

Balachandran, K. P., & Oldroyd, K. G. (2004). Medical management of coronary heart disease. In G. Lindsay & A. Gaw (Eds.), *Coronary heart disease prevention: A handbook for the health-care team* (2nd ed., pp. 237–270). London: Churchill Livingstone.

Barefoot, J. C., & Schroll, M. (1996). Symptoms of depression, acute myocardial infarction, and total mortality in a community sample. *Circulation, 93*, 1976–1980.

Billings, J. H., Scherwitz, L. W., Sullivan, R., Sparler, S., & Ornish, D. (1996). The Lifestyle Heart Trial: Comprehensive treatment and group support therapy. In R. Allen & S. Scheidt (Eds.), *Heart and mind: The practice of cardiac psychology* (pp. 233–253). Washington, DC: American Psychological Association.

Bogg, J., Thornton, E., & Bundred, P. (2000). Gender variability in mood, quality of life, and coping following primary myocardial infarction. *Coronary Health Care, 4*, 163–168.

Carlisle, D. M., Leake, B. D., & Shapiro, M. F. (1997). Racial and ethnic disparities in the use of cardiovascular procedures: Associations with type of health insurance. *American Journal of Public Health, 87*, 263–267.

Carney, R. M., Blumenthal, J. A., Freedland, K. E., Youngblood, M., Veith, R. C., Burg, M. M., et al. for the ENRICHD Investigators (2004). Depression and late mortality after myocardial infarction in the Enhancing Recovery in Coronary Heart Diseases (ENRICHED) Study. *Psychosomatic Medicine, 66*, 466–474.

Carney, R. M., & Freedland, K. E. (2000). Depression and medical illness. In L. F. Berkman & I. Kawachi (Eds.), *Social epidemiology* (pp. 191–212). New York: Oxford University Press.

Centers for Disease Control & Prevention (2003). *A public health action plan to prevent heart disease and stroke.* Atlanta, GA: Centers for Disease Control and Prevention. Retrieved November 23, 2005, from http://www.cdc.gov/dhdsp/library/action_plan/index.htm

Chesney, M. A. (1996). New behavioral risk factors for coronary heart disease: Implications for intervention. In K. Orth-Gomer & N. Schneiderman (Eds.), *Behavioral medicine approaches to cardiovascular disease prevention* (pp. 169–182). Mahwah, NJ: Lawrence Erlbaum Associates.

Cohen, H. W., Madhavan, S., & Alderman, M. H. (2001). History of treatment for depression: Risk factor for myocardial infarction in hypertensive patients. *Psychosomatic Medicine, 63*, 203–209.

Daly-Nee, C., Brunt, H., & Jairath, N. (1990). Risk and coronary heart disease. In N. Jairath (Ed.), *Coronary heart disease and risk factor management: A nursing perspective* (pp. 3–19). Philadelphia: W. B. Saunders Company.

Doering, L. V., Dracup, K., Caldwell, M. A., Moser, D. K., Erickson, V. S., Fonarow, G., et al. (2004). Is coping style linked to emotional states in heart failure patients? *Journal of Cardiac Failure, 10*, 344–349.

Donker, F. J. S. (2000). Cardiac rehabilitation: A review of current developments. *Clinical Psychology Review, 20*, 923–943.

Duru, F., Candinas, R., Dziekan, G., Goebbels, U., Myers, J., & Dubach, P. (2000). Effect of exercise training on heart rate variability in patients with new onset left ventricular dysfunction after myocardial infarction. *American Heart Journal, 140*, 157–161.

Dusseldorp, E., van Elderen, T., Maes, S., Meulman, J., & Kraaij, V. (1999). A meta-analysis of psychoeducational programs for coronary heat disease patients. *Health Psychology, 18*, 506–519.

Earle, A., Ayanian, J. Z., & Heymann, J. (2006). Work resumption after newly diagnosed coronary heart disease: Findings on the importance of paid leave. *Journal of Women's Health, 15*, 430–441.

Engblom, D., Korpilahti, K., Hamalainen, H., Ronnemaa, T., & Puukka, P. (1997). Quality of life and return to work 5 years after coronary artery bypass surgery: Long-term results of cardiac rehabilitation. *Journal of Cardiopulmonary Rehabilitation, 17*, 29–36.

ENRICHD Investigators (2003). The effects of treating depression and low perceived social support on clinical events after myocardial infarction: The Enhancing Recovery in Coronary Heart Disease Patients (ENRICH) randomized trial. *Journal of the American Medical Association, 289*, 3106–3116.

Fitchet, A., Doherty, P. J., Bundy, C., Bell, W., Fitzpatrick, A. P., & Garrett, C. J. (2003). Comprehensive cardiac rehabilitation programme for implantable cardioverter-defibrillator patients: A randomized trial. *Heart, 89,* 155–160.

Frasure-Smith, N. (1991). In-hospital symptoms of psychological stress as predictors of long-term outcome after acute myocardial infarction in men. *American Journal of Cardiology, 67,* 121–127.

Frasure-Smith, N., Lesperance, F., Prince, R. H., Verrier, P., Garber, R. A., Juneau, M., et al. (1997). Randomised trial of home-based psychosocial nursing intervention for patients recovering from myocardial infarction. *The Lancet, 350,* 473–479.

Frasure-Smith, N., Lesperance, F., & Talajic, M. (1995a). Coronary heart disease/myocardial infarction: Depression and 18-month prognosis after myocardial infarction. *Circulation, 91,* 999–1005.

Frasure-Smith, N., Lesperance, F., & Talajic, M. (1995b). The impact of negative emotions on prognosis following myocardial infarction: Is it more than depression? *Health Psychology, 14,* 388–398.

Frasure-Smith, N., & Prince, R. (1989). Long-term follow-up of the Ischemic Heart Disease Life Stress Monitoring Program. *Psychosomatic Medicine, 51,* 485–513.

Friedman, M., & Rosenman, R. (1959). Association of specific overt behavioral pattern with blood and cardiovascular findings: Blood cholesterol, blood clotting time, incidence of arcus senilis, and clinical coronary artery disease. *Journal of the American Medical Association, 169,* 1286–1296.

Friedman, M., Thoreson, C., Gill, J., Powell, L., Ulmer, D., Thompson, L., et al. (1984). Alteration of Type A behavior and reduction in cardiac recurrences in post-myocardial infarction patients. *American Heart Journal, 108,* 237–248.

Giles, W. H., Anda, R. F., Casper, M. L., Escobedo, L. G., & Taylor, H. A. (1995). Race and sex differences in rates of invasive cardiac procedures in US hospitals: Data from the National Hospital Discharge Survey. *Archives of Internal Medicine, 155,* 318–324.

Hallman, T., Thomsson, H., Burell, G., Lisspers, J., & Setterlind, S. (2003). Stress, burnout and coping: Differences between women with coronary heart disease and healthy matched women. *Journal of Health Psychology, 8,* 433–445.

Harenstam, A., Theorell, T., & Kaijser, L. (2000). Coping with anger-provoking situations, psychosocial working conditions, and ECG-detected signs of coronary heart disease. *Journal of Occupational Health Psychology, 5,* 191–203.

Havik, O. E., & Maeland, J. G. (1988). Verbal denial and outcome in myocardial infarction patients. *Journal of Psychosomatic Research, 32,* 145–157.

Hughes, J. W., Tomlinson, A., Blumenthal, J. A., Davidson, J., Sketch, M. H., Jr., & Watkins, L. L. (2004). Social support and religiosity as coping strategies for anxiety in hospitalized cardiac patients. *Annals of Behavioral Medicine, 28,* 179–185.

Kaplan, G. A., & Keil, J. E. (1993). Socioeconomic factors and cardiovascular disease: A review of the literature. *Circulation, 88,* 1973–1998.

Kessler, R. C., Berglund, P., Demler, O., Jin, R., & Walters, E. E. (2005). Lifetime prevalence and age-of-onset distributions of DSM-IV disorders in the National Comorbidity Survey Replication. *Archives of General Psychiatry, 62,* 593–602.

Kinne, G., Droste, C., Fahrenberg, J., & Roskamm, H. (1999). Symptomatic myocardial ischemia and everyday life: Implications for clinical use of interactive monitoring. *Journal of Psychosomatic Research, 46,* 369–377.

Kristofferzon, M., Lofmark, R., & Carlsson, M. (2003). Myocardial infarction: gender differences in coping and social support. *Journal of Advanced Nursing, 44,* 360–374.

Kristofferzon, M., Lofmark, R., & Carlsson, M. (2005a). Coping, social support, and quality of life over time after myocardial infarction. *Journal of Advanced Nursing, 52,* 113–124.

Kristofferzon, M., Lofmark, R., & Carlsson, M. (2005b). Perceived coping, social support, and quality of life 1 month after myocardial infarction: A comparison between Swedish women and men. *Heart and Lung, 34,* 39–50.

Kubzansky, L. D., & Kawachi, I. (2000). Affective states and health. In L. F. Berkman & I. Kawachi (Eds.), *Social epidemiology* (pp. 213–241). New York: Oxford University Press.

Lavie, C. J., & Milani, R. V. (1999a). Effects of cardiac rehabilitation and exercise training on peak aerobic capacity and work efficiency in obese patients with coronary artery disease. *American Journal of Cardiology, 83,* 1477–1480.

Lavie, C. J., & Milani, R. V. (1999b). Effects of cardiac rehabilitation and exercise training programs on coronary patients with high levels of hostility. *Mayo Clinic Proceedings, 74,* 959–966.

Lesperance, F., Frasure-Smith, N., & Talajic, M. (1996). Major depression before and after myocardial infarction: Its nature and consequences. *Psychosomatic Medicine, 58,* 99–110.

Levenson, J. L., Mishra, A., Hamer, R. M., & Hastillo, A. (1989). Denial and medical outcome in unstable angina. *Psychosomatic Medicine, 51,* 27–35.

Levine, J., Warrenburg, S., Kerns, R., Schwartz, G., Delaney, R., & Fontana, A. (1987). The role of denial in recovery from coronary heart disease. *Psychosomatic Medicine, 49,* 109–117.

Linden, W. (2000). Psychological treatments in cardiac rehabilitation: Review of rationales and outcomes. *Journal of Psychosomatic Research, 48,* 443–454.

Livneh, H. (1999). Psychosocial adaptation to heart diseases: The role of coping strategies. *Journal of Rehabilitation, 65,* 24–32.

Lynch, J. W., Kaplan, G. A., & Salonen, J. T. (1997). Why do poor people behave poorly? Variation in adult health behaviours and psychosocial characteristics by stages of the socioeconomic lifecourse. *Social Science Medicine, 44,* 809–813.

Maes, S., & Bruggemans, E. (1990). Approach-avoidance and illness behaviour in coronary heart patients. In L. R. Schmidt, P. Schwenkmezger, J. Weinman, & S. Maes (Eds.), *Health psychology: Theoretical and applied aspects* 297–308). London: Harwood.

Maines, T. Y., Lavie, C. J., Milani, R. V., Cassidy, M. M., Gilliland, Y. E., & Murgo, J. P. (1997). Effects of cardiac rehabilitation and exercise programs on exercise capacity, coronary risk factors, behavior, and quality of life in patients with coronary artery disease. *Southern Medical Journal, 90,* 43–49.

McInnes, G. T., Curzio, J. L., & Kennedy, S. S. (2004). Hypertension and antihypertensive therapy. In G. Lindsay & A. Gaw (Eds.), *Coronary heart disease prevention: A handbook for the health-care team* (2nd ed., pp. 75–129). London: Churchill Livingstone.

McIntosh, L. (2004). Cardiac rehabilitation. In G. Lindsay & A. Gaw (Eds.), *Coronary heart disease prevention: A handbook for the health-care team* (2nd ed., pp. 271–286). London: Churchill Livingstone.

Miller, T. D., Balady, G. J., & Fletcher, G. F. (1997). Exercise and its role in the prevention and rehabilitation of cardiovascular disease. *Annals of Behavioral Medicine, 19,* 220–229.

Miller, T. Q., Smith, T. W., Turner, C. W., Guijarro, M. L., & Hallet, A. J. (1996). A meta-analytic review of research on hostility and physical health. *Psychological Bulletin, 119*, 322–348.

Mital, A., Shrey, D. E., Govindaraju, M., Broderick, T. M., Colon-Brown, K., & Gustin, B. W. (2000). Accelerating the return to work (RTW) chances of coronary heart disease (CHD) patients: Part 1—Development and validation of a training programme. *Disability and Rehabilitation, 22*, 604–620.

Morrin, L., Black, S., & Reid, R. (2000). Impact of duration in a cardiac rehabilitation program on coronary risk profile and health-related quality of life outcomes. *Journal of Cardiopulmonary Rehabilitation, 20*, 115–121.

Ornish, D., Brown, S. E., Scherwitz, L. W., Billings, J. H., Armstrong, W. T., Ports, T. A., et al. (1990). Can lifestyle changes reverse coronary heart disease? The Lifestyle Heart Trial. *The Lancet, 336*, 129–133.

Ornish, D., Scherwitz, L. W., Doody, R. S., Derten, D., McLanahan, S. M., Brown, S. E., et al. (1983). Effects of stress management training and dietary changes in treating ischaemic heart disease. *Journal of the American Medical Association, 249*, 54–60.

Pargament, K. I., Ano, G. G., & Wachholtz, A. B. (2005). *The religious dimension of coping: Advances in theory, research, and practice.* New York: Guilford Press.

Petrie, K. J., Weinman, J., Sharpe, N., & Buckley, J. (1996). Role of patients' view of their illness in predicting return to work and functioning after myocardial infarction: Longitudinal study. *British Medical Journal, 312*, 1191–1194.

Porter, R. R., Krout, L., Parks, V., Gibbs, S., Luers, E. S., Nolan, M. T., et al. (1994). Percieved stress and coping strategies among candidates for heart transplantation during the organ waiting period. *Journal of Heart and Lung Transplantation, 13*, 102–107.

Saab, P. G. (1997). Influence of ethnicity and gender on cardiovascular responses to active coping and inhibitory-passive coping challenges. *Psychosomatic Medicine, 59*, 434–446.

Sapolsky, R. M. (2004). *Why zebras don't get ulcers: The acclaimed guide to stress, stress-related diseases, and coping* (3rd ed.). New York: Henry Holt and Company.

Scheidt, S. (1996). A whirlwind tour of cardiology for the mental health professional. In R. Allen & S. Scheidt (Eds.), *Heart and mind: The practice of cardiac psychology* (pp. 15–62). Washington, DC: American Psychological Association.

Schneiderman, N., Saab, P. G., Catellier, D. J., Powell, L. H., DeBusk, R. F., Williams, R. B., et al. for the ENRICHD Investigators (2004). Psychosocial treatment within sex by ethnicity subgroups in the Enhancing Recovery in Coronary Heart Disease clinical trial. *Psychosomatic Medicine, 66*, 475–483.

Shen, B., McCreary, C. P., & Myers, H. F. (2004). Independent and mediated contributions of personality, coping, social support, and depressive symptoms to physical functioning outcome among patients in cardiac rehabilitation. *Journal of Behavioral Medicine, 27*, 39–62.

Shen, B., Myers, H. F., & McCreary, C. P. (2006). Psychosocial predictors of cardiac rehabilitation quality of life outcomes. *Journal of Psychosomatic Research, 60*, 3–11.

Sher, L. (2004). Type D personality, cortisol, and cardiac disease. *Australian and New Zealand Journal of Psychiatry, 38*, 652–653.

Shrey, D. E., & Mital, A. (2000). Accelerating the return to work (RTW) chances of coronary heart disease (CHD) patients: Part 2—Development and validation of a vocational rehabilitation programme. *Disability and Rehabilitation, 22*, 621–626.

Siegrist, J., Peter, R., Junge, A., Cremer, P., & Seidel, D. (1990). Low status control, high effort at work and ischemic heart disease: Prospective evidence from blue-collar men. *Social Science and Medicine, 31*, 1127–1134.

Sirois, B. C., & Burg, M. M. (2003). Negative emotion and coronary heart disease: A review. *Behavior Modification, 27*, 83–102.

Soloff, P. H. (1980). Effects of denial on mood, compliance, and quality of functioning after cardiovascular rehabilitation. *General Hospital Psychiatry, 2*, 307–313.

Soloff, P. H., & Bartel, A. G. (1979). Effects of denial on mood and performance in cardiovascular rehabilitation. *Journal of Chronic Disease, 32*, 307–313.

Stewart, M. J., Hirth, A. M., Klassen, G., Makrides, L., & Wolf, H. (1997). Stress, coping, and social support as psychosocial factors in readmissions for ischaemic heart disease. *International Journal of Nursing Studies, 34*, 151–163.

Suls, J., & Fletcher, B. (1985). The relative efficacy of avoidant and non-avoidant coping strategies: A meta-analysis. *Health Psychology, 11*, 249–288.

Taylor-Piliae, R. E. (2001). An exploration of the relationships between uncertainty, psychological distress and type of coping strategy among Chinese men after cardiac catheterization. *Journal of Advanced Nursing, 33*, 79–88.

Terry, D. J. (1992). Stress, coping, and coping resources as correlates of adaptation in myocardial infarction patients. *British Journal of Clinical Psychology, 31*, 215–225.

Vaccarino, V., Rathore, S. S., Wenger, N. K., Frederick, P. D., Abramson, J. L., Barron, H. V., et al. (2005). Sex and racial differences in the management of acute myocardial infarction, 1994–2002. *New England Journal of Medicine, 353*, 671–682.

van Elderen, T., Maes, S., & Dusseldorp, E. (1999). Coping with coronary heart disease: A longitudinal study. *Journal of Psychosomatic Research, 47*, 175–183.

van Rijen, E. H. M., Utens, E. M. W. J., Roos-Hesselink, J. W., Meijboom, F. J., van Domburg, R. T., Roelandt, J. R. T. C., et al. (2004). Styles of coping and social support in a cohort of adults with congenital heart disease. *Cardiology in the Young, 14*, 122–130.

Walker, N., & Lorimer, A. R. (2004). Coronary heart disease: Epidemiology, pathology, and diagnosis. In G. Lindsay & A. Gaw (Eds.), *Coronary heart disease prevention: A handbook for the health-care team* (2nd ed., pp. 1–27). London: Churchill Livingstone.

Whitmarsh, A., Koutantji, M., & Sidell, K. (2003). Illness perceptions, mood and coping in predicting attendance at cardiac rehabilitation. *British Journal of Health Psychology, 8*, 208–221.

Yarzebski, J. (2004). Recent and temporal trends (1975–1999) in the treatment, hospital, and long-term outcomes of Hispanic and non-Hispanic white patients hospitalized with acute myocardial infarction: A population-based perspective. *American Heart Journal, 147*, 690–697.

Young, R. F., & Kahana, E. (1993). Gender, recovery from late life heart attack, and medical care. *Women and Health, 20*, 11–31.

14
Coping with Multiple Sclerosis: Considerations and Interventions

Kristy McNulty

Description

Multiple sclerosis (MS) is a chronic, immune-mediated disease that affects the central nervous system (CNS). It is the most common cause of chronic neurological disability in young adults in North America and Europe, with onset commonly between ages 20 and 40 years. The reported prevalence in the United States varies from 30 to 100 per 100,000 people (Herndon, 2000; Smith & Schapiro, 2004). A study for the World Federation of Multiple Sclerosis Societies estimates that 1.1 million people world-wide have the disease (Dean, 1994). Two to three females are afflicted for every male. The disease appears more frequently in Caucasians than in Hispanics or African Americans and is relatively rare among Asians and the black peoples of Africa. MS is more common in temperate areas of the world and is relatively unusual in the tropics.

Like many other chronic illnesses and disabilities (CID), MS almost always has a downward illness trajectory, becoming more severe with the passage of time. The rate of progression of the disease is unpredictable (Matthews, 1993). The person typically experiences cyclical periods of new or worsening symptoms (exacerbations), alternating with periods of symptom stability or decrement (remissions) (Boyden, 2000; Pakenham, Stewart, & Rogers, 1997). Except in relatively rare cases, and individual's life span is not greatly affected (Sadovnick, Eisen, Ebers, & Paty, 1991).

Etiology

The cause of MS is currently unknown. However, decades of research suggest that it is the result of an abnormal autoimmune response to some infectious agent (e.g., viral or bacterial) or environmental trigger in a genetically-susceptible individual (Smith & Schapiro, 2004). Myelin (the covering of the nerve fibers) is treated as foreign by the body's defenses and is attacked, resulting in scattered areas of *demyelination*, or scar tissue (plaques), in the brain and spinal cord, which delay or block the passage of nerve impulses. Although the etiology of MS remains unclear, epidemiological studies have identified demographic characteristics that increase the risk for developing the disease as female gender, Caucasian race, and geographic location (Smith & Schapiro, 2004).

Characteristics and Symptoms

Because different areas of the brain and spinal cord are responsible for different kinds of movements and sensations, the neurologic deficit that results from an area of scarring is dependent on the exact location of the lesion (Smith & Schapiro, 2004). Due to dependence of symptoms on the area of scarring, no two cases of MS are exactly alike, and symptoms vary considerably from one individual to another, as well as within the person from time to time. Symptoms can include slurred speech, coordination problems, neurogenic pain, impaired mobility, paralysis, fatigue, visual impairments (e.g., double vision, eye-muscle jerking, blurred vision, problems of depth perception), cognitive deterioration, dizziness and vertigo, bladder and bowel dysfunction, sexual dysfunction, spasticity, and intolerance to heat (Cavallo & McLaughlin, 1997).

Neuropsychological Features

Because MS is a disease that produces demyelination of the nerves in the brain and spinal cord, it is not surprising that many individuals with the disease show some neuropsychological features when properly evaluated (Rao, 1995). Cognitive dysfunction and affective disorders are common neuropsychological manifestations of the disease, which can have a significant impact on daily living and employment status (Schiffer, 2002).

Cognitive Dysfunction

Upwards of 50% of individuals with MS show evidence of some cognitive impairment, with a spectrum of mild to severe involvement (LaRocca & Sorensen, 2004). The occurrence of cognitive symptoms is only weakly related to the disease course and duration of the disease. In other words, a person can experience cognitive changes at any point over the course of the disease, regardless of the severity of physical symptoms.

The cognitive functions that are most often affected are recent memory, sustained attention and concentration, and executive functioning, such as impairment in planning, abstract reasoning, sequential thinking, and conceptualization. The impact of such impairment, even if relatively mild, can have a profound effect on a person's ability to perform important daily activities, including those related to driving, social interactions, and work.

Affective Disorders

A sizable portion of the overall emotional impact of MS can be viewed in terms of affective disorders that have been shown to accompany the illness. Foremost among these is depression (Minden, Orav, & Reich, 1987; Pakenham et al., 1997; Schiffer, 2002; Siegert & Abernethy, 2005), with an estimated 25–50% experiencing major depression at some time following MS onset (Aikens, Fischer, Namey, & Rudick, 1997; Feinstein, 1997; Minden & Schiffer, 1990; Mohr & Cox, 2001; Patten, Beck, & Williams, 2003; Rao, Huber, & Bornstein, 1992; Sadovnick, Remick, & Allen, 1996), which significantly exceeds the rates found in samples of individuals with other medical conditions (Minden et al., 1987) or neurological disorders (Rao et al., 1992; Schubert & Foliart, 1993; Whitlock & Siskind, 1980).

Of further concern is the finding that depression in people with this disease is often not detected and treated. If left untreated, depression in people with MS is likely to worsen (Siegert & Abernethy, 2005). Although existing studies have established depression as a major psychological symptom of MS, it has yet to be determined whether depressive episodes are psychosocial reactions to the progressive, unpredictable, and chronic nature of the disease, or are clinical manifestations of neurobiological impairments that are attributable to the disease process itself (Rao, 1986; Siegert & Abernethy, 2005).

Although research on affective disorders in MS tends to focus on depression, individuals with MS have also been found to have high levels of anxiety (Maurelli et al., 1992). Other psychological sequelae include emotional and psychological problems that do not meet diagnostic criteria (Feinstein, Feinstein, Gray, & O'Connor, 1997; Feinstein, O'Connor, Gray, & Feinstein, 1999), such as pathological laughing and crying, mood swings, anger, and distress (LaRocca, Kalb, Foley, & McGann, 1993).

Disease Course

The extremely variable progression of MS makes it difficult to predict the course of the disease (Matthews, 1993). Approximately 65–70% of affected individuals experience *relapsing-remitting multiple sclerosis*, in which symptoms intensify suddenly and subsequently subside, often with little or no residual deficit or effect. Approximately 15–20% experience a *progressive* course of illness (differentiated into primary-, secondary-, and relapsing-progressive variants), in which the disease activity is generally uninterrupted. The remainder experiences a *benign* course, in which the disease does not progress and neurologic systems remain unaffected long after diagnosis (Lublin & Reingold, 1996). For the vast majority of people with the disease, the trend is one of progressive deterioration and disability (Smith & Schapiro, 2004).

Diagnosis

The diagnosis of MS remains as a clinical judgment at present, based on a person's medical history, an assessment of the symptoms experienced and reported, and the existence of signs detected during a neurologic examination (Smith & Schapiro, 2004). Both symptoms and signs are necessary because symptoms are subjective complaints that can vary tremendously from one individual to another, while signs are more measurable, objective observations. Tests currently used as major adjuncts to the clinical examination include an analysis of cerebrospinal fluid that is obtained from a lumbar puncture, tracing patterns of evoked electrical activity of the brain, and imaging techniques (i.e., magnetic resonance imaging [MRI]). Recent advances in imaging techniques have improved the accuracy and efficiency of a clinical diagnosis over the past decade (Fox, 2006).

Medical Management

Management strategies utilized to treat MS may be divided into two general categories: (a) Those used to treat the underlying disease, and (b) those used to minimize and control specific symptoms (Schapiro & Schneider, 2002).

Treating the Underlying Disease

The most common approach in current treatment regimens for MS is to systematically regulate immune activation (Vollmer, 2005). In the presence of relapsing-remitting multiple sclerosis, this is best achieved by the use of the immunomodulatory drugs. Although none of these drugs can stop or reverse the disease, they can be highly effective in managing its course by reducing the frequency and severity of attacks. They have also been shown to alter disease features that are measured by a MRI. Studies suggest these agents are most effective in the early relapsing-remitting phase of the disease and are much less effective with progressive disease (Comi, 2000; Comi, Columbo, & Martinelli, 2000; Kalb, 2004).

Although the immunomodulating agents represent advancement in therapeutic options, the drugs are costly and may cause side effects, including flu-like symptoms, abnormal liver function, injection-site reactions (Gottber, Cardulf, & Fredrikson, 2000), and possible depression (Feinstein, 2000). Although side effects may undermine treatment adherence for some, the availability and efficacy of these agents have brought new hope to individuals with relapsing-remitting multiple sclerosis and their families (Hadjimichael, 1999).

A variety of immunosuppressive, therapeutic regimens have been tried in individuals with progressive variants of MS in hopes of retarding disease progression. The aim of these treatments is to indiscriminately eliminate or reduce the cells involved in the immune response (Vollmer, 2005). Immunosuppressive therapies have potentially serious toxicities and are only indicated for individuals with active severe disease (Kalb, 2004).

Symptomatic and Supportive Therapies

Spasticity may also be reduced with the use of medications. Medications have also been beneficial in treating bladder problems, including urgency, frequency, and incontinence. In addition to the assortment of MS medications to treat the underlying disease, a variety of therapies is available to treat the specific symptoms that can also occur. Occupational therapy is helpful in managing hand tremors, lack of coordination, fatigue, and sensory symptoms in the upper extremities (Schapiro & Schneider, 2002). Physical therapy is valuable in treating muscle weakness, and also improves mobility and spasticity.

A person with mild symptoms (e.g., muscle stiffness, mild pain) of MS, which do not require conventional medications, might choose to try an intervention such as yoga, tai chi, or meditation. To improve the functioning of individuals who have cognitive impairment due to MS, cognitive rehabilitation may be offered by a neuropsychologist, speech/language pathologist, and/or occupational therapist (LaRocca & Sorensen, 2004). Siegert and Abernethy (2005) underscore that screening for depression and monitoring of mood should be a feature of the medical management of all clients with MS. Depression responds well to psychotherapy that emphasizes the development of active coping skills (i.e., cognitive-behavioral therapy), or to antidepressant medications (Mohr et al., 2001).

Coping with Multiple Sclerosis

Psychosocial Impact

MS can have wide ranging effects on individuals (and on family life), ranging from mild interruption in daily routine to complete disruption of everyday life. By virtue of the disease pattern, individuals must not only make an initial adjustment to disability, but are required to make a continual process of readjustment due to the erratic nature of the symptoms (Strauss et al., 1984). Sullivan, Mikail, and Weinshenker (1997) noted that the individual diagnosed with MS must struggle with the reality of being diagnosed with an incurable, debilitating disease, even though in the early stages of the illness, the individual may suffer from little or no functional impairment. In addition, the early stages of the disease are often marked by the threat of loss, while the more advanced stages of the illness are primarily focused on coping with the actual loss.

Salient features of MS include its long-term nature, uncertainty, unpredictability, and financial burden (e.g., loss of earnings, cost of care) (Scheinberg et al., 1998; Williamson, 2000). Associated problems, such as symptom control, the prevention and management of medical crises, failure of therapy, unpredictable symptom control, and physical deterioration, despite adherences to the prescribed regimen, may result in a perception of lack of control in all its aspects (Strauss et al., 1984).

Certain psychological reactions, reflecting a process of adaptation, are often expressed by individuals following the onset of MS. These reactions can include anxiety, denial, depression, anger, and reintegration or adjustment (Livneh & Antonak, 1997, 2005). Disability-triggered reactions are also likely to occur each time the person with MS encounters disease-related changes (Strauss et al., 1984). Although psychological reactions parallel those typically observed among people who have experienced major personal losses, most clinicians and researchers seldom agree on the nature and sequencing of these reactions or on the necessity of experiencing certain reactions, in order to ultimately accept or adjust to a changed life situation (Livneh & Cook, 2005).

Coping Research about Multiple Sclerosis

Like many other CIDs, the intrusion of MS can be a stressful condition as a result of its potential physical, psychological, social, vocational, economic, and recreational impact (O'Brien, 1993). The role played by coping in adapting to life stresses engendered by chronic illness and its wide-ranging effects has received growing attention in the scientific literature. In particular, numerous research efforts have been spent on articulating which ways of coping are beneficial in adapting to the individual's constantly changing needs (e.g., Billings & Moos, 1981; Maes, Leventhal, & de Ridder, 1996). The vast majority of coping research in MS had been guided by Lazarus and Folkman's (1984) stress-coping model, which defines coping as "constantly changing cognitive and behavioral efforts to manage specific external and/or internal demands that are appraised as taxing or exceeding the resources of the person" (p. 141).

A coping model, which is derived from the Lazarus and Folkman theory and applied to chronic illness, is based on the premise that adjustment is determined by illness parameters and three hypothesized mediational processes: namely, cognitive appraisal, coping strategies, and coping resources (Maes et al., 1996). Both cross-sectional and longitudinal studies have supported the utility of this model in explaining adjustment to MS (e.g., Pakenham, 1999; Pakenham et al., 1997).

Illness Parameters

Illness measures in MS coping research vary widely, but typically include illness duration, disability, and disease severity (neurological impairment). Some studies have found illness duration to be unrelated to adjustment (e.g., Maybury & Brewin, 1984; Rudick, Miller, Clough, Gragg, & Farmer, 1992), whereas others have found longer duration related to better adjustment (Fisk, Pontfract, Ritvo, Archibald, & Murry, 1994; Pakenham et al., 1997) .

Although several studies have found that severity of MS is unrelated to adjustment (Devins, Seland, Klein, Edworthy, & Saary, 1993; Devins et al., 1996; Fisk et al., 1994; Pakenham et al., 1997; Rudick et al., 1992), others have found a positive relationship (e.g., McIvor, Riklan, & Reznikoff, 1984). Greater levels of physical disability have also been related to poorer adjustment and quality of life (Devins et al., 1993; Nortvedt, Ruse, Myhr, & Nyland, 2000; Wineman, 1990; Zeldow & Pavlou, 1984) .

Cognitive Appraisal

As defined by Lazarus and Folkman (1984), cognitive appraisal is an evaluative process that reflects the person's subjective interpretation of the event. Events are appraised in terms of threat, challenge, and controllability. The appraisal of an illness-related event, as threatening and limiting opportunities for personal growth and/or as uncontrollable, is likely to generate stress that may exceed the coping skills and resources available to the person, thus negatively influencing adjustment to MS.

In a study examining relations between appraisals and adjustment to MS, Wineman, Durand, and Steiner (1994) found that higher illness uncertainty and threat appraisals were related to more distress, whereas challenge appraisals were related to lower distress. Pakenham et al. (1997) found similar links between threat appraisals and adjustment, but found that challenge appraisals and adjustment were unrelated.

Coping Resources

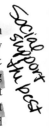

Coping resources are relatively stable characteristics of a person's disposition and environment and refer to what is available to individuals when they select their coping strategies (e.g., personality factors, social support) (Moos & Billings, 1982). A commonly reported and highly effective modality for reducing psychological distress and facing challenging situations is social support. At its most simplistic level, social support refers to interpersonal transactions that include some combination of aid or instrumental assistance, affirmation, and affection (Gulick, 1994).

Several studies have shown that social support is related to better adjustment to MS, although the relation is not a simple linear one (Foote, Piazza, Holcombe, Paul, & Dappin, 1990; Gulick, 1994; Long & Miller, 1991; Miller, 1997; Pakenham, 1999; Wineman, 1990). For example, Pakenham (1999) examined the stress and coping model of chronic illness in people with MS and found that social support had a beneficial effect on adjustment, but only under circumstances of high perceived threat. Additional research is needed to clarify the complex relation between social support and adjustment to MS.

Coping Style

Within the context of coping with MS, two major styles of coping with stressors are identified in the literature: Problem-focused and emotion-focused. Problem-focused coping involves cognitive actions such as problem-solving or confrontive coping, which are directed at reducing or modifying the source of stress. Emotion-focused coping, such as wishful thinking and avoidance, are directed at reducing the emotional distress elicited by the stressful situation (Lazarus, 1993).

Problem-Focused Coping

Problem-focused coping tends to be associated with well-being in people without chronic physical illness (Folkman & Lazarus, 1986; Lazarus & Folkman, 1984; Zeidner & Saklofske, 1996). In MS, this relationship is less clear, with some studies finding a positive relationship between adaptation and problem-focused coping (Aikens et al., 1997; O'Brien, 1993; Pakenham et al., 1997) and others finding no relationship (Beatty et al., 1998; Hickey & Greene, 1989; Jean, Paul, & Beatty, 1999). The differences in these findings may have been an artifact of small sample size (i.e., limiting generalizability), cultural differences, and/or instrumentation weaknesses.

Specific forms of problem-focused coping may be more helpful than others. Behavioral coping strategies, which are focused on achievable health maintenance goals (e.g., moderate levels of exercise tailored to the person's physical capacities, maintaining a healthy diet and appropriate weight, adherence to medical regimens) or behavioral compensation (e.g., compensating for fatigue by building rest periods into one's daily schedule, proper use of ambulation aids or other adaptive devices, shopping at nonpeak hours), are associated with higher quality of life (QOL) in cross-sectional studies of MS subjects (Mathiowetz, Matuska, & Murphy, 2001; Stuifbergen 1995; Stuifbergen, Becker, Blozis, Timmerman, & Kullberg, 2003). Mediational analyses suggest that health behaviors mediate the effects of disability on QOL (Stuifbergen & Roberts, 1997). However, when behavioral strategies are focused on alleviating problems that cannot be resolved (e.g., attempts to return physical functioning to a pre-MS baseline, despite progressed disability), coping efforts are likely to result in frustration (Maes et al., 1996).

Cognitive coping strategies, such as cognitive reframing, information gathering, planning, and goal setting, have generally been associated with better adaptation to MS (Aikens et al., 1997; Baker, 1998). Cognitive reframing is a way of reconceptualizing a problem, from something that is considered impossible to solve into something for which other coping strategies may be helpful (Aikens et al., 1997).

A specific form of cognitive coping, positive reframing, is related to better adjustment in MS (Aikens et al., 1997; Mohr & Goodkin, 1999; Mohr et al., 1999; Pakenham, 2005). Positive reframing reflects efforts on the part of the individual to uncover the positive aspects of the condition, and to view the condition as an opportunity for further growth. In a study by Mohr et al. (1999), individuals reported not only a variety of demoralizing consequences to how MS had affected their lives, but also benefits they had derived from the illness. The benefits included such things as improved relations with family and enhanced appreciation of life.

A study by Pakenham (2005) examined the direct and stress-buffering effects of benefit-finding on positive and negative outcomes, after controlling for relevant demographics, illness (e.g., subjective health status), and appraisal. Hierarchical regressions revealed that benefit-finding played an important role in sustaining positive psychological states in individuals with MS, but had little or no direct impact on distress. This study provides support for the role of benefit-finding in sustaining and promoting well-being in the context of an ongoing stressor. That individuals with MS report perceived benefits from their illness experience is consistent with a growing body of literature on benefit-finding as an adaptation to adversity (Affleck & Tennen, 1996; Tennen & Affleck, 2002). More research is needed, however, to further clarify the role of benefit-finding in coping processes that are involved in adapting to chronic illness.

Emotion-Focused Coping

In the majority of studies of coping and adjustment, emotion-focused coping has been associated with higher levels of distress. Both cross-sectional and longitudinal studies in MS have found that passive, avoidant, emotion-focused coping strategies (e.g., wishful thinking, self-blame, avoidance) are related to poorer outcomes across multiple adjustment domains (Aikens et al., 1997; Buelow, 1991; McCabe & McKern, 2002; Mohr & Goodkin, 1999; O'Brien, 1993; Pakenham, 1999; Pakenham et al., 1997).

Emotion-focused coping may be beneficial however. Folkman and Lazarus (1988) suggest that selecting an emotion-focused coping style may serve a protective function for the individual. For example, denial of illness, an emotion-focused attempt to disavow the threatening implications of disease exacerbations, may be helpful to the individual as a diversional strategy that temporarily hides an unpleasant reality, while allowing the individual to maintain awareness of the seriousness of the disease (Livneh & Antonak, 1997). Indeed, Sullivan et al. (1997) suggests that denial, avoidance, and a focus on the present may be adaptive ways in which some individuals initially cope with a diagnosis of MS. Denial and avoidance may become problematic only when these strategies interfere with illness prevention, with health promoting behaviors, or when they increase the intensity of intrusive thoughts.

Physical and Psychosocial/Behavioral Interventions

Eliminating or reducing emotional distress and increasing overall adjustment to life with MS may be facilitated by physical and psychosocial adjustment interventions (Livneh & Woosley-George, 1997). Physical adjustment concerns the body's capacity for successful negotiation of the physical environment, and emphasizes physical barrier-removal as the target of intervention. Psychosocial adjustment concerns the capacity to function appropriately in the personal and interpersonal spheres, and is facilitated through psychosocial and behavioral interventions.

Physical Barrier Removal

Ambulation aids may assist the person to improve function and remain walking as long as possible. The appropriate use of an aid, specific to the needs of the individual can increase endurance, decrease energy cost, and improve safety while ambulating (Schapiro, 1991). Common ambulation aids include one or two canes, a quad cane, lightweight forearm crutches, ankle-foot orthoses, a walker, wheelchair, or scooter (Blake & Bodine, 2002). Fatigue, not impaired walking, may be the main driving factor in determining the need for a wheelchair or scooter.

In addition to mobility aids, there are tools available to assist in removing or reducing physical obstacles in the home environment (Blake & Bodine, 2002). Voice-activated remote controls are available for TV's and CD players. Sensory assistive technology (AT) ranges from magnifiers and self-threading needles to currency-recognition devices and beeping liquid level-indicators for pouring drinks. With the current advances in AT, performing insurmountable tasks in daily living, such as meal preparation, cleanup, bathing, grooming and other daily duties, are now possible.

Augmentative and alternative communication (AAC) aids pertain to all electronic or non-electronic devices, which enable expressive, receptive communication for those who are unable to communicate fully through natural speech and/or writing (Blake & Bodine, 2002). Computer-access technology offers voice recognition software, screen magnification, various input and output devices, including Braille, modified or alternative keyboard, and more. The goal of AAC is to enable individuals to experience the social, emotional, recreational, and employment benefits that accrue from communication.

Psychosocial/Behavioral Interventions

Given the scope of life domains that can be affected by MS, the facilitation of efforts, to adapt and live as full and satisfying a life as possible, is a common goal across clinical interventions. More specifically, these interventions provide clients (and their families) with emotional, cognitive, and/or behavioral support. Intervention strategies, which have been commonly applied to help individuals with MS, and which represent a sense of the breadth of potential approaches, include those involving psychotherapy, disease self-management, and client and family education.

Psychotherapy

Commonly administered clinical interventions for people with MS include individual psychotherapy and group psychotherapy. Individual psychotherapy is used to help clients develop skills, in order to better cope with emotions, thoughts, and adjustment to MS diagnosis and symptoms (Minden, 1992). Group psychotherapy is commonly used to decrease the alienation that may be experienced by people with chronic illness, to facilitate expression of emotions related to the disease, to provide support, and to help clients learn from one another (Stuber, Sullivan, Kennon, & Nobler, 1988). Specific individual or group psychotherapeutic strategies are generally regarded as either: (a) Supportive, affective-insightful, or psychodynamic in nature (e.g., person-centered therapy, Gestalt therapy, Jungian therapy), or (b) active-directed, goal-oriented, or cognitive-behavioral in nature (e.g., cognitive therapy, behavioral therapy, coping skills training) (Livneh & Antonak, 2005).

Studies on the effects of psychotherapeutic strategies, which are regarded as supportive, or affective-insightful in nature, have recently been shown to provide little or no consistent improvement in QOL, or mental health functioning in clients with MS (Uccelli, Mohr, Battaglia, Zagami, & Mohr, 2004). An emerging literature suggests that clinical interventions that actively teach clients adaptive coping strategies (e.g., cognitive therapy, behavioral therapy, cognitive-behavioral therapy [CBT], coping skills training) are more effective at reducing depression and improving mood, than interventions involving supportive, affective-insightful therapy (Uccelli et al., 2004). In MS research, coping-focused, cognitive-behavioral strategies have been shown to provide strong improvements in affective distress and depression (Crawford & McIvor, 1987; Larcombe and Wilson, 1984; Mohr et al., 2000; Mohr & Goodkin, 1999), as well as enhancing QOL (Mathiowetz et al., 2001; Schwartz, 1999; Stuifbergen et al., 2003; Uccelli et al., 2004).

Larcombe and Wilson (1984) described the first controlled, randomly assigned treatment study employing a six-week group-administered CBT. Although the study was small, with nine active clients and ten controls, results revealed a large reduction in depression for CBT, compared to an increase in depression for the control group with MS. A randomized trial by Crawford and McIvor (1985) documented that insight-oriented group psychotherapy was effective in reducing depression in MS, enhancing sense of control, and improving mood. Yet, a cross-study comparison of outcomes found this treatment to be less effective than coping-focused interventions (Mohr & Goodkin, 1999). Crawford and McIvor (1987) compared a 13-session group CBT stress-management program administered to 23 clients and 21 control clients. Similar to Larcombe and Wilson's findings, the CBT treatment group exhibited a reduction in depression and anxiety, while the control group worsened.

Teaching coping skills to people with MS was found by Schwartz (1999) to be associated with a greater number of aspects of well-being, in comparison to a program that involved telephone support from peers. In a study by Mohr and colleagues (2001), it was revealed that individual CBT was more effective than supportive-expressive group therapy in treating MS clients with a coexisting diagnosis of major depressive disorder.

Researchers at a Veteran's Administration in the U.S. (Mohr et al., 2005) reported positive conclusions from a study of the effectiveness of telephone-administered cognitive-behavioral therapy (T-CBT) for people with MS. The T-CBT was tested against a randomized control group that received telephone-administered, supportive, emotion-focused therapy. Results indicated significant improvements in depression and positive affect during the 16 weeks of T-CBT. Furthermore, the specific cognitive-behavioral components of T-CBT produced improvements above and beyond the emotion-focused therapy.

Interventions partially based on the behavioral principles of social cognitive theory (Bandura, 1986; 1998) have reported positive psychological and physical changes. For example, Mathiowetz et al. (2001) used a six-week, energy-conservation course in a quasi-experimental study, for which 54 subjects with MS served as their own controls. The researchers' intervention resulted in significant improvements in fatigue impact, self-efficacy, and several aspects of QOL (i.e., vitality, social functioning, mental health).

Disease Self-Management

Devins (1994; Devins and Shnek, 2000) and others (Lorig & Holman, 2003; Lorig, Sobel, Ritter, Laurent, & Hobbs, 2001; Uccelli et al., 2004) have suggested the importance of self-management, or actively taking responsibility and informed control over managing one's disability or chronic illness. The aim of self-management education is to help people acquire skills to cope with, or better adapt to, their illness. Through a variety of alternative experiential and didactic methods, it seeks to enhance self-efficacy to perform these effectively (Lorig & Holman, 2003).

The Gateway to Wellness Program for Individuals with Multiple Sclerosis is one prototype (Neufeld, 1999). A number of component interventions are combined with the objective of training affected individuals to manage symptoms, collaborate with the health-care team, and minimize illness-induced life-style disruptions, thereby enhancing QOL. Although the application of this intervention to MS is still at an early stage, such programs can effect the desired behaviors, which will support health and minimize the negative features of a chronic, potentially disabling disease, such as MS.

Client and Family Education

The need for factual information about MS is the most basic element for enhancing QOL for the person with MS, his or her family, and significant others (Holland, 2002). Educational strategies can assist individuals, in anticipating the potential impact of the condition across life domains, and can introduce positive steps, which can be taken to manage symptoms and to adjust lifestyles, in order to maximize health and wellness. Modalities, which people with MS have found helpful for learning, include one-to-one in-person, print, videotape, audiotape, educational groups, and the internet.

Vocational Implications for Individuals with MS

MS is an adult-onset disability that commonly occurs at a time in which individuals are just beginning to participate and be productive in the worker role. This role is also one of the most valued in American and western society. In addition to providing income and economic stability, work helps to define who that person is and their role in the community (Rumrill & Hennessey, 2004).

Most adults with MS are an experienced, qualified, and capable group of workers. In fact, more than 90% of Americans with MS have employment histories (i.e., they have worked in the past; LaRocca, 1995; Rumrill & Hennessey, 2004). They are also typically solidly educated (LaRocca & Hall, 1990). About two-thirds are still employed at the time of diagnosis (Rumrill & Hennessey, 2004). This represents higher occupational functioning than that of the general population (Fraser, 2002).

However, as time and illness progress, individuals with MS experience a precipitous decline in employment. In fact, between 70% and 80% of individuals with the disease are unemployed five years after diagnosis, despite advances in medical treatment, the availability of adaptive technology, and passage of federal laws including the 1990 Americans with Disabilities Act, and the Family and Medical leave Act of 1993 (O'Day, 1998). The vast majority of unemployed people with MS voluntarily make the choice to leave the work force. Yet, once they have stopped working, about 75% of unemployed people with MS feel that they would like to return to work, while more than 80% believe they are able to work (Rumrill & Hennessey, 2004).

Despite numerous research studies that have been conducted over the years concerning employment and MS, it is still unclear why one person with MS keeps his or her job, while another, with a similar degree of disability, leaves the work force (Rumrill & Hennessey, 2004). Factors that have been identified as predictors of employment difficulty and/or job loss for people with MS include: Female gender, limited formal education, employed spouse, poor relationship with one's employer, negative attitudes on the part of co-workers, job requiring significant physical exertion, cognitive dysfunction, and severe physical symptoms that affect mobility (Fraser, 2002; Rumrill, 1996; Rumrill & Hennessey, 2004).

Gordon, Lewis and Wong (1994) noted that "vocational planning for people with multiple sclerosis is complicated due to the progressive and unpredictable nature of the disorder" (p. 34). Indeed, not only is the individual with MS unable to predict when an exacerbation will occur, but as Rumrill, Roessler and Cook (1998) noted, an individual cannot anticipate with any certainty which symptomatology to expect. Fear of disease progression is a common response for individuals with MS (Selder & Breunig, 1991). This can lead to an early departure from employment, if interventions are not considered (Kornblith, LaRocca, & Baum, 1986).

Interventions by professionals need to be timely, because there also may be a risk of people with MS for developing a sense of stress or apprehension, related to work demands exceeding their personal resources. This may further decrease work effectiveness and satisfaction, leading to premature work-cessation (Johnson et al., 2004; Roessler, Rumrill, & Fitzgerald, 2004). In addition, interventions are generally facilitated when the disability situation is perceived by both employee and employer as potentially manageable (Johnson et al., 2004).

Vocational Implications for Professionals

There are a number of ways that professionals can assist individuals with MS in returning to work. Job-retention interventions can be designed for people with disabilities. They are most effective when priority is placed on helping the person to continue in his or her present position or a related job, as quickly as possible, particularly if a client enjoyed the work (Matkin, 1995; Rumrill, Roessler, Battersby, & Schuyler, 1998). Diverse computer software, such as Occupational Awareness System (OASYS, 2003), can actually identify companies within one's county or city with related jobs.

In promoting successful employment, Gordon et al. (1994) recommended providing counseling either before individuals leave their jobs, or at least in the early stages of the illness, concerning fear and apprehension about continuing employment. Involving the family in assessment and intervention, when the individual is seriously impacted by the emotional and psychosocial aspects of the disease, is also important (Long, Glueckauf, & Rasmussen, 1998). The response to opportunities by an individual with MS will be limited, if he or she has not made a successful adaptation to the illness.

Patterns of relapse need to be examined, in conjunction with methods that may be utilized to maintain employment during and/or continue employment after relapses (Illan, 1999). Assessment needs to take into account that individuals with the benign form of MS may have minimal disability. Individuals with relapsing-remitting multiple sclerosis may be unable to work during specific periods of relapse, and/or formal functional levels may be impaired, requiring retraining to accommodate increasing disability.

Importantly, the last decade has brought changes in medical management, with the introduction of disease-modifying drugs that reduce exacerbations in relapsing-remitting multiple sclerosis. These drugs result in less unpredictability in the early stages of the disease. Those with progressive variants of MS might best benefit from an assessment of the rate of progression and subsequently trained for less demanding employment, in order to prepare them for possible increased disability (Gordon et al., 1994; Illan, 1999; Kraft, 1981).

Functional Limitations

Functional limitations associated with MS, which are commonly cited reasons for job-loss, include problems with mobility, manual dexterity, vision, fatigue, memory, and information-processing (Roessler & Rumrill, 1995). Professionals (e.g., rehabilitation workers) can assist individuals with MS deal with direct physical effects of the disease (e.g., problems with fatigue, mobility, spasticity, vision), as they impinge upon vocational functioning, by consulting on the job modifications and restructuring. For example, an individual with numbness of hands and problems with coordination can continue his or her essential job function related to a dictation machine by an installation of a foot pedal to control the machine. Both rehabilitation professionals and employees, therefore, need access to information on accommodative strategies by obtaining technical assistance from rehabilitation engineers, and consulting resources, such as the Job Accommodation Network (JAN), which is a national repository of information and consultation on adaptive technology (Rumrill, 1996).

According to Kraft (1981), individuals with MS are not likely to retain employment unless rehabilitation professionals give major consideration to the physical demands of the individual's occupation. Vocational interests that require heightened physical activity, such as walking, prolonged standing, and exertion of physical force, should not be encouraged. Rather, the individual with MS should be directed toward sedentary work. In addition, maintaining employment may involve curtailing activities outside of work, due to reduced energy and endurance (Johnson et al., 2004).

Because one neuropsychological consequence of the disease may be cognitive dysfunction, rehabilitation professionals should consider having a cognitive assessment performed in the absence of previous assessment. The potential impact of even "mild" cognitive symptoms in the workplace needs to be analyzed and addressed. Formal evaluation should include an assessment of the cognitive and communication requirements of job tasks (LaRocca & Sorensen, 2004).

Reasonable Accommodations

Reasonable accommodations at the worksite constitute a central theme of contemporary MS research on career maintenance (Gordon et al., 1994; Jackson & Quaal, 1991; Roessler & Rumrill, 1995; Rumrill, 1996). "Reasonable accommodation is a modification or adjustment to a job, the work environment, or the way things usually are done that enables a qualified individual with a disability to enjoy an equal employment opportunity" (Patterson, Bruyere, Szymanski, & Jenkins, 2005, p. 38).

Accommodations may involve minimal financial and organizational costs and, in fact, often cost nothing. An example may be moving an employee's desk closer to an exit to reduce walking (Gordon et al., 1994). Additional accommodations that have been found to be work-enhancing for people with MS include: Adjusted or modified work-schedule, intermittent rest-periods, conveniently arranged equipment, providing offices near restrooms, reduced room temperature, and telecommuting (Fraser, 2002). It is also important to educate clients to competently discuss their accommodation needs and rights, in a manner which promotes employer and co-worker cooperation (Johnson et al., 2004).

Conclusion

MS is a relatively common, progressive, neurological disease with an onset that is most often in young adulthood. People with MS must confront and attempt to cope with profound stressors, including the unknown etiology of the disease, variability of symptoms, unpredictability of exacerbations and remissions, and lack of a cure. The vast majority of the literature on coping with MS has been guided by the coping model of Lazarus and Folkman. Within the context of this model, coping processes are differentially used in adapting to the individual's constantly changing physical, psychosocial, economic, and environmental needs.

Psychosocial and/or behavioral interventions may improve the psychological and physical well-being of individuals with MS by treating affective disorders (e.g., depression), by reducing stress, improving self-management of symptoms, enhancing self-efficacy, and improving coping skills and general quality of life. The most effective clinical interventions for individuals with MS have been based on actively teaching adaptive coping strategies.

Individiuals with MS provide a challenge to rehabilitation professionals. Unemployment rates are high, despite the fact that people with MS, on average, have a positive work history, a strong work-ethic, and a desire to resume employment. Employment barriers confronting people with MS arise from a complex set of interacting variables, including disease characteristics, and environmental and social factors. To help preserve employment, the literature supports approaches to job retention, which include focusing on technical assistance for on-the-job modifications, and the timely provision of workplace accommodations.

References

Affleck, G., & Tennen, H. (1996). Construing benefits from adversity: Adaptational significance and dispositional underpinnings. *Journal of Personality, 64*, 899–922.

Aikens, J. E., Fischer, J. S., Namey, M., & Rudick, R. A. (1997). A replicated prospective investigation of life stress, coping, and depressive symptoms in multiple sclerosis. *Journal of Behavioral Medicine, 20*, 433–445.

Baker, L. M. (1998). Sense making in multiple sclerosis: The information needs of people during acute exacerbation. *Qualitative Health Research, 8*, 106–120.

Bandura, A. (1986). *Social foundations of thought and action: A social cognitive theory.* Englewood Cliffs, NJ: Prentice Hall.

Bandura, A. (1998). Health promotion from the perspective of social cognitive theory. *Psychology and Health, 13*, 623–649.

Beatty, W. W., Hames, K. A., Blanco, C. R., Williamson, S. J., Wilbanks, S. I., & Olson, K. A. (1998). Correlates of coping style in patients with multiple sclerosis. *Multiple Sclerosis, 4*, 440–443.

Billings, A. G., & Moos, R. H. (1981). The role of coping responses and social resources in attenuating the stress of life events. *Journal of Behavioral Medicine, 4*, 139–157.

Blake, D. J., & Bodine, C. (2002). An overview of assistive technology for persons with multiple sclerosis. *Journal of Rehabilitation Research and Development, 39*(2), 299–312.

Boyden, K. M. (2000). The pathophysiology of demyelination and the ionic basis of nerve conduction in multiple sclerosis: An overview. *Journal of Neuroscience Nursing, 32*(1), 9–53.

Buelow, J. M. (1991). A correlational study of disabilities, stressors and coping methods in victims of multiple sclerosis. *Journal of Neuroscience Nursing, 23*, 247–252.

Cavallo, P. G., & McLaughlin, C. M. (1997). *Improving care for persons with multiple sclerosis: Nursing in the new millennium*. New York: National Multiple Sclerosis Society.

Comi, G. (2000). Why treat early multiple sclerosis patient? *Current Opinion in Neurology, 13*, 235–240.

Comi, G., Columbo, B., & Martinelli, V. (2000). Prognosis-modifying therapy in multiple sclerosis. *Neurological Sciences, 21*, 893–899.

Corbin, J., & Strauss, A. (1998). *Unending work and care: Managing chronic illness at home*. San Francisco: Jossey-Bass.

Crawford, J. D., & McIvor, G. P. (1985). Group psychotherapy: Benefits in multiple sclerosis. *Archives of Physical Rehabilitation, 66*, 810–813.

Crawford, J. D., & McIvor, G. P. (1987). Stress management for multiple sclerosis patients. *Psychological Reports, 61*, 423–429.

Dean, G. (1994). How many people in the world have multiple sclerosis? *Neuroepidemiology, 13*, 1–7.

Devins, G. M. (1994). Illness intrusiveness and the psychosocial impact of lifestyle disruptions in chronic life-threatening disease. *Advances in Renal Replacement Therapy, 1*, 251–263.

Devins, G. M., Seland, T. P., Klein, G., Edworthy, S. M., & Saary, M. J. (1993). Stability and determinants of psychosocial well-being in multiple sclerosis. *Rehabilitation Psychology, 38*, 11–26.

Devins, G. M., & Shnek, Z. M. (2000). Multiple sclerosis. In R. G. Frank & T. R. Elliott (Eds.), *Handbook of rehabilitation psychology* (pp. 163–184). Washington, DC: American Psychological Association.

Devins, G. M., Styra, R., O'Connor, P., Gray, T., Seland, T. P., Klein, G., et al. (1996). Psychosocial impact of illness intrusiveness moderated by age in multiple sclerosis. *Psychology, Health, and Medicine, 1*, 179–191.

Feinstein, A. (1997). Multiple sclerosis, depression, and suicide. *British Medical Journal, 315*, 691–692.

Feinstein, A. (2000). Multiple sclerosis, disease modifying treatments and depression: A critical methodological review. *Multiple Sclerosis, 6*, 343–348.

Feinstein, A., Feinstein, K., Gray, T., & O'Connor, P. (1997). Prevalence and neurobehavioral correlates of pathological laughing and crying in multiple sclerosis. *Archives of Neurology, 54*, 1116–1121.

Feinstein, A., O'Connor, P., Gray, T., & Feinstein, K. (1999). Pathological laughing and crying in multiple sclerosis: A preliminary report suggesting a role for the prefrontal cortex. *Multiple Sclerosis, 5*, 69–73.

Fisk, J. D., Pontefract, A., Ritvo, P. G., Archibald, C. J., & Murray, T. J. (1994). The impact of fatigue on patients with multiple sclerosis. *Canadian Journal of Neurological Science, 21*, 9–14.

Folkman, S., & Lazarus, R. S. (1986). Stress processes and depressive symptomatology. *Journal of Abnormal Psychology, 95*, 107–113.

Folkman, S., & Lazarus, R. S. (1988). *Manual for the Ways of Coping Questionnaire: Research edition.* Palo Alto, CA: Consulting Psychologists Press.

Foote, A. W., Piazza, D., Holcombe, J., Paul, P., & Dappin, P. (1990). Hope, self-esteem and social support in persons with multiple sclerosis. *Journal of Neuroscience Nursing, 22*, 155–159.

Fox, R. J. (2006). Imaging MS: A window into the disease. *Multiple Sclerosis Quarterly Report, 25*(1), 5–11.

Fraser, R. T. (2002). Vocational rehabilitation intervention. In R. T. Fraser, D. C. Clemmons, & F. Bennett (Eds.), *Multiple sclerosis: Psychosocial & vocational interventions* (45–82). New York: Demos.

Gordon, P. A., Lewis, M. D., & Wong, D. (1994). Multiple sclerosis: Strategies for rehabilitation counselors. *Journal of Rehabilitation, 60*(3), 34–38.

Gottber, K., Cardulf, A., & Fredrikson, S. (2000). Interferon-beta treatment for patients with multiple sclerosis: The patient's perceptions of side-effects. *Multiple Sclerosis, 6*, 349–354.

Gulick, E. (1994). Social support among persons with multiple sclerosis. *Research in Nursing and Health, 17*, 195–206.

Hadjimichael, O. (1999). Adherence to injection therapy in multiple sclerosis. *Neurology, 52*, 549–556.

Herndon, R. M. (2000). Pathology and pathophysiology. In J. S. Burkes & K. P. Johnson (Eds.), *Multiple sclerosis: Diagnosis, medical management, and rehabilitation* (pp. 35–45). New York: Demos.

Hickey, A., & Greene, S. M. (1989). Coping with multiple sclerosis. *Irish Journal of Psychological Medicine, 6*, 118–124.

Holland, N. J. (2002). Patient and family education. In J. Halper & N. J. Holland (Eds.), *Comprehensive nursing care in multiple sclerosis* (2nd ed., pp. 191–203). New York: Demos.

Illan, H. (1999). Neuromuscular disorders. In M. G. Eisenberg, R. L. Glueckauf, & H. H. Zaretsky (Eds.), *Medical aspects of disability: A handbook for the rehabilitation professional* (pp. 312–328). New York: Springer.

Jackson, M., & Quaal, C. (1991). Effects of multiple sclerosis on occupational and career patterns. *Axon, 13*(1), 16–22.

Jean, V. M., Paul, R. H., & Beatty, W. W. (1999). Psychological and neuropsychological predictors of coping patterns by patients with multiple sclerosis. *Journal of Clinical Psychology, 55*, 21–26.

Johnson, K. L., Yorkston, K. M., Klasner, E. R., Kuehn, C. M., Johnson, E., & Amtmann, D. (2004). The cost and benefits of employment: A qualitative study of experiences of persons with multiple sclerosis. *Archives of Physical Medicine and Rehabilitation, 85*, 201–209.

Kalb, R. C. (2004). *Multiple sclerosis: The questions you have the answers you need* (3rd ed.). New York: Demos.

Kornblith, A. B., LaRocca, N. G., & Baum, H. M. (1986). Employment in individuals with multiple sclerosis. *International Journal of Rehabilitation Research, 9*, 1555–1165.

Kraft, G. H. (1981). Multiple sclerosis. In W. C. Stolov & M. R. Clowers (Eds.), *Handbook of severe disability* (pp. 111–118). Washington, DC: U.S. Department of Education, Rehabilitation Services Administration.

Larcombe, N. A., & Wilson, P. H. (1984). An evaluation of therapy cognitive-behavioral therapy for depression in patients with multiple sclerosis. *British Journal of Psychiatry, 145,* 366–371.

LaRocca, N. G. (1995). *Employment and multiple sclerosis.* New York: National Multiple Sclerosis Society.

LaRocca, N. G., & Hall, H. L. (1990). Multiple sclerosis program: A model for neuropsychiatric disorders. *New Directions for Mental Health Services, 45,* 49–64.

LaRocca, N. G., Kalb, R. C., Foley, F. W., & McGann, C. M. (1993). Psychosocial, affective, and behavioral consequences of multiple sclerosis: Treatment of the "whole" patient. *Neuro-rehabilitation, 3,* 30–38.

LaRocca, N. G., & Sorensen, P. M. (2004). Cognition. In R. C. Kalb (Ed.), *Multiple sclerosis: The questions you have the answers you need* (3rd ed., pp. 205–232). New York: Demos.

Lazarus, R. S. (1993). Coping theory and research: Past, present, and future. *Psychosomatic Medicine, 55,* 234–247.

Lazarus, R. S., & Folkman, S. (1984). *Stress, appraisal, and coping.* New York: Springer Publishing.

Livneh, H., & Antonak, R. F. (1997). *Psychosocial adaptation to chronic illness and disability.* Gaithersburg, MD: Aspen Publishers.

Livneh, H., & Antonak, R. F. (2005). Psychological adaptation to chronic illness and disability: A primer for counselors. *Journal of Counseling & Development, 83,* 12–20.

Livneh, H., & Cook, D. (2005). Psychosocial impact of disability. In R. M. Parker, E. M. Szymanski, & J. B. Patterson (Eds.), *Rehabilitation counseling: Basics and beyond* (4th ed., pp. 187–224). Austin, TX: Pro-Ed.

Livneh, H., & Wosley-George, E. T. (1997). Counseling clients with disabilities. In D. Capuzzi & D. R. Gross (Eds.), *Introduction to the counseling profession* (2nd ed., pp. 463– 495). Needham Heights, MA: Allyn & Bacon.

Long, M. P., Glueckauf, R. L., & Rasmussen, J. L. (1998). Developing family counseling interventions for adults with episodic neurological disabilities. Presenting problems, persons involved, and problem severity. *Rehabilitation Psychology, 43*(2), 101–117.

Long, D. D., & Miller, B. J. (1991). Suicidal tendency and multiple sclerosis. *Health and Social Work, 16,* 104–109.

Lorig, K. R., & Holman, H. R. (2003). Self-management education: History, definition, outcomes, and mechanisms. *Annals of Behavioral Medicine, 26*(1), 1–7.

Lorig, K. R., Sobel, D. S., Ritter, P. L., Laurent, D., & Hobbs, M. (2001). Effect of a self-management program on patients with chronic disease. *Effective Clinical Practice, 4*(6), 256–262.

Lublin, F. D., & Reingold, S. C. (1996). Defining the clinical course of multiple sclerosis: Results of an international survey. *Neurology, 46,* 907–911.

Maes, S., Leventhal, H., & de Ridder, D. (1996). Coping with chronic diseases. In M. Zeidner & N. S. Endler (Eds.), *Handbook of coping: Theory, research, applications* (pp. 221–251). New York: Wiley.

Mathiowetz, V., Matuska, K. M., & Murphy, M. E. (2001). Efficacy of an energy conservation course for persons with multiple sclerosis. *Archives of Physical Medicine and Rehabilitation, 82,* 449–456.

Matkin, R. E. (1995). Private sector rehabilitation. In S. E. Rubin & R. T. Roessler (Eds.), *Foundations of the vocational rehabilitation process* (pp. 375–398). Austin, TX: Pro-Ed.

Matthews, S. (1993). *Multiple sclerosis: The facts* (3rd ed.). New York: Oxford University Press.

Maurelli, M., Marchioni, E., Cerretano, R., Bosone, D., Bergamaschi, R., & Citterio, A. (1992). Neuropsychological assessment in MS: Clinical, neurophysiological and neuroradiological relationships. *Acta Neurologica Scandinavica, 86*, 124–128.

Maybury, C. P., & Brewin, C. R. (1984). Social relationships, knowledge and adjustment to multiple sclerosis. *Journal of Neurology, Neurosurgery, and Psychiatry, 47*, 372–376.

McCabe, M. P., & McKern, S. (2002). Quality of life and multiple sclerosis: Comparison between people with MS and people from the general population. *Journal of Clinical Psychology in Medical Settings, 9*(4), 287–295.

McIvor, G. P., Riklan, M., & Reznikoff, M. (1984). Depression in multiple sclerosis as a function of length and severity of illness, age, remissions, and perceived social support. *Journal of Clinical Psychology, 40*, 1029–1033.

Miller, C. M. (1997). The lived experience of relapsing multiple sclerosis: A phenomenological study. *Journal of Neuroscience Nursing, 29*, 294–304.

Minden, S. L. (1992). Psychotherapy for people with multiple sclerosis. *Neuropsychiatry, 4*, 198–213.

Minden, S. L., Orav, J., & Reich, P. (1987). Depression in multiple sclerosis. *General Hospital Psychiatry, 9*, 426–434.

Minden, S. L., & Schiffer, R. B. (1990). Affective disorders in multiple sclerosis: Review and recommendations for clinical research. *Archives of Neurology, 47*, 98–104.

Mohr, D. C., Boudewyn, A. C., Goodkin, D. E., Bostrom, A., Siskin, L., Epstein, L., et al. (2001). Comparative outcomes for individual cognitive-behavior therapy, supportive-expressive group psychotherapy, and sertraline for the treatment of depression in multiple sclerosis. *Journal of Counseling and Clinical Psychology, 69*(6), 942–949.

Mohr, D. C., & Cox, D. (2001). Multiple sclerosis: Empirical literature for the clinical health psychologist. *Journal of Clinical Psychology, 57*, 479–499.

Mohr, D. C., Dick, L. P., Russo, D., Pinn, J., Boudewyn, A. C., Likosky, W., et al. (1999). The psychosocial impact of multiple sclerosis: Exploring the patient's perspective. *Health Psychology, 18*, 376–382.

Mohr, D. C., & Goodkin, D. E. (1999). Treatment of depression in multiple sclerosis: Review and meta-analysis. *Clinical Psychology: Science and Practice, 6*(1), 1–9.

Mohr, D. C., Hart, S. L., Julian, L., Catledge, C., Honos-Webb, L., Vella, L., et al. (2005). Telephone administered psychotherapy for depression. *Archives of General Psychiatry, 62*(9), 1007–1014.

Mohr, D. C., Likosky, W., Dick, L. P., Van Der Wende, J., Dwyer, P., Bertagnolli, D., et al. (2000). Telephone-administered cognitive-behavioral therapy for the treatment of multiple sclerosis. *Journal of Consulting and Clinical Psychology, 68*, 356–361.

Moos, R. H., & Billings, A. G. (1982). Conceptualizing and measuring coping resources and processes. In L. Goldberger & S. Breznitz (Eds.), *Handbook of stress: Theoretical and clinical aspects.* New York: Free Press.

Neufeld, P. (1999). *Leader's manual for leaders, co-leaders, and chapter staff to administer the Gateway to Wellness Course for individuals with multiple sclerosis.* Program in Occupational Therapy, Washington University, St. Louis, MO.

Nortvedt, M. W., Ruse, T., Myhr, K. M., & Nyland, H. I. (2000). Quality of life as a predictor for change in disability in MS. *Neurology, 55*(1), 51–54.

O'Brien, M. T. (1993). Multiple sclerosis: The relationship among self-esteem, social support and coping behavior. *Applied Nursing Research, 2*, 54–63.

Occupational Awareness System (OASYS) (2003). Bellevue, WA: VERTEK, Inc.

O'Day, B. (1998). Barriers for people with multiple sclerosis who want to work: A qualitative study. *Journal of Neurologic Rehabilitation, 12*(3), 139–146.

Pakenham, K. I. (1999). Adjustment to multiple sclerosis: Application of a stress and coping mode. *Health Psychology, 18*, 383–392.

Pakenham, K. I. (2005). Benefit finding in multiple sclerosis and associations with positive and negative outcomes. *Health Psychology, 24*(2), 123–132.

Pakenham, K. I., Stewart, C. A., & Rogers, A. (1997). The role of coping in adjustment to multiple sclerosis-related adaptive demands. *Psychology, Health & Medicine, 3*(3), 197– 211.

Patten, S. B., Beck, C. A., & Williams, J. V. A. (2003). Major depression in multiple sclerosis: A population-based perspective. *Neurology, 61*, 1524–1527.

Patterson, J. B., Bruyere, S., Szymanski, E. M., & Jenkins, W. (2005). Philosophical, historical, and legislative aspects of the rehabilitation counseling profession. In R. M. Parker, E. M. Szymanski, & J. B. Patterson (Eds.), *Rehabilitation counseling: Basics and beyond* (4th ed., pp. 27–53). Austin, TX: Pro-ed.

Rao, S. M. (1986). Neuropsychology of multiple sclerosis. A critical review. *Journal of Clinical and Experimental Neuropsychology, 8*(5), 503–542.

Rao. S. M. (1995). Neuropsychology of multiple sclerosis. *Current Opinion Neurology, 8*(3), 216–220.

Rao, S. M., Huber, S. J., & Bornstein, R. A. (1992). Emotional changes with multiple sclerosis and Parkinson's disease. *Journal of Consulting and Clinical Psychology, 60*, 369–378.

Roessler, R. T., & Rumrill, P. D. (1995). The relationship of perceived work site barriers to job mastery and job satisfaction for employed people with multiple sclerosis. *Rehabilitation Counseling Bulletin, 39*(1), 2–14.

Roessler, R. T., Rumrill, P. D., & Fitzgerald, S. M. (2004). Factors affecting job satisfaction of employed adults with multiple sclerosis. *Journal of Rehabilitation, 70*, 42–50.

Rudick, R. A., Miller, D., Clough, J. D., Gragg, L. A., & Farmer, R. G. (1992). Quality of life in multiple sclerosis. *Archives of Neurology, 49*, 1237–1242.

Rumrill, P. D. (1996). *Employment issues and multiple sclerosis.* New York: Demos.

Rumrill, P. D., & Hennessey, M. L. (2004). Employment issues. In R. C. Kalb (Ed.), *Multiple sclerosis: The questions you have the answers you need* (3rd ed., pp. 347–376). New York: Demos.

Rumrill, P. D., Roessler, R. T., Battersby, J., & Schuyler, B. (1998). Situational assessment of the accommodation needs of employees with visual impairments and blindness. *Journal of Visual Impairment and Blindness, 92*(1), 42–54.

Rumrill, P. D., Roessler, R. T., & Cook, B. G. (1998). Improving career re-entry outcomes for people with multiple sclerosis: A comparison of two approaches. *Journal of Vocational Rehabilitation, 10*(3), 241–252.

Sadovnick, A. D., Eisen, K., Ebers, G. C., & Paty, D. W. (1991). Cause of death in patients attending multiple sclerosis clinics. *Neurology, 41*, 1193–1198.

Sadovnick, A. D., Remick, R. A., & Allen, J. (1996). Depression and multiple sclerosis. *Neurology, 46*, 628–632.

Schapiro, R. T. (1991). *Multiple sclerosis: A rehabilitation approach to management.* New York: Demos.

Schapiro, R. T., & Schneider, D. M. (2002). Symptom management in multiple sclerosis. In J. Halper & N. J. Holland (Eds.), *Comprehensive nursing care in multiple sclerosis* (2nd ed., pp. 31–52). New York: Demos.

Scheinberg, L. C., Pfennings, L., Pouwer, F., Cohen, L., Ketelaer, P., Polman, C., et al. (1998). Psychological functioning in primary progressive versus secondary progressive multiple sclerosis. *British Journal of Medical Psychology, 71,* 99– 106.

Schiffer, R. B. (2002). Neuropsychiatric problems in patients with multiple sclerosis. *Psychiatric Annals, 32*(2), 128–132.

Schubert, D. S., & Foliart, R. H. (1993). Increased depression in multiple sclerosis patients: A meta-analysis. *Psychosomatics, 34,* 124–130.

Schwartz, C. E. (1999). Teaching coping skills enhances quality of life more than peer support: Results of a randomized trial with multiple sclerosis patients. *Health Psychology, 18*(3), 211–220.

Selder, F. E., & Breunig, K. A. (1991). Living with multiple sclerosis. The gradual transition. *Loss-Grief-and-Care, 4,* 89–98.

Siegert, R. J., & Abernethy, D. A. (2005). Depression in multiple sclerosis: A review. *Journal of Neurology, Neurosurgery, and Psychiatry, 76*(4), 469–475.

Smith, C. R., & Schapiro, R. T. (2004). Neurology. In R. C. Kalb (Ed.), *Multiple sclerosis: The questions you have the answers you need* (3rd ed., pp. 7–42). New York: Demos.

Strauss, A. L., Corbin, J., Fagerhaugh, S., Glasser, B. G., Maines, D., Suczek, B., et al. (1984). *Chronic illness and the quality of life* (2nd ed.). St. Louis: CV Mosby.

Stuber, M. L., Sullivan, G., Kennon, T. L., & Nobler, H. (1988). Group therapy for chronic medical illness: A multidiagnosis group. *General Hospital Psychiatry, 10*(5) 360–366.

Stuifbergen, A. K. (1995). Health promoting behaviors and quality of life among individuals with multiple sclerosis. *Scholarly Inquiry for Nursing Practice: An International Journal, 9*(1), 31–50.

Stuifbergen, A. K., Becker, H., Blozis, S., Timmerman, G., & Kullberg, V. (2003). A randomized clinical trial of a wellness intervention for women with multiple sclerosis. *Archives of Physical Medicine and Rehabilitation, 84,* 467–476.

Stuifbergen, A. K., & Roberts, G. J. (1997). Health promotion practices of women with multiple sclerosis. *Archives of Medical Rehabilitation, 78,* S3–S9.

Sullivan, M. J., Mikail, S., & Wenshenker, B. (1997). Coping with a diagnosis of multiple sclerosis. *Canadian Journal of Behavioral Science, 29,* 249–257.

Tennen, H., & Affleck, G. (2002). Benefit-finding and benefit-reminding. In C. R. Snyder & S. J. Lopex (Eds.), *Handbook of Positive Psychology* (pp. 584–597). London: Oxford University Press.

Uccelli, M. M., Mohr, L. M., Battaglia, M. A., Zagami, P., & Mohr, D. C. (2004). Peer support groups in multiple sclerosis: Current effectiveness and future directions. *Multiple Sclerosis, 10*(1), 80–84.

Vollmer, T. V. (2005). MS medications in the pipeline. *Multiple Sclerosis Quarterly Report, 24*(3), 5–12.

Whitlock, F. A., & Siskind, M. M. (1980). Depression as a major symptom of multiple sclerosis. *Journal of Neurology, Neurosurgery & Psychiatry, 43,* 861–865.

Williamson, K. (2000). A review of the psychosocial aspects of multiple sclerosis. *British Journal of Community Nursing, 5*(3), 132–138.

Wineman, N. M. (1990). Adaptation to multiple sclerosis: The role of social support, functional disability, and perceived uncertainty. *Nursing Research, 39*, 294–299.

Wineman, N. M., Durand, E. J., & Steiner, R. P. (1994). A comparative analysis of coping behaviors in persons with multiple sclerosis or a spinal cord injury. *Research in Nursing & Health, 17*, 185–194.

Zeidner, M., & Saklofske, D. (1996). Adaptive and maladaptive coping. In M. Zeidner & N. S. Endler (Eds.), *Handbook of coping: Theory, research, applications* (pp. 505–531). New York: Wiley.

Zeldow, P. B., & Pavlou, M. (1984). Physical disability, life stress and psychosocial adjustment in multiple sclerosis. *Journal of Nervous and Mental Disease, 172*, 80–84.

15
Coping with Chronic Pain:
A Stress-Appraisal Coping Model

Beverly E. Thorn and Kim E. Dixon

Estimations of the number of individuals, who are suffering with chronic pain, vary widely from a low of 20% to over 60% (American Pain Foundation [APF], 2006). Chronic pain is the primary contributor to long-term disability for almost 50 million people (Brookoff, 2000). It contributes to over 50 million lost work-days in the United States alone (APF). Thus, it is not surprising that chronic pain has been heralded as the most expensive and burdensome health condition in North America (Harstall & Ospina, 2003), producing high incidences of physical and emotional disability and suffering.

Living with intractable chronic pain and the related disability taxes coping resources of even the most stoic individuals. While individuals with chronic pain are desperate for relief, health-care providers are also challenged to "do something," even though in many instances there is little that can be done biomedically to bring substantial pain-relief. Indeed, usual medical care often fails to meet the needs of many chronically ill individuals, although they require the greatest bulk of care. This may be due in part to the structure of the present U.S. health-care system, which was designed largely to address acute illnesses, rather than to serve as a chronic care system (Wagner et al., 2001). Individuals with chronic pain face the very real problem of long-term management of their condition, and day-to-day care responsibilities fall most heavily on the individuals themselves and their families (Von Korff, Gruman, Schaefer, Curry, & Wagner, 1997).

Because many different physical conditions result in chronic pain, this is a difficult, but important chapter to write. Even though there are numerous conditions that contribute to chronic pain syndromes (e.g., arthritis, fibromyalgia, low back pain), the overall treatment model is, for the most part, more similar than different. Because chronic pain is not disease-specific, traditionally it has not been viewed as a disability. However, based upon the prevalence statistics shown above, it is evident that chronic pain disorders are a major contributor to a downward spiral of disability and dysfunction that is experienced by so many individuals with chronic, unrelenting pain.

This chapter provides a brief overview of important theoretical issues that are related to the current understanding of chronic pain, its diagnosis, and treatment. The primary focus of this chapter is on discussing factors that directly affect the ways in which individuals attempt to cope with chronic pain. First, a short discussion of the empirical examination of coping strategies that are used by individuals with chronic pain is provided. Then, psychological interventions that promote adaptive coping in this population are reviewed. This chapter concludes by providing suggestions for incorporating this information into a model of pain self-management and by offering a brief look at future directions of pain-coping treatment and research.

What Is Chronic Pain?

Defining Chronic Pain

The definition of "chronic pain" is rather imprecise. However, it is often described as pain lasting more than a few months, lacks diagnostic specificity, and persists beyond the normal tissue healing time (usually taken to be three months) (Turk & Okifuji, 2001). Distinctions between acute pain and chronic pain may include arbitrary chronological demarcations (e.g., three months, six months), and are often based on subjective judgments about whether the pain extends beyond the expected healing period.

For the purpose of this chapter, the following distinctions are made: *Acute pain* is pain that is elicited by injury and activation of pain receptors (e.g., trauma, surgery), usually lasts a short time, and remits when tissue is healed. In the acute pain situation, biomedical health-care interventions are typically sought and are often effective. *Chronic pain* is often (but not always) elicited by an injury, but is worsened by factors that are removed from the original cause, usually lasts a long time, and is oftentimes not explained by underlying pathology; thus biomedical interventions are usually ineffective (Turk & Okifuji, 2001). *Recurrent pain* (e.g., cancer pain, migraine headache) is pain that is episodic in nature, but that recurs across an extended time-period, thus sharing characteristics of both acute and chronic pain.

A myriad of physical conditions can lead to chronic pain, but in many cases the exact etiology for the pain remains elusive. The absence of a clear physical basis for persistent pain often contributes to presumptions that the root cause of the pain is psychogenic (or even malingered) and that its intensity is exaggerated, either intentionally or unconsciously. Because pain is such a subjective experience with a multitude of psychosocial influences, health-care providers may harbor negative attitudes regarding chronic pain in general, and individuals with chronic pain in particular. These attitudes are contrary to the mounting empirical evidence that permanent physiological and chemical changes in neural pathways occur in individuals after prolonged exposure to painful stimuli, but are not overtly evident during physical exam (Brookoff, 2000; Covington, 2000; Hampton, 2005).

Theories of Pain

The evolution of scientific thought regarding what constitutes "pain," takes us from a biomedical framework (the dominating illness conceptualization for almost 300 years) to a biopsychosocial model. The biomedical view of pain held that the amount of tissue pathology should correspond to the amount of pain experienced. When the two sides of that biomedical equation did not balance out, questions such as "is it organic or psychogenic?" were asked.

Until the early 1960s, the standard of care for nonmalignant chronic pain was to offer extant biomedical approaches, basing treatment decisions on physiological evidence for pain etiology and on associated physical sequelae (e.g. muscle spasms, sleep disturbance). Treatment itself consisted primarily of medications, various medical interventions, oftentimes surgery; in many instances, such treatments were ineffective. Presently available evidence suggests that medical treatments based on an acute care model are often ineffective in chronic conditions (Wagner et al., 2001). Furthermore, biomedical approaches largely ignore psychosocial issues, which are known to be important in the pain experience.

The understanding and treatment of chronic pain was revolutionized by the seminal work of Ronald Melzack and Patrick Wall (1965) in the mid-1960s, with introduction of the Gate Control Theory of Pain. This theory proposed that pain is more than simply a physiological response to a nociceptive (pain-producing) stimulus. Rather, Melzack and Wall argued that pain is multifaceted and is influenced by sensory-discriminative, evaluative-cognitive, and affective-motivational factors. The Gate Control Theory prompted researchers and clinicians alike to begin to recognize the complexity of the pain experience, and launched a movement that ultimately legitimized the need to assess psychological factors when considering treatment options for pain (Keefe, Dixon, & Pryor, 2005).

In more recent years, Melzack (1999) expanded the Gate Control Theory to include a more sophisticated Neuromatrix Model of Pain. In this model, it is hypothesized that a widespread neural network extends throughout the central nervous system (i.e., the spinal cord, thalamus, limbic system, and cortex), which processes pain-related information. This network receives both phasic (e.g., attention, anxiety, expectations) and tonic (e.g., memory, personality, cultural influences) cognitive inputs, which contribute strongly to the pain experience. In this model, pain is viewed as having a genetic component (neural matrix), which is also influenced by experiences unique to the individual. There is recent evidence that acute-pain experiences actually sensitize the brain for the future development of chronic pain (Covington, 2000) and that painful experiences may lead to encoding of pain "memories" (Hampton, 2005).

Pain "Memories" and Their Contribution to Chronic Pain

In recent years, surprising evidence has arisen suggesting that the experience of pain produces permanent changes in brain structures. This phenomenon in which neurons change their structure, their function, or even their chemical profile is called *neural plasticity* (Woolf & Salter, 2000).

Brain-related pain processing can be temporarily altered (or modulated) in a way that increases the sensitivity of neurons to even mild pain signals. For example, tissue injury causes chemical signals to be released from injured cells, leading to an increased sensitivity of the free nerve-ending to other chemicals, and creating a change in the way the nerve-ending processes a pain stimulus. When the tissue heals, the hypersensitivity usually returns to normal. However, alterations in neurons that are more permanent can also result from the experience of pain, and these changes are called modifications. These include structural changes, such as an increase in the number of pain receptors in the spinal cord following tissue damage, and a reduction in brain inhibitory processes following nerve injury (Woolf & Salter, 2000).

It is also known that neural regions, which are associated with processing of physical pain stimuli, are different from neural regions associated with pain anticipation. With repeated presentations of pain stimuli, pain sensory-processing areas remain the same size over time, while pain anticipation areas actually recruit other neurons (the area becomes larger) (Ploghaus et al., 1999). An example of this is found in research on individuals with Fibromyalgia (FM). Those who scored high on a measure of pain catastrophizing ("my pain is awful, horrible, unbearable") showed increased activity in brain areas that are related to anticipation of pain (medial frontal cortex, cerebellum), attention to pain (dorsal anterior cingulate cortex, dorsolateral prefrontal cortex), emotional aspects of pain (claustrum, closely connected to amygdala), and motor control (Gracely et al., 2004). Individuals with FM, who scored high on depressive symptoms, showed increased activity in brain areas associated with affective pain-processing (amygdala, contralateral anterior insula), thus demonstrating that depression has a qualitatively different influence on neural-pain processing, compared to pain catastrophizing (Giesicke et al., 2005). Certainly, functional imaging studies confirm the multidimensional nature of pain (sensation, affect, cognitive), and validate a physiological (neural) substrate for pain cognition and affect.

Short-term and long-term neural plasticity may lead to conditions that have previously had no adequate physiological explanation. Some examples include allodynia, a condition in which non-painful stimulation (e.g., light touch) produces pain; hyperalgesia, a situation where a mildly painful stimulus produces intense pain; and referred pain, the perception of pain spread to non-injured tissue (Covington, 2000; Iadarola & Caudle, 1997). These conditions often persist after healing of the damaged tissue. An additional illustration of pathological alteration of the nervous system via the experience of pain is neuropathic pain, the sensation of pain long after injured nerve tissue has healed. For example, herpes zoster ("shingles") can produce long-lasting, excruciating, neuropathic pain.

Although the biomedical model is slowly changing, the assessment of individuals with chronic pain is still heavily biomedical. This presents a conundrum. Although it is important to diagnose and treat pathological conditions by all available evidence-based means, reliance on physical evidence to validate pain leaves the individual in the untenable position of trying to convince those around him that "my pain is real!" For example, an individual experiencing low back pain may feel that his pain (and passive reliance on biomedical treatments) is well-justified, if imaging studies reveal a bulging vertebral disc; whereas he may feel defensive, angry, and insistent on more or different tests, if the diagnostic work-up reveals "only" muscle tension and atrophy. When physical diagnostic means do not provide the necessary etiological explanation for the pain, mental health-care providers (particularly psychologists) are often consulted to make "functional/organic" distinctions in individuals complaining of chronic pain.

Biomedical Approaches to Treating Chronic Pain

While multidisciplinary approaches to pain management are now the gold standard, many individuals in pain are initially seen by their primary-care physicians; thus, early treatment tends to follow the traditional biomedical model. The biomedical management of pain differs somewhat by the status or classification of the pain type. Numerous guidelines have been published regarding pain management of various painful conditions. While there is some measure of specificity in each depending on the medical condition, in general, traditional medical approaches to pain management progress from very conservative treatments up to, and including, surgery.

When a patient comes to a physician with an acute pain event, he or she is usually prescribed an analgesic initially and may be told to rest for a few days. In cases such as low back pain, a short-term trial of physical therapy may also be ordered and might include back-strengthening exercises and/or treatment with heat therapies or massage. Individuals who do not gain relief from these more conservative treatments may be referred to a pain specialist for an evaluation for more aggressive pain-management interventions, such as epidural steroid injections. If no relief is obtained from non-surgical interventions, individuals may be offered surgery as an option.

With advances in understanding of pain as a multidimensional experience came a trend toward a multidisciplinary approach to pain management. Multidisciplinary clinics, which integrated psychological treatment with medical, surgical, and other types of pain interventions, sprang up in the 1970's. Unfortunately, despite strong empirical evidence of the efficacy of such programs (Flor, Fydrich, & Turk, 1992; Karjalainen et al., 2006), the trend towards managed care has all but eliminated these programs, due to ill-founded fears on the part of third-party payors of inefficiency and added expense (Keefe, Dixon, et al., 2005; Thomsen, Sorensen, Sjogren, & Eriksen, 2001).

Regardless of the setting in which pain treatment is offered, the most important treatment goal should be early resolution of symptoms and a return to physical activity, in order to decrease the likelihood of development of a chronic pain condition. This is particularly important in light of convincing evidence regarding the structural changes described earlier. The individual's perception of pain severity predicts significant and unique variance in perceived disability, both in the short- and the long-term (Sieben, 2005). Thus, to ignore the individual's reported pain severity is ill-advised, especially in the acute pain phase.

Oftentimes, minimal effort on the part of the treating physician will go a long way in preventing chronic pain. Simply informing individuals about the limited nature of an acute pain episode, coupled with medication management, may be sufficient in preventing development of a pessimistic outlook for recovery, which can adversely affect recuperation and ultimately lead to the development of chronic pain (Gatchel, 2005). Although rest is often advised for acute pain conditions, substantial decreases in activity may exacerbate chronic pain by leading to muscle atrophy and dysfunction, and may increase the likelihood that the individual will avoid physical activity, for fear of increasing pain or causing re-injury. These beliefs and avoidance behaviors have been associated with increased chronic pain and disability, even after adjusting for age, sex, and pain intensity (Vlaeyen and Linton, 2000; Woby, Watson, Roach, & Urmston, 2004), and drive coping responses.

Coping with Chronic Pain

Pain and Disability

The *Americans with Disabilities Act of 1990* defines a person with a disability in part as someone with "a physical or mental impairment that substantially limits one or more of the major life activities of such individual." For the individual with chronic pain, the level of impairment (abnormal functioning of body part or organ system) oftentimes does not easily translate into the level of disability (alteration in one's ability to meet personal, social, or occupational responsibilities, secondary to an impairment), which is experienced by a person (Aronoff & Feldman, 2000).

Further, the amount of disability exhibited is frequently incongruent with the intensity of reported pain. That is, many individuals, who report high levels of pain, experience very little actual disability, while others display marked disability in the absence of significant pain (Waddell, 2004). Such discrepancies suggest that there are other important factors unique to the individual, which may ameliorate or exacerbate the magnitude of a disability. With conditions resulting in persistent pain, psychological factors, such as beliefs and cognitions, previous experiences with pain, and fear of pain/(re)injury, ultimately influence the level of disability; and the magnitude of disability is strongly influenced by the coping strategies employed by the individual (Johansson, Dahl, Jannert, Melin, & Anderson, 1998).

Pain as a Stressor

Just as with any serious life stressor, coping with pain on an on-going basis requires cognitive and behavioral resources to manage pain flares and other significant situations, which at times may exceed an individual's resources. In the case of chronic pain, there are two important factors that affect pain coping: the primary issue of living with persistent pain and the secondary issues that are related to the pain interfering with one's life (e.g., family/spouse issues, emotional distress, financial/work issues). Therefore, coping with pain becomes especially challenging, because the stressor is not simply the physical pain, but the additional effects of persistent pain on a number of important areas of an individual's functioning (Boothby, Thorn, Jensen, & Stroud, 1999).

Across individuals with chronic pain, there is a great deal of well-documented variability in coping abilities. Both *intrinsic* and *extrinsic* factors influence one's coping abilities, although these two categories are somewhat confluent and should not be conceptualized as independent of each other. Intrinsic factors reflect individual difference variables, such as age, sex, and ethnicity, and purportedly provide a relatively stable coping profile; whereas extrinsic factors (e.g, appraisal of the situation, ability to control pain, or average pain intensity) are more contextual and require coping strategies that differ across stressful situations (Novy, Nelson, Hetzel, Squitieri, & Kennington, 1998).

Building on the conceptualization of pain as being stress-related, Thorn (2004) proposed the Stress-Appraisal-Coping Model of Pain, which is an adaptation of Lazarus and Folkman's (1984) Transactional Model of Stress. At first glance, the idea of pain as a stressor may seem puzzling, because pain is commonly considered to be a sensory event brought about by a nociceptive stimulus. However, as Lazarus and Folkman point out, stress is not an event or stimulus, but rather, a *judgment* that an event or stimulus taxes or exceeds one's resources, thereby endangering one's well-being.

Thus, neither a painful stimulus, nor the biological response to the stimulus is considered "stress," although they may well be potential *stressors*. Rather, the cognitive process, which translates the stimulus and response into "threatening," and "unmanageable," is the actual stress response. Research findings clearly point to the importance of these cognitive processes in predicting outcome or adjustment to chronic painful states.

As stated earlier in Chapter 2 (Section I), according to Lazarus and Folkman's (1984) model, dispositional variables, such as personality, stable social roles and/or biological parameters, can affect a person's interaction with a stressor. Furthermore, peoples' appraisal of a potential stressor influences their response to the stressor, including whether, and which, coping responses will be attempted. Stress appraisals are categorized as "primary" or "secondary."

Primary Appraisals

Primary appraisals are those relating to judgments about whether a potential stressor is irrelevant, benign-positive, or stressful. Three types of primary appraisals are particularly relevant to chronic pain: (a) Threat (a perception that the danger posed by the situation outweighs the individual's ability to cope); (b) harm/loss (a perception that damage has occurred as a result of the stimulus);

and (c) challenge (a perception that the ability to cope is not outweighed by the potential danger of the stimulus).

If a pain stimulus is appraised as threatening, it is likely to focus one's attention toward the stimulus, as well as giving rise to certain emotional responses. A hypervigilant focus on pain stimuli (or *anticipated* pain stimuli) may reduce the person's ability to concentrate and attend to other tasks, and may impair their ability to remember important information (Kuhajda, Thorn, & Klinger, 1998; Kuhajda, Thorn, Klinger, & Rubin, 2002). Threat appraisals may give rise to certain emotional responses (e.g., anxiety, worry, fear of pain and re-injury) and behavioral responses (e.g., discontinuance or avoidance of activities that may be associated with pain).

Fear of pain may further increase the individual's focus of attention on pain-related stimuli (Asmundson, Kuperos, & Norton, 1997; McCracken, 1997) and increase one's reluctance to engage in activities that might produce discomfort (Crombez, Vervaet, Lysens, Baeyens, & Eelen, 1998; Vlaeyen & Linton, 2000). Avoidant behaviors add to the physical deconditioning of the individual, thereby greatly compounding the disability from the pain itself. Although the pain stimulus (or anticipated pain) is likely to elicit a threat appraisal, the secondary stressors associated with chronic pain are likely to bring forth a primary appraisal of loss. The primary appraisal of loss is likely to give rise to depressed affect, a perceived sense of helplessness, and a reduced likelihood of engaging in adaptive coping behaviors.

Appraisals that an environmental stressor is a challenge are by far the more adaptive type of primary appraisal, particularly when the person believes that effective coping responses are possible. It is probably not surprising that challenge appraisals do not appear to be common among individuals with chronic pain (Unruh & Ritchie, 1998). However, there is some evidence that in experimentally-induced pain, men have more challenge appraisals, and women report more threat appraisals (Sanford, Kersh, Thorn, Rich, & Ward, 2002).

Secondary Appraisals

Beliefs

Beliefs about coping options, and their possible effectiveness, are called secondary appraisals in a transactional model of stress. For individuals with chronic pain, these are acquired beliefs about the pain condition and automatic thoughts that arise in anticipation of, or in response to the pain. People experiencing chronic pain develop a set of beliefs about the cause of their pain and the way it should be treated. These acquired beliefs are not only personally formed beliefs, but also often culturally-shared beliefs (e.g., "With pain, one should rest and avoid re-injury"). Individuals with chronic pain also hold beliefs about how much control they have over their condition, whether they can execute certain coping responses, and whether particular coping responses will have any impact on their pain.

Cognitions

Whereas a belief has been described as a cognitive understanding of a condition or event (Wrubel, Benner, & Lazarus, 1981), cognitions, which arise somewhat mechanistically in response to a circumstance, have been termed automatic thoughts (Beck, 1976; Thorn, 2004). Research suggests that with pain disorders, the greater the tendency to display overly negative, distorted, automatic thoughts, the greater the individual's report of pain, dysfunction, depression, and overall poor adjustment to the pain condition (Jensen, Turner, Romano, & Karoly, 1991).

Furthermore, poor adjustment has been found to be related to specific pain-related cognitive errors, and not just general cognitive errors (Flor & Turk, 1988). The cognitive thought process labeled "catastrophizing" has been studied more than any other cognitive variable thought to influence pain perception and adjustment to pain. Catastrophizing has repeatedly been shown to predict functioning, over and above other psychosocial and physical predictors (Sullivan et al., 2001). Catastrophic pain-related thoughts can occur as part of the primary or secondary appraisal process, or as part of an attempt to cope with the stressors that are brought about by chronic pain (Thorn, Rich, & Boothby, 1999).

Coping

Coping involves both cognitive and behavioral efforts to manage stress, and ultimately influences important adaptational outcomes, such as social functioning, morale, and somatic health (Lazarus and Folkman, 1984). Cognitive coping techniques might influence one's perception of pain intensity, or the impact of stressors related to pain, via one's thoughts. Behavioral coping techniques modify overt behavior in an effort to alleviate pain, mitigate the interference in one's life due to pain, or manage pain-related stressors. Although coping strategies are often categorized as "behavioral," or "cognitive," the distinction between the two categories of coping is not rigid, and thus, they should be considered relative, rather than fixed, categories.

Coping need not be linked with mastery or with an adaptive response. For example, even if relaxation exercises do not result in reduced muscle tension and an increased sense of calm, they are still considered coping efforts because they are an attempt at reducing the impact of a chronic painful condition (Keefe, Lefebvre, & Smith, 1999). Even more important, some coping efforts, such as expressive pain behaviors that solicit emotional support, may actually be non-adaptive; yet, if they are used as an attempt to manage stressors, they are still included under the category of coping (Hewson, 1997).

The majority of the early research on pain-coping strategies used rationally-derived categories from which to differentiate styles of coping. Lazarus and Folkman (1984) distinguished between *emotion-focused* versus *problem-focused* coping. Within a chronic pain paradigm, problem-focused coping involves strategies that aim to change or control a stressor (e.g. activity-rest cycling), whereas emotion-focused coping functions to address emotional responses to a stressor (e.g., catastrophizing, positive self-affirmations).

Brown and Nicassio (1987) referred to *passive pain* coping strategies as those in which the individual delegates responsibility for managing his pain to an external source (e.g., doctor, higher power), or when the individual allows pain to interfere in a number of areas of her life. *Active coping* strategies reflect an assumption of responsibility for managing one's pain and allow the individual to attempt to reduce pain, but also to go on with her life despite the pain. Pain coping has also been distinguished by *illness-focused* coping versus *wellness-focused* coping (Jensen, Turner, Romano, & Strom, 1995). Most pain treatment approaches encourage wellness-focused coping by stressing the use of coping strategies consistent with health, such as physical activity and relaxation. Conversely, illness-focused coping occurs when the individual with chronic pain assumes the "sick role" and continues to approach a chronic pain condition with coping strategies that are more appropriate for acute pain (e.g., bed-rest, use of medication).

Regardless of the particular terminology or conceptualization used to distinguish coping styles, the choice of coping strategies is dependent upon a number of factors. As a group, coping strategies are generally conceptualized as being either active (e.g., distraction, activity-pacing) and adaptive, or passive (e.g., taking pain medications, praying and hoping) and non-adaptive. Most of the research suggests that the use of "active," "problem-focused," and "wellness-focused" coping strategies (e.g., exercise, activity despite the presence of pain, positive coping self-statements) is associated with better psychological and physical functioning. On the other hand, "non-adaptive" coping strategies, which include types of strategies described as "passive," "emotion-focused," or "illness-focused" (e.g., pain-contingent rest, seeking solicitous responses from others, catastrophizing, medication use), often predicts poorer functioning.

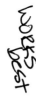

Interventions to Promote Coping with Pain

From a Curative Approach for Pain to a Pain Self-Management Approach

An overarching assumption in this next section is that working with individuals with chronic pain has less to do with changing the perception of the pain itself, than it has to do with helping the individual minimize the impact of pain on his or her life (i.e., increase functioning). Helping the individual with chronic pain to maintain functioning, or to change behavior in order to regain functioning, can be a daunting task. Some of the barriers to this goal include individual motivation issues, depression, anxiety, and a sense of helplessness.

Nevertheless, the bulk of the available research suggests that efforts to increase functioning, rather than continuing a quest to find a physical cause and cure for one's pain, predict better adjustment to the chronic pain condition. It is

Self-care active approach.

evident that the goal of increasing or maintaining one's functioning is more dependent upon self-care or self-management behaviors than on care from others. In fact, Von Korff (1999) asserted that positive adjustment to chronic pain is "more dependent on *effective self-care* [italics added] (e.g., exercise, sustaining work activities, appropriate use of pain medications), than on the quality of the diagnostic or therapeutic interventions of the physicians." (p. 363).

Reasonable pain self-management behaviors might include the following: (a) Restore or maintain work/family activities; (b) get regular physical activity; (c) pace physical activity; (d) use effective body mechanics; (e) use health-care services and pain medications *appropriately*; (f) adopt an attitude of acceptance (willingness to accept presence of pain), and self-identity as a "well-person with pain" (if appropriate); and (g) manage the effects of pain on thoughts and emotions, in terms of one's interaction with others (see Gatchel, 2005, p. 185; Turk, 2002).

Cognitive-Behavioral Therapy to Promote Pain Self-Management

There is good empirical support for the efficacy of cognitive-behavioral therapy (CBT) for chronic pain (Gil, et al., 1996). Furthermore, CBT is cost-effective relative to medication and/or hospitalization (Turk, 2001). Thus, CBT has become the gold standard for psychosocial interventions for pain.

A number of meta-analyses have found CBT to be quite successful, albeit, not always on the same outcome measures. In a meta-analytic review of CBT for chronic pain conditions other than headaches, Morley, Eccleston, and Williams (1999) found CBT to be superior to wait-list control groups on all outcome measures. When compared to alternative treatments, CBT proved better on outcomes related to pain severity, positive cognitive coping, and behavioral expression of pain, but not significantly different on outcomes measuring negative cognitive coping, and social-role functioning. Various meta-analyses of behavior therapy or CBT for headaches found these therapies to be at least equivalent to pharmacological interventions, and superior to placebo controls on various outcomes including frequency, intensity, and duration (Bogaards & ter Kuile, 1994; Goslin et al., 1999; Holroyd & Penzien, 1990).

More recent meta-analyses for specific types of pain confirm the conclusions from previous systematic reviews. Dixon, Keefe, Scipio, Perri, and Abernethy (in press) reported that for osteoarthritis and rheumatoid arthritis, CBT produced a significant decrease in pain; but the strongest positive findings were for non-physical variables, such as self-efficacy, mood, and pain coping. Conversely, Hoffman, Papas, Chatkoff, and Kerns (2007) found CBT with individuals with low back pain to be superior to wait-list controls in reducing pain intensity, but not superior to control in improving outcomes, such as quality of life and depressive symptoms. Finally, in a meta-analysis of CBT for irritable bowel syndrome, psychosocial treatments were found to be superior to control groups in reducing abdominal pain, bowel dysfunction, depression, and anxiety (Lackner, Mesmer, & Morley, 2004).

Applying CBT techniques with individuals with chronic pain uses a structured (often manualized) treatment, aimed at behavior change or maintenance of functioning, and treatment related to individuals' thoughts and emotions. CBT assumes that both cognitions and behaviors are crucial aspects of adjusting to chronic pain. CBT differs from traditional biomedical management of chronic pain in that the biomedical focus is on reducing the perception of the pain itself, whereas the CBT goal is to help the individual minimize the impact of pain on his or her life (i.e., to functioning despite the pain). Parenthetically, CBT often does result in reductions of perceived pain, but that is not the main focus of this treatment approach. The cognitive aspects of CBT are often incorporated to remove barriers that might otherwise prevent appropriate behavioral change.

What are the Important Components of CBT?

It is not known which components of CBT are the most critical for inclusion in pain management. CBT-pain treatment studies have sometimes compared "behavioral" components with "cognitive" components. Components most often categorized as behavioral include relaxation, biofeedback, and behavioral pacing strategies; whereas, the major cognitive components of CBT are cognitive restructuring and cognitive coping – skills training. Cognitive coping – skills training for pain includes such techniques as attention-diversion strategies, reinterpreting pain sensations, positive self-statements, and imagery techniques. Cognitive restructuring involves the identification and modification of dysfunctional thinking. When applied to the treatment of pain, cognitive restructuring typically focuses on identifying and decreasing dysfunctional pain-related cognitions.

Cognitive Components of CBT

Cognitive Restructuring

The efficacy of cognitive therapy for mood disorders has been well-established, and the details of treatment are well-articulated in numerous sources (cf., Beck, 1995). Cognitive components of CBT for chronic pain have also been established as efficacious (Kerns, Turk, Holzman, & Rudy, 1986; Knapp & Florin, 1981; Mitchell &White, 1977).

Thorn (2004) described a structured cognitive therapy program for chronic pain centered on three main phases. The first phase introduces the importance of stress appraisal, and the perspective that one's judgment regarding a situation influences one's coping (thoughts, images, feelings, behaviors, and pain). The second phase teaches clients to recognize, challenge, and then reconstruct, if necessary, non-adaptive automatic thoughts. The point of focusing on thought distortions is not so much to change the *content* of the thought, as it is to "decouple" the emotion from the thought. The thought becomes "just a thought" by removing the power of "truth" from it. Phase three teaches recognition of thought processes that are more deeply ingrained than situation-specific, automatic thoughts. As individuals begin to realize that beliefs are also *just thoughts* and not necessarily complete truths, they may become more receptive to the idea of taking more responsibility for pain self-management behaviors, rather than relying on the belief of a cure and the attitude that their health and well-being is in the hands of physicians.

Core pain-related beliefs reflect the individual's sense of self as a person in pain. Unfortunately, with increasing pain duration and mounting associated problems, individuals with chronic pain oftentimes take on the identity of a *disabled, chronic-pain individual*, and assume the role commensurate with such a core belief. These individuals, caught in a downward spiral of disability, continue to rest and seek medical diagnosis and cure, with little success. The goal, in helping individuals examine their core pain-related beliefs, is to develop a more wellness-focused identity, even in the face of chronic pain.

Cognitive Coping Strategies

There are numerous studies that have tried to determine whether certain cognitive coping strategies are relatively more useful than other strategies for individuals with chronic pain (e.g., Edwards & Fillingim, 2005; Jensen, Nielson, Turner, Romano, & Hill, 2003; Keefe, Affleck, et al., 1997). Research investigating the interactions between individual personality or appraisal variables and coping strategies may provide the most precise answers regarding the efficacy of particular coping strategies. The question seems to be which coping strategies work for which kinds of individuals, rather than globally assessing the efficacy of coping strategies without considering the individual's temperament or appraisal processes. Thus, the more research that is conducted, the more that researchers discover that individual and appraisal variables interact with treatment variables to influence their ultimate effectiveness. Perhaps for these reasons, the presently-available findings are rather inconsistent.

Nevertheless, some generalizations can be made. As was emphasized above, the use of distorted negative cognitions (catastrophic thinking, negative self-statements, and negative reflections regarding social interactions with others) can be considered non-adaptive cognitive strategies. Numerous studies have found strong and consistent relations between cognitive errors and poor adjustment to pain. Likewise, the use of wishful thinking, praying, and hoping (at least as these concepts are currently defined) have been associated with greater dysfunction, although the findings are not nearly as strong as the findings about cognitive errors (Dozois, Dobson, Wong, Hughes, & Long, 1996; Geisser, Robinson, & Henson, 1994). Examples of these cognitive strategies are "I wish that the situation would go away, or somehow be over," "I pray for the pain to stop," and "I have faith in doctors that someday there will be a cure for my pain," respectively.

Furthermore, cognitive strategies involving distraction or diverting attention (e.g., "I watch TV to distract myself from the pain") have not been found to be particularly useful techniques for individuals with chronic pain. Although some studies have found a relation between distraction strategies and positive outcome, many have not found any relation; recent reports indicate that distraction strategies may exacerbate pain in individuals with chronic pain (Hill, 1993; Riley, Robinson, & Geisser, 1999; Robinson et al., 1997). A final generalization that can be made is that the use of positive coping self-statements (e.g., "I concentrate on convincing myself that I will deal with the pain and that it will get better in the near future") has been associated with better adjustment in individuals with chronic pain (Hill, 1993; Riley et al., 1999; Van Lankveld, Van't Pad Bosch, Van De Putte, Naring, & Van Der Straak, 1994).

Acceptance of Pain as a Cognitive Coping Strategy

A growing body of research shows that individuals who have chronic pain and who accept their pain as a chronic condition, have *lower* perceived pain levels, *less* pain-related distress and depression, *less* avoidance of activities, *lower* levels of disability, and *greater* daily functioning (McCracken, 1997). "Acceptance" here is defined as recognizing that one has a chronic condition that cannot necessarily be cured, letting go of fruitless attempts to rid oneself of the pain, working towards living a satisfying life despite the pain, and not equating chronic pain with disability. In fact, it has been suggested that one of the main aims of CBT should be to facilitate acceptance of the pain, and in doing so, broaden a person's identity to beyond that of an individual who has chronic pain and who is "disabled" (Morley, Shapiro, & Biggs, 2004). McCracken (2004) proposed a CBT approach for chronic pain, in which a major component of the treatment involves helping individuals to accept (but not resign to) the chronic pain and thereby free themselves to pursue those aspects of their lives that have personal meaning and value, rather than chasing an elusive cure.

Conceptually related to McCracken's approach to acceptance of pain are mindfulness-based stress-reduction programs, such as those promulgated by Kabat-Zinn (1990). Mindfulness-based stress-reduction programs teach the individual to observe physical sensations in the body as moment-by-moment occurrences, which have no more importance or accuracy than other transient mental phenomenon. Several uncontrolled studies reported positive results of mindfulness training in individuals with chronic pain (Chang et al., 2004; Kabat-Zinn, Lipworth, & Burney, 1985). A meta-analysis of 20 studies, meeting acceptable quality criterion and covering a broad spectrum of clinical populations (including pain), concluded that mindfulness-based stress reduction may improve both mental and physical well-being in individuals with both clinical and non-clinical problems (Grossman, Niemann, Schmidt, & Walach, 2004).

Enhancing Behavioral Coping Strategies

Individuals with chronic pain often develop an entrenched pattern of non-adaptive coping behaviors, which contributes to increased pain and poor overall functioning. There are a number of behavioral coping skills which are extremely effective for reducing pain interference and, oftentimes, pain intensity as well. Several of these skills are discussed below.

It is well known that muscle tension and anxiety exacerbate pain intensity; therefore, perhaps the most important behavioral skill for individuals with chronic pain to learn is progressive muscle relaxation (PMR). Individuals are provided with the rationale for PMR and are guided through the relaxation of each of the major muscle groups with verbal instruction, demonstration, and feedback. Individuals are encouraged to practice PMR at least twice daily, with the goal of learning through "mini practices" to recognize muscle tension and to relax very quickly with minimal effort (Waters, McKee, & Keefe, 2004).

Relaxation skills can also be taught via the use of ancillary physiological feedback methods such as biofeedback, EMG, or skin conductance. While each of these modalities is somewhat different in their specific approach, all provide feedback regarding physiological correlates of tension, such as muscle tone, skin temperature, or skin conductance (Andrasik, 2004). Individuals learn to quickly identify physiological symptoms of tension, which signal a need to relax and to readily distinguish between a tense and relaxed state.

Many individuals with chronic pain attempt to avoid their pain by remaining inactive. Indeed, fear of pain and (re)injury has been identified as a major psychosocial variable that contributes to disability in individuals with chronic pain (Boersma & Linton, 2005). Preliminary trials with small samples suggest that individuals reporting substantial pain-related fear can benefit from individually-tailored, in vivo exposure to physical activity. The prescribed (and supervised) physical movements are hierarchically ordered and fear-eliciting; it is reported that such exposure treatment results in decreases in pain-related fear and pain vigilance, and increases in adaptive functioning (Boersma et al., 2004; Vlaeyen, de Jong, Geilen, Heuts, & Breukelen, 2002).

On the other hand, sometimes individuals with chronic pain begin feeling better and then get *too* active for too long of a period, which almost guarantees a significant pain flare. Teaching individuals activity-rest cycling breaks the cycle of inactivity, overexertion, and pain exacerbation. Individuals are taught to plan their day to include periods of moderate activity, followed by a scheduled period of rest, with the goal of increasing the intensity and length of time spent engaging in activity, while maintaining adequate rest periods and minimizing time spent reclining or in bed (Keefe, Jacobs, & Edwards, 1997).

The disruption in activity associated with chronic pain also contributes to social isolation and relinquishing of pleasurable and rewarding activities. All too often, individuals with chronic pain assume that they cannot participate in the very activities that once brought them pleasure. They quickly label certain pleasant activities, such as going to a movie or babysitting a grandchild, as off-limits. Thus, it becomes important to encourage individuals to purposefully schedule participation in pleasant activities. This technique provides an avenue for positive reinforcement from the enjoyment that is garnered by participating in valued activities. It is not sufficient to simply *tell* individuals to participate in such activities, because the limitations of the chronic pain condition (e.g., pain, fatigue) decrease the likelihood of self-initiated pleasant activities (Williams, Gehrman, Ashmore, & Keefe, 2003).

Individuals who lack assertive communication skills may exhibit pain behaviors that represent indirect attempts to convey information to others that they are in pain (Sullivan, Martel, Tripp, Savard, & Crombez, 2006). However, this method of communication is often met with much resentment on the part of the receiver. Therefore, such individuals will benefit from learning assertive communication skills, which include ways to more directly relay information regarding pain to others (Turner, Clancy, McQuade, & Cardenas, 1990).

Set Goals

In order to ensure use of these and other behavioral coping skills, goal-setting becomes particularly important. Helping individuals to develop and implement reasonable goals for all aspects of their lives (e.g., work, social, domestic) is useful for moving them in the direction of pain self-management. Both short- and long-term goals for gradually increasing the amount and intensity of activities are set and monitored (Johansson et al., 1998; Keefe, Abernethy, & Campbell, 2005). Examples of long-term goals might be building up to a certain level of daily physical activity, whereas more short-term goals might be to spend more time out of bed.

Any learned skill is subject to disuse if not kept upfront in a repertoire of coping techniques. It is important that individuals with chronic pain adopt regular practice and monitor for the possibility of relapse (Keefe, Beaupre, Gil, Rumble, & Aspnes, 2002). This process should be considered early and often during treatment by setting of specific goals for monitoring symptoms and observing for signs of relapse (Keefe, Abernethy, et al., 2005).

Implications and Future Directions

The traditional biomedical model, which guided the assessment and treatment of persistent pain for many years, is obsolete. The clinical and scientific understanding of the mechanisms underlying an individual's ability to live a fulfilling life with persistent pain has vastly increased in recent years. Clearly, individual variability in cognitive appraisals, thoughts, beliefs, and attitudes about pain are important to consider when planning and implementing interventions for individuals with chronic pain.

In addition, individuals' preferences regarding their treatment options are an important consideration. Approaching individuals as if they were a homogeneous group and prescribing a rote, manualized intervention ignore the valuable information provided by assessment and treatment-outcome research regarding individual variability in cognitions and the importance of individuals' preferences. Furthermore, when the individual characteristics influencing the selection of coping strategies, such as primary appraisals, automatic thoughts, beliefs, and attitudes about pain, are ignored by the practitioner, individuals with chronic pain may become frustrated or conclude that a biopsychosocial approach to pain management is not appropriate for them. Fortunately, there are a number of interesting recent advances in identifying individual characteristics that are important to pain coping, which may be used to guide treatment in the future.

The recent development and initial psychometric testing of a new assessment instrument, *The Pain Solutions Questionnaire* (De Vlieger, Van den Bussche, Eccleston, & Crombez, 2006), provides an avenue for exploring several important pain-related coping strategies, such as how hard one strives to resolve his or her pain (Solving Pain subscale), the extent to which one strives for meaning in a life with pain (Meaningfulness of Life Despite Pain subscale), and the ability one has to detach from trying to solve the pain and acknowledge that pain is not controllable (Acceptance of the Insolubility of Pain subscale). Two important findings from this initial validation study are relevant to pain interventions. First, individuals with chronic pain, who focus their efforts on attempting to resolve their pain, report high levels of attention to pain sensations, as well as high levels of catastrophizing about pain. Comparatively, individuals with chronic pain, who report that they can find meaning in their life despite the pain, report less attention to pain, less catastrophizing, and less distress and disability. When sufficiently validated, the *Pain Solutions Questionnaire* may provide another means for identifying, early in treatment, the specific ways in which individuals with chronic pain cope with their pain, thus providing useful information for tailoring treatment.

A promising new treatment method is to identify preferred coping styles early in treatment and then tailor the interventions, in order to take advantage of the individual's strengths and preference for treatment (Heapy, Stroud, Higgins, & Sellinger, 2006). Such "tailoring" of interventions may ultimately increase an individual's adherence and satisfaction with treatment and improve outcomes. Using such an approach ensures that time and effort are not wasted on interventions, which the individual ultimately will not find useful, but which may increase the likelihood that the individual will become frustrated and drop out of treatment.

Incorporating motivational enhancement strategies in CBT is another promising way of engaging individuals and potentially improving adherence (Jensen, 2005; Jensen, Nielsen, & Kerns, 2003). Motivational interviewing (MI), originally developed to enhance treatment success in individuals with substance-abuse problems, has been shown to be effective in facilitating change in a variety of health behavior-problems (Miller & Rollnick, 2002). Recently, the application of MI techniques to the treatment of chronic pain has shown promising results (Habib, Morrissey, & Helmes, 2005; Jensen, 2005).

As mentioned earlier in the chapter, a number of coping strategies that produce higher levels of functioning and quality of life have been identified. Thus, while it is impossible to offer individuals a *cure* for their pain, interventions, such as coping – skills training, can and should be offered to them, providing them with the requisite skills to maximize functioning and increase the likelihood of return to work, or at least to minimize the magnitude of disability that they experience.

Summary

All individuals with chronic pain are not alike. Some bring to the table a full cadre of adaptive coping strategies, while others seem to languish in a sea of despair, helplessness, and hopelessness. One distinguishing factor in these two outcomes may be in the choice of coping strategies which are implemented in attempts to live with unrelenting pain. There is ample empirical evidence that beliefs and appraisals underlie the choice of coping responses, and thus affect the overall level of impairment or disability that is experienced by the individual.

Regardless of choice of appproaches, the ultimate goal for any pain-management intervention should be to promote pain *self*-management to ensure that individuals with chronic pain maximize the resources that they have. Perhaps they will be encouraged to add a few new skills, which will allow them to move from an endless pursuit of a cure toward a mindset of acceptance and living a full life, despite having pain. Relinquishing the identity of being an "individual with chronic pain" (Point A) and claiming the identity of a "well person with pain" (Point B) underlie the ultimate success of pain treatment. Nevertheless, helping the individual with chronic pain move from Point A to Point B is no small therapeutic challenge.

References

American Pain Foundation. (2006). *Pain Facts*. Retrieved April 29, 2006, from http://www.painfoundation.org/page.asp?file=Library/PainSurveys.htm

Americans with Disabilities Act of 1990, 42 U.S.C.A. § 12101 et seq.

Andrasik, F. (2004). The essence of biofeedback, relaxation, and hypnosis. In R. H. Dworkin & W. S. Breitbart (Eds.). *Progress in pain research and management:, Vol. 27. Psychosocial aspects of pain: A handbook for health care providers* (pp. 285–305). Seattle: IASP Press.

Aronoff, G. M., & Feldman, J. B. (2000). Preventing disability from chronic pain: A review and reappraisal. *International Review of Psychiatry, 12*, 157–169.

Asmundson, G. J. G., Kuperos, J. L., & Norton, G. R., (1997). Do patients with chronic pain selectively attend to pain-related information? Preliminary evidence for the mediating role of fear. *Pain, 72*, 27–32.

Beck, A. T. (1976). *Cognitive therapy and the emotional disorders.* New York: International Universities Press.

Beck, J. S. (1995). *Cognitive therapy: Basics and beyond.* New York: Guilford Publications.

Boersma, K., & Linton, S. (2005). How does persistent pain develop? An analysis of the relationship between psychological variables, pain and function across stages of chronicity. *Behaviour Research and Therapy, 43*, 1495–1507.

Boersma, K., Linton, S., Overmeer, T., Jannson, M., Vlaeyen, J., & de Jong, J. (2004). Lowering fear avoidance and enhancing function through exposure in vivo: A multiple baseline study across six patients with back pain. *Pain, 108*, 8–16.

Bogaards, M.C., & ter Kuile, M. M. (1994). Treatment of recurrent tension headache: A meta-analytic review. *Clinical Journal of Pain, 10*, 174–190.

Boothby, J. L., Thorn, B. E., Jensen, M., & Stroud, M. (1999). Coping with chronic pain. In R. J. Gatchel & D. J. Turk (Eds.), *Psychosocial factors in pain: Critical perspectives* (pp. 343–359). New York: Guilford.

Brookoff, D. (2000). Chronic pain: 1. A new disease? *Hospital Practice, 35,* 45–52.

Brown, G. K. & Nicassio, P. M. (1987). Development of a questionnaire for the assessment of active and passive coping strategies in chronic pain patients. *Pain, 31,* 53–63.

Chang, V. Y., Palesh, O., Caldwell, R., Glasgow, N., Abramson, M., Lusking, F., et al. (2004). The effects of a mindfulness-based stress reduction program on stress, mindfulness self-efficacy, and positive states of mind. *Stress and Health, 20,* 141–147.

Covington, E. C. (2000). The biological basis of pain. *International Review of Psychiatry, 12,* 128–147.

Crombez, G., Vervaet, L., Lysens, R., Baeyens, F., & Eelen, P. (1998). Avoidance and confrontation of painful back straining movement in chronic back pain patients. *Behavior Modification, 22,* 62–77.

De Vlieger, P., Van den Bussche, E., Eccleston, C., & Crombez, G. (2006). Finding a solution to the problem of pain: Conceptual formulation and the development of the Pain Solutions Questionnaire (PaSol). *Pain,123,* 285–293.

Dixon, K. E., Keefe, F. J., Scipio, C. D., Perri, L. M., & Abernethy, A. P. (in press). Psychological interventions for arthritis pain management in adults: A meta-analysis. *Health Psychology.*

Dozois, D. J. A., Dobson, K. S., Wong, M., Hughes, D., & Long, A. (1996). Predictive utility of the CSQ in low back pain: Individual vs. composite measures. *Pain, 66,* 251–259.

Edwards, R. R., & Fillingim, R. B. (2005). Styles of pain coping predict cardiovascular function following cold pressor test. *Pain Research and Management, 10,* 219–222.

Flor, H., Fydrich, T., & Turk, D. C. (1992). Efficacy of multidisciplinary pain treatment centers: a meta-analytic review. *Pain, 49,* 221–230.

Flor, H., & Turk, D. C. (1988). Chronic back pain and rheumatoid arthritis: Predicting pain and disability from cognitive variables. *Journal of Behavioral Medicine, 11,* 251–265.

Gatchel, R. J. (2005). *Clinical essentials of pain management.* Washington, DC: American Psychological Association.

Geisser, M. E., Robinson, M. E., & Henson, C. D. (1994). The Coping Strategies Questionnaire and chronic pain adjustment: A conceptual and empirical reanalysis. *Clinical Journal of Pain, 10,* 98–106.

Giesicke, T., Gracely, R. H., Williams, D. A., Geisser, M. E., Petzke, F. W., et al. (2005). The relationship between depression, clinical pain, and experimental pain in a chornic pain cohort. *Arthritis and Rhuematism, 52,* 1577–1584.

Gil, K. M., Wilson, J. J., Edens. J. L., Webster, D. A., Abrams, M. A., Orringer, E., et al. (1996). The effects of cognitive coping skills training on coping strategies and experimental pain sensitivity in African American adults with sickle cell disease. *Health Psychology, 15,* 3–10.

Goslin, R. E., Gray, R. N., McCrory, D. C., Penzien, D., Rains, J., & Hasselblad, V. (1999). Behavioral and physical treatments for migraine headache. Technical review 2.2. February 1999. (Prepared for the Agency for Health Care Policy and Research under Contract No. 290-94-2025. Available from the National Technical Information Service; NTIS Accession No. 127946).

Gracely, R. H., Geisser, M. E., Giesecke, T., Grant, A. B., Petzke, F. & Williams, D. A. (2004). Pain catastrophizing and neural responses to pain among persons with fibromyalgia. *Brain, 127*, 835–843.

Grossman, P., Niemann, L., Schmidt, S., & Walach, H. (2004). Mindfulness-based stress reduction and health benefits: A meta-analysis. *Journal of Psychosomatic Research, 57*, 35–43.

Habib, S., Morrissey, S., & Helmes, E. (2005). Preparing for pain management: A pilot study to enhance engagement. *Journal of Pain, 6*, 48–54.

Hampton, T. (2005). Pain and the brain: researchers focus on tackling pain memories. *Journal of the American Medical Association, 293*, 2845–2846.

Harstall C., & Ospina, M. (2003). How prevalent is chronic pain? *Pain Clinical Updates, XI*, 1–4.

Heapy, A. A., Stroud, M. W., Higgins, D. M., & Sellinger, J. J. (2006). Tailoring Cognitive-Behavioral Therapy for chronic pain: A case example. *Journal of Clinical Psychology: In Session, 62*, 1345–1366.

Hewson, D. (1997). Coping with loss of ability: "Good Grief" or episodic stress response. *Social Science Medicine, 44*, 1129–1139.

Hill, A. (1993). The use of pain coping strategies by patients with phantom limb pain. *Pain, 55*, 347–353.

Hoffman, B. M., Papas, R. K., Chatkoff, D. K., & Kerns, R. D. (2007). Meta-analysis of psychological interventions for chronic back pain. *Health Psychology, 26*, 1–9.

Holroyd, K. A., & Penzien, D. B. (1990). Pharmacological versus non-pharmacological prophylaxis of recurrent migraine headache: A meta-analytic review of clinical trials. *Pain, 42*, 1–13.

Iadarola, J. M., & Caudle, R. M. (1997). Good pain, bad pain [comment]. *Science. 278*, 239–240.

Jensen, M. P. (2005). Enhancing motivation to change in pain treatment. In D. C. Turk & R. J. Gatchel (Eds.), *Psychological approaches to pain management: A practitioner's handbook* (2nd ed., pp. 71–93). New York: Guilford Press.

Jensen, M. P., Nielsen, W. R., & Kerns, R. D. (2003). Toward the development of a motivational model of pain self-management. *Journal of Pain, 4*, 477–492.

Jensen, M. P., Nielson, W. R., Turner, J. A., Romano, J. M. & Hill, M. L. (2003). Readiness to self-manage pain is associated with coping and with psychological and physical functioning among patients with chronic pain. *Pain, 104*, 529–537.

Jensen, M. P., Turner, J.A., Romano, J. M., & Karoly, P. (1991). Coping with chronic pain: A critical review of the literature. *Pain. 47*, 249–283.

Jensen, M. P., Turner, J. A., Romano, J. M., & Strom, S. E. (1995). The Chronic Pain Coping Inventory: Development and preliminary validation. *Pain, 60*, 203–216.

Johansson, C., Dahl, J., Jannert, M., Melin, L., & Anderson, G. (1998). Effects of a cognitive-behavioral pain-management program. *Behavior Research and Therapy, 36*, 915–930.

Kabat-Zinn, J. (1990). *Full catastrophe living: Using the wisdom of your body and mind to face stress, pain, and illness.* New York: Dell.

Kabat-Zinn, J., Lipworth, L., & Burney, R. (1985). The clinical use of mindfulness meditation for the self-regulation of chronic pain. *Journal of Behavioral Medicine, 8*, 163–190.

Karjalainen, K., Malmivaara, A., van Tulder, M, Roine, R., Jauhiainen, M., Hurri, H., Kaes B.(2003). Multidisciplinary biopsychosocial rehabilitation for subacute low-back pain among working age adults. *Cochrane Database of Systematic Reviews* Issue 2. Art No: CD002193.DOI: 10.1002/14651858.CD002193.

Keefe, F. J., Abernethy, A. P., & Campbell, L. C. (2005). Psychological approaches to treating pain. *Annual Review of Psychology, 56*, 601–630.

Keefe, F.J., Affleck, G., Lefebvre, J.C., Starr, K., Caldwell, D.S., & Tennen, H. (1997). Pain coping strategies and coping efficacy in rheumatoid arthritis: a daily process analysis. *Pain, 69*, 35–42.

Keefe, F. J., Beaupre, P. M., Gil, K. M., Rumble, M., & Aspnes, A. (2002). Group therapy for patients with chronic pain. In D. C. Turk & R. J. Gatchel (Eds.), *Psychological Approaches to Pain Management* (pp. 234–255). New York: Guilford.

Keefe, F. J., Dixon, K. E., & Pryor, R. W. (2005). Psychological contributions to understanding and treatment of pain. In H. Merskey, J. D. Loeser, & R. Dubner (Eds.), *The Paths of Pain: 1975–2005* (pp. 403–420). Seattle: IASP Press.

Keefe, F. J., Jacobs, M., & Edwards, C. (1997). Persistent pain: Cognitive-behavioral approaches to assessment and treatment. *Seminars in Anesthesia, 16*, 117–126.

Keefe, F. J., Lefebvre, J. C., & Smith, S. J. (1999). Catastrophizing research: Avoiding conceptual errors and maintaining a balanced perspective. *Pain Forum, 8*, 176–180.

Kerns, R.D., Turk, D.C., Holzman, A.D., & Rudy, T.E. (1986). Comparison of cognitive-behavioral and behavioral approaches to the outpatient treatment of chronic pain. *Clinical Journal of Pain, 1*, 195–203.

Knapp, T.W., & Florin, I. (1981). The treatment of migraine headache by training in vasoconstriction of the temporal artery and a cognitive stress-coping training. *Behavioral Analysis and Modification, 4*, 267–274.

Kuhajda, M. C., Thorn, B. E., & Klinger, M. (1998). The effect of pain on memory for affective words. *Annals of Behavioral Medicine, 20*, 31–35.

Kuhajda, M. C., Thorn, B. E., Klinger, M., & Rubin, N. (2002). The effects of headache pain on attention (encoding) and memory (recognition). *Pain, 97*, 213–221.

Lackner, J. M., Mesmer, C., & Morley, S. (2004). Psychological treatments for irritable bowel syndrome: A systematic review and meta-analysis. *Journal of Consulting and Clinical Psychology, 72*, 1100–1113.

Lazarus, R. S., & Folkman, S. (1984). *Stress, appraisal and coping.* New York: Springer.

McCracken, L. M. (1997). "Attention" to pain in persons with chronic pain. *Behavior Therapy, 28*, 283–289.

McCracken, L. M. (2004). *Contextual cognitive behavioral therapy for chronic pain.* Seattle: IASP.

Melzack, R. (1999). From the gate to the neuromatrix. *Pain* (Suppl. 6 August), S121–S126.

Melzack, R., & Wall, P. D. (1965). Pain mechanisms: A new theory. *Science, 150*, 971–979.

Miller, W. R., & Rollnick, S. (2002). *Motivational interviewing: Preparing people to change* (2nd ed.). New York: Guilford.

Mitchell, K. R., & White, R. G. (1977). Behavioral self-management: An application to the problem of migraine headaches. *Behavior Therapy, 8*, 213–221.

Morley, S., Eccleston, C., & Williams, A. (1999). Systematic review and meta-analysis of randomized controlled trials of cognitive behavior therapy for chronic pain in adults, excluding headache. *Pain, 80*, 1–13.

Morley, S., Shapiro, D. A., & Biggs, J. (2004). Developing a treatment manual for attention management in chronic pain. *Cognitive Behavior Therapy, 33*, 1–11.

Novy, D. M., Nelson, D. V., Hetzel, R. D., Squitieri, P., & Kennington, M. (1998). Coping with chronic pain: Sources of intrinsic and contextual variability. *Journal of Behavioral Medicine, 21*, 19–34.

Ploghaus, A., Tracey, I., Gati, J. S., Clare, S., Menon, R. S., Matthews, P. M., et al. (1999). Dissociating pain from its anticipation in the human brain. *Science, 284*, 1979–1981.

Riley, J. L., Robinson, M. E., & Geisser, M. E. (1999). Empirical subgroups of the Coping Strategies Questionnaire – Revised: A multi-sample study. *The Clinical Journal of Pain, 15*, 111–116.

Robinson, M. E., Riley, J. L., Myers, C. D., Sadler, I. J., Kvaal, S. A., Geisser, M. E., et al. (1997). The Coping Strategies Questionnaire: A large sample, item level factor analysis. *Clinical Journal of Pain, 13*, 43–49.

Sanford, S. D., Kersh, B. C., Thorn, B. E., Rich, M. A., & Ward, L. C. (2002). Psychosocial mediators of sex differences in pain responsivity. *Journal of Pain, 3*, 58–64.

Sieben, J.M. (2005). A longitudinal study on the predictive validity of the fear-avoidance model in low back pain. *Pain, 117*, 162–170.

Sullivan, M. J. L., Martel, M. O., Tripp, D., Savard, A., & Crombez, G. (2006). The relation between catastrophizing and the communication of pain experience. *Pain, 122*, 282–288.

Sullivan, M. J. L., Thorn, B. E., Haythornthwaite, J. A., Keefe, F. J., Martin, M., Bradley, L. A., et al. (2001). Theoretical perspectives on the rlation between catastrophizing and pain. *Clinical Journal of Pain, 17*, 52–64.

Thomsen, A. B., Sorensen, J., Sjogren, P., & Eriksen, J. (2001). Economic evaluation of multidisciplinary pain management in chronic pain patients: A qualitative systematic review. *Journal of Pain and Symptom Management, 22*, 688–698.

Thorn, B. E. (2004). *Cognitive therapy for chronic pain: A step-by-step guide.* New York: Guilford.

Thorn, B. E., Rich, M. A., & Boothby, J. L. (1999) Pain beliefs and coping attempts. *Pain Forum, 8*(4), 169–171.

Turk, D. C. (2001). Treatment of chronic pain: Clinical outcomes, cost-effectiveness, and cost benefits. *Drug-Benefit-Trends, 13*, 36–38.

Turk, D. C. (2002). A cognitive-behavioral perspective on treatment of chronic pain patients. In D. C. Turk & R. J. Gatchel (Eds.), *Psychological approaches to pain management: a practitioner's handbook* (2nd ed., pp. 138–158). New York: Guilford.

Turk, D. C., & Okifuji, A. (2001). Pain terms and taxonomies of pain. In J. D. Loeser, S. H. Butler, C. R. Chapman, & D. C. Turk (Eds.), *Bonica's management of pain* (3rd ed., pp. 17–35). New York: Lippincott, Williams, and Williams.

Turner, J. A., Clancy, S., McQuade, K. J., & Cardenas, D. D. (1990). Effectiveness of behavioral therapy for chronic low back pain: A component analysis. *Journal of Consulting and Clinical Psychology, 58*, 573–579.

Unruh, A. M. & Ritchie, J. A. (1998). Development of the Pain Appraisal Inventory: Psychometric properties. *Pain Research and Medicine, 3*, 105–110.

Van Lankveld, W., Van't Pad Bosch, P., Van De Putte, L., Naring, G., & Van Der Straak, C. (1994). Disease-specific stressors in rheumatoid arthritis: Coping and well-being. *British Journal of Rheumatology, 33*, 1067–1073.

Vlaeyen, J., de Jong, J., Geilen, M., Heuts, P., & Breukelen, G. (2002). The treatment of fear of movement/(re)injury in chronic low back pain: Further evidence eon the effectiveness of exposure in vivo. *Clinical Journal of Pain, 18*, 251–261.

Vlaeyen, J. W. S., & Linton, S. J. (2000). Fear-avoidance and its consequences in chronic musculoskeletal pain: a state of the art. *Pain, 85*, 331–332.

Von Korff, M. (1999). Pain management in primary care: An individualized stepped-care approach. In R. J. Gatchel & D. J. Turk (Eds.), *Psychosocial factors in pain: Critical perspectives* (pp. 360–373). New York: Guilford.

Von Korff, M., Gruman, J., Schaefer, J., Curry, S. J., & Wagner, E. H. (1997). Collaborative management of chronic illness. *Annals of Internal Medicine, 127,* 1097–1102.

Waddell, G. (2004). *The back pain revolution.* Edinburgh: Churchill Livingstone.

Wagner, E. H., Austin, B. T., Davis, C., Hindmarsh, M., Schaefer, J., & Bonomi, A. (2001). Improving chronic illness care: Translating evidence into action. *Health Affairs, 20,* 64–78.

Waters, S. J., McKee, D. C., & Keefe, F. J. (2004, Spring). Cognitive behavioral approaches to the treatment of pain. *Chronic Comorbidity in CNS Medicine: Applied Psychiatry in the Medically Ill, 1,* 45–51.

Williams, D. A., Gehrman, C., Ashmore, J., & Keefe, F. J. (2003). Psychological considerations in the surgical treatment of patients with chronic pain. *Techniques in Neurosurgery, 8,* 168–175.

Woby, S. R., Watson, P. J., Roach, N. K., & Urmston M. (2004). Adjustment to chronic low back pain – the relative influence of fear-avoidance beliefs, catastrophizing, and appraisals of control. *Behaviour Research & Therapy, 42,* 761–774.

Woolf, C. J., & Salter, M. W. (2000). Neuronal plasticity: Increasing the gain in pain. *Science, 288,* 1765–1772.

Wrubel, J., Benner, P., & Lazarus, R. S. (1981). Social competence from the perspective of stress and coping. In J. Wine & M. Syme (Eds.), *Social competence* (pp. 61–99). New York: Guilford Press.

16
Coping with Severe Mental Illness: A Multifaceted Approach

Shlomo Kravetz and David Roe

Overview of Severe Mental Illness

Coping within the Context of Severe Mental Illness

Over the last 20 years, numerous articles (e.g., Andres Pfammatter, Fries, & Brenner, 2003; Cohen & Berk, 1985; Dittmann & Schuttler, 1990; Falloon & Talbot, 1981) have been published, whose titles include severe mental illness (SMI) and coping. Such research has been invaluable in informing individuals with SMI, their families and friends, and their mental-health service-provider of ways of dealing with the negative consequences of SMI. Many other books, articles, and other media sources have been written by individuals with SMI, which described how they have individually coped with SMI (e.g., the "Coping with" column in the *Psychiatric Rehabilitation* journal).

One definition of coping is that it is a "special category of adaptation elicited in normal individuals by unusually taxing circumstances" (Costa, Sommerfield, & McCrae, 1996, p. 45). Such a definition implies that the term, coping, does not include individuals, who are considered by society as "abnormal." Further, such a definition does little to articulate an understanding of how these individuals struggle with mental-health difficulties. For many, the word "abnormal" is associated with psychopathology and psychiatry, due to the perspectives taught in basic psychology courses or the viewpoint propagated by the "medical model" of disability (i.e., the organ or system-disorder is the focus of services). Accordingly, Costa et al.'s (1996) definition of coping seems to imply, perhaps unintentionally, that the term, coping is only appropriate for the problems of normal individuals and that coping will not help "abnormal" individuals with their difficulties.

However, this chapter makes no such assumptions. Empirical studies indicate that 72–100% of the individuals with a SMI claimed that they used coping strategies to deal with their SMI (Garcelan & Rodriguez, 2002). Thus, it can be stated that *coping is a potentially empowering activity that is a major part of the behavioral and experiential repertoire of individuals with SMI*. The purpose of this chapter is to examine coping with SMI research and interventions and to propose a new multidimensional and multifaceted framework to deal with the issues raised by the above review, after briefly covering such topics as definitions and labels.

Definitions of Severe Mental Illness

Professionals, who specialize in general psychiatry and in psychiatric rehabilitation, often use the Diagnostic and Statistical Manual-IV-TR (DSM; American Psychiatric Association, 2000) and the International Classification of Diseases, 10th Revision (ICD; World Health Organization, 1992) to define mental illness. According to the DSM, a mental disorder is "a clinically significant behavioral or psychological syndrome or pattern that occurs in an individual... [and that] is associated with present stress... or disability... or with a significant increased risk of suffering" (APA, 2000, p. xxxi). The DSM classifies disorders by sets of symptoms and places these disorders along a seriousness continuum, according to symptom duration and severity. Effort has been invested in matching the DSM with the ICD, so that the DSM includes the ICD diagnoses.

From an analysis of the definitions of mental illness to be used in state parity laws, Peck and Scheffler (2002) concluded that states' laws use a variety of definitions of mental illness. The most comprehensive term, which refers to all of the mental illnesses in the *DSM-IV*, is "broad-based mental illness." More restrictive terms, which are contained in state parity laws, are "serious mental illness" and "biologically-based mental illness." Torrey and Miller (2001) claim that the current denotation of "insanity" refers to the various subtypes of schizophrenia, schizoaffective disorder, manic-depressive illness, delusional disorder, and major depression with psychotic features. In discussions of psychiatric rehabilitation, the term "SMI" is generally reserved for schizophrenia, major depression, and mania-depression (Dicky, 2005).

If SMI is defined as having at some time, during the last 12 months, a diagnosable mental, behavioral, or emotional disorder that meets the criteria of the *DSM-IV-R* and results in significant functional impairment, then the incidence for SMI in the United States has been estimated as 8.3% (Epstein, Barker, Vorburger, & Murtha, 2002). The World Health Organization (2006a) indicated that the world-wide prevalence of mental, neurological, or behavioral problems is an estimated 450 million people. These large numbers suggest that there is a great need to better understand how individuals with SMI cope with their various consequences of their illness.

Coping with a Label or Diagnosis

In the field of psychology and psychiatry, there is a sometimes bitter controversy about whether labeling individuals, who have severe and persistent cognitive, emotional, and behavioral problems, as having a "mental illness" is meaningful or even helpful (Horowitz, 2002; Roth & Krull, 1986). However, the problematic and controversial nature of the mental illness diagnosis notwithstanding, this chapter's authors believe that, when presented from a biopsychosocial perspective, a SMI diagnosis can be meaningful and helpful. One reason for such an assertion is the assumption of the biopsychosocial approach that any conceptualization of the etiology and treatment will significantly emphasize the interaction among brain, behavior, and the environment (Engel, 1977, 1980). This assumption can potentially free the person with the SMI and his or her family from the responsibility for causing the illness, while allowing them to be responsible for coping with the wide array of the negative consequences of the illness.

Generally speaking, many professionals attribute a major role to the central nervous system in both the etiology and treatment of SMI. Some individuals with SMI and mental-health professionals argue that the focus on the medical causes of SMI is misleading. In this chapter, a more holistic model of SMI will be presented, which includes multiple facets of SMI. This approach should form a conceptual map, which is sufficiently comprehensive to incorporate the broad spectrum of perspectives about the human problems underlying SMI and to provide a framework for research into the substance and structure of coping with SMI. This conceptual map could also serve as a source of coping-focused interventions and of measures for assessing these interventions' effectiveness.

A Multifaceted Approach to Coping with Severe Mental Illness

As discussed in this book's initial chapters, many efforts have been made to identify, assess, and classify the ways that individuals cope with stressful life events, such as the onset of a physical or mental disability. A number of theories, which integrate the coping taxonomies produced by these by these efforts, have also been proposed. Despite the theoretical and research efforts generated by the construct of coping, the results of the efforts have been criticized for not adequately specifying and clarifying which variables are included in various conceptualizations of coping (Gol & Cook, 2004). A similar argument has been raised with regard to the study of the variety of behaviors adapted by individuals with SMI to deal with their disorders and the limitations imposed by these disorders. On the basis of a critical survey of research into the coping strategies used by individuals with psychosis, Garcelan and Rodriguez (2002) claim that arriving at a global and comprehensive view of this research is difficult, due to the multitude of approaches that this research has generated.

To develop the model of coping with SMI that is presented in this chapter, facet theory was used to identify the major domains of variables that comprise the ways in which individuals cope with the broad range of phenomena associated with SMI. Facet theory is a formal research methodology for sampling variables and constructing measures to analyze multidimensional phenomena, such as the coping strategies of individuals with SMI (Guttman & Greenbaum, 1998).

Within facet theory, a *facet* is defined formally as a set of variables representing the conceptual and semantic content of a universe. Facets are made-up of elements that spell-out the different values that logically pertain to the variations within a facet. The technical term, *mapping sentences*, is used for the designation of both the facets that represent multidimensional phenomena, such as the strategies used to cope with the SMI, and the relations between these facets. These sentences include three kinds of general facets: (1) population, (2) content, and (3) range.

Individuals with a diagnosis of schizophrenia will be used to illustrate the model, after it is explained; hence, persons with schizophrenia is the *population* of interest. The coping *content* domains, which are examined in this chapter, respond to the following questions:

Facet A. How does a person cope with the problems and challenges of SMI?

Facet B. With what problems and challenges of SMI does a person cope?

Facet C. In what context does a person cope with the problems and challenges of SMI?

The *range* of coping responses ranges from very infrequent use to very frequent use of a coping strategy (i.e., for an example of the use of a similar response range, see the *Ways of Coping Questionnaire* by Folkman and Lazarus, *1988*).

Figure 16.1 presents a structural model of this chapter's multifaceted theory of coping with SMI. This model is based on the following mapping sentence, which includes three content facets and one range facet:

A response can be considered coping with SMI if it is:

[Facet A] {a1. assimilative, a2. accommodative, a3. engaged, a4. disengaged} response to the *[Facet B]* {b1. impairments and symptoms, b2. disabilities, b3. stress, b4. stigma, b5. reduced quality of life and meaning in life, b6. mental illness diagnosis} in a *[Facet C]* {c1. personal, c2. interpersonal} context and that ranges from *[Range]* {very infrequent to very frequent}.

The following sections explicate the facets and facet elements that appear in Figure 16.1 and in the above mapping sentence. They also provide a rationale for the selection of the particular facet and facet elements as well as for the relations that are depicted between the facets and facet elements in the three-dimensional figure. After a research-based explanation of the model, the diagnosis of schizophrenia will be used to illustrate the clinical applications of this model.

Ways of Coping with the Problems and Challenges of SMI

This content-facet was the most challenging and problematic in the multifaceted model of coping with SMI. A great deal of the theoretical and empirical research, which has been conducted to clarify the nature of coping in general and of coping with SMI in particular, consists of attempts to describe and classify the

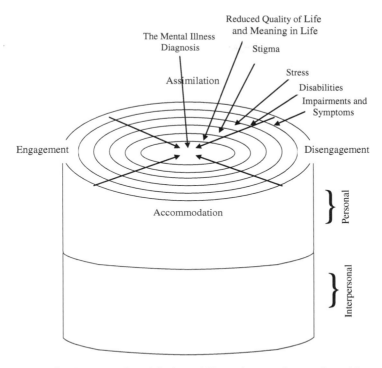

FIGURE 16.1. A structural model of a multifaceted approach to coping with severe mental illness.

way by which individuals cope with negative life-events. These attempts, which have been carried-out at different levels of abstraction (i.e., the abstract term of problem-solving versus the more concrete term of confronting the voices), have produced a plethora of coping responses.

In their critical review of studies of various classifications of coping responses and strategies, Skinner, Edge, Altman, and Sherwood (2003) examined more than a hundred non-overlapping category systems and provide a list of 400 category labels. This abundance of terms may indicate that scientific and professional use of the term coping has not rescued it from its every-day language "fuzziness." Acton and Revelle (2002) claim that multidimensional and multifaceted models, such as the one suggested here, are attempts to portray precisely this lack of definitional clarity. On the one hand, a broad range of definitions may be advantageous, because it may reflect the linguistic imprecision of natural language (Zhang, 1998), which individuals with a physical or mental illness use to describe their attempts at coping. On the other hand, this lack of precision could seriously compromise efforts to differentially assess and increase the effectiveness of such attempts.

Skinner et al. (2003, p. 219) apply a list of seven desiderata for category systems (i.e., "Category definitions are conceptually clear. The criteria for category membership are precise and unambiguous."). An examination of the results of a number of hierarchical confirmatory factor analyses reduced the more than 100 categories of coping responses to 14 families of coping (e.g., Problem-solving, Information-Seeking, Helplessness). However, Skinner et al. (2003) did not include considerations of meaning overlap and of utility in their analysis of the large number of coping classifications that appears in the literature. Thirteen families of coping and their associated lower-level coping responses may prove to be unwieldy, especially with regard to their use in guiding assessment and interventions.

Investigations of coping with SMI have also uncovered a relatively large variety of ways of coping with number, kind, and level of abstraction of these ways varying across studies (Garcelan & Rodriguez, 2002). The number of coping strategies, presented by Garcelan and Rodriguez (2002) varies from two (i.e., Boker, Brenner, & Wurgler, 1989) to nine (i.e., Cohen & Berk, 1985). Coping strategies also ranged from specific and concrete coping strategies, such as speaking to a friend and adjusting medication (Kumar, Thara, & Rajkumar, 1989) to general and abstract coping strategies such as cognitive coping (Mueser, Valentine, & Agresta, 1997).

In their literature review, Garcelan and Rodriguez (2002) distinguished between structural and functional approaches to coping with SMI. Structural approaches consist of descriptions of what a person does when faced with a problematic situation created by the SMI, whereas functional approaches refer to coping strategies that are conceptualized in terms of the role they play in the process of adaptation. According to this review, from the structural point of view, the most frequently reported coping strategies were behavioral (i.e., watching television, going for walks, participating in sports, playing a musical instrument). The functional coping strategies that had a pervasive influence on the study of coping with SMI were problem-oriented coping and emotion-oriented coping. With regard to these two ways of coping, Garcelan and Rodriguez (2002) conclude from their review that problem-solving is used by individuals who are the most cognitively competent and, as a consequence, experience less stress. In contrast, emotion-focused coping is used by individuals with greater psychiatric difficulties. They also suggest that the extensive use of behavioral coping strategies is due to the lower cognitive cost involved in the use of such strategies.

Whereas there are a number of theoretical paradigms that are more widely accepted in the domain of general coping, the coping responses and strategies in the domain of coping with SMI seem to be non-paradigmatic and relatively non-theoretical. Empirical research in this area also seems to have been relatively unsophisticated. Even the wide-spread adoption of the higher level coping categories of problem-focused and emotion-focused coping among SMI coping researchers may be more the product of the popularity of Lazarus and Folkman's Ways of Coping Scale rather than the serious commitment to a theoretical stance

(Snyder, 1999). This lack of theory may result in piecemeal, bottom-up research that cannot deal adequately with the complexity of the phenomena of coping with SMI. Therefore, the first facet of the multifaceted model of coping with SMI will be tentatively formulated in terms of a higher-level coping strategy, borrowed from a normative, developmental, self-regulation theory of human behavior (Brandstädter & Greve, 1994).

Brandstädter and Renner (1990) posited assimilation and accommodation as two processes central to theories of developmental self-control, which readily translate into coping strategies. According to theories of developmental self-regulation, individuals throughout their life-span invest effort in influencing their development and adapting psychologically to the requirements of the context in which they live (Lackovic-Grgin, Grgin, Penezic, & Soric, 2001). Individuals coordinate the above efforts by means of assimilative and accommodative processes. *Assimilation* refers to processes that direct efforts to transform the developing circumstances, in order that they are in line with the individuals' preferences; whereas *accommodation* consists of channeling efforts to transform the individuals' preferences to bring them more in line with the developing circumstances (Brandstädter and Renner, 1990). In Figure 16.1, these processes are applied to classifying ways of coping with the symptoms of a SMI. Examples of this application would be categorizing, quieting, or silencing hallucinatory voices (Wahass & Kent, 1997) as assimilative coping; while accepting hallucinatory voices as neutral aspects of the self (Romme & Escher, 1996) as accommodative coping.

Assimilative and accommodative coping are two elements of the first facet of this chapter's multifaceted model of coping with SMI. Individuals with SMI also cope with the problems and challenges by distancing and avoidance (Takai, Uekmatsu, Kaiya Inoue, & Ueki, 1990). Engagement and disengagement are two additional elements of the question about how individuals cope with the problems and challenges of SMI. For logical and semantic reasons, Skinner et al. (2003) criticize the use of approach-avoidance and engagement-disengagement as higher-level coping strategies. They argue that these distinctions are neither clear nor exhaustive. Nevertheless because assimilative and accommodative coping are different ways of relating to control over life-span tasks, coping strategies that increase or decrease opportunities for different kinds of control could prove to be valuable and informative. Thus, according to the multifaceted model presented here, individuals can cope with these problems and challenges by assimilation, by accommodation, by engagement, and by disengagement.

Figure 16.1 represents Facet A as a circle with assimilation opposite accommodation, with engagement posited opposite with disengagement, and assimilation and accommodation adjacent to engagement and disengagement. This configuration has theoretical implications. Accordingly, assimilative and accommodative coping strategies are putatively mutually exclusive, as are engagement and disengagement coping strategies. However, coping strategies can combine either assimilation or accommodation with either engagement or disengagement.

Coping with the Problems and Challenges of SMI

As can be seen from Figure 16.1 and the accompanying mapping sentence, the content Facet B specifies the kinds of problems and challenges confronting a person with a SMI. This facet's elements are the impairments and symptoms, disabilities, stigma, stress, low quality and meaning of life, and the mental illness diagnosis associated with SMI. In fact, Figure 16.1 represents Facet B as a simplex, which orders the problems and challenges of SMI from coping with relative specific symptoms and disabilities, located at the periphery of the figure, to coping with the relatively comprehensive and complex core of the mental illness diagnosis, located at the figure's center.

As pointed out above, many consumers and caregivers are uncomfortable with traditional mental illness diagnosis of SMI. Throughout this chapter, coping with this discomfort is referred to as coping with the mental illness diagnosis. As is discussed later in this chapter (see the section on coping and recovery), coping with a mental illness diagnosis concerns negotiating the meaning of the experience of SMI with the care-providers, who are often designated by society as the unofficial and official "gatekeepers" (i.e., those who make decisions about services) of individuals with a SMI. This element may significantly impact all of the other elements of Facet B, just as the other more general elements of this facet portrayed in Figure 16.1 putatively impact the more specific elements.

Proposing that the other specific problems and challenges faced by individuals with a SMI as one of the three facets of a multifaceted coping model is a step toward creating a hierarchical coping model. This model combines a higher-level coping category, which is the relatively abstract problems and challenges facet, with a lower-level coping category, which includes the relatively concrete, situation-oriented elements of this facet (see Chapter 3 for examples of other hierarchical coping models). Thus, it is consistent with a recommendation of a recent comprehensive and critical review of category systems for classifying ways of coping (Skinner et al., 2003). According to this recommendation, at least two levels of coping categories of intermediate abstraction are required to construct a complete and coherent set of categories, which organizes innumerable situation-specific, highly personal responses to stress.

The psychological and social consequences of SMI are potentially very stressful. Individuals with SMI frequently report low levels of quality of life (Rosenfeld, 1999; Shepherd, Muijen, Dean, & Cooney, 1996). They are often unemployed (Anthony & Blanch, 1987), live in substandard housing or are homeless (Susser, Struening, & Conover, 1989), and have little social support (Cresswell, Kuipers, & Power, 1992). In addition, their dependence on their families for assistance and social support can place a heavy burden of care-taking on family members (Leflley, 1996). The World Health Organization (2006b) has compiled multi-leveled statistics (i.e., policies, programs, services, financial resources) from numerous countries, in order to examine the resources available to individuals with SMI world-wide.

According to the traditional mental illness model of SMI, a reduction in quality of life is a direct consequence of the impairments, symptoms, and disabilities that are correlates of SMI (Anthony & Liberman, 1986). However, the stigma and prejudice that follow SMI also seriously limit access to the social resources that are necessary for the maintenance of acceptable standards of quality of life.

Survey research has shown that the general attitudes toward individuals with SMI are that they are considered to be dangerous and violent, developmentally delayed, unable to function and hold a job, weak and lazy, unpredictable, uncommunicative, and responsible for their own condition (Canadian Mental Health Association, 1994; Corrigan, 1998; Crisp, Gelder, Rix, Melttzer, & Rowlans, 2001; Miles, 1987). Due to such stereotypes and the prejudice that they produce, Byrne (2000) claims that discrimination against individuals with SMI is prevalent throughout the social and economic domains of life. However, Fischler and Booth's (1999) book is full of suggestions about accommodations that can help individuals with SMI function in the employment setting and maintain their jobs. Boston University (2006) also provides information about accommodations for SMI in the workplace.

The Context of Coping with the Problems and Challenges of SMI

People may cope with the impairments, symptoms, disabilities, stigma, stress, low quality of life, and the mental illness diagnosis by themselves, or they may cope with these problems and challenges with the help of other individuals. The latter may include family members, friends, or professionals. Consequently, the elements of the facet include personal coping and interpersonal coping. Personal coping refers to coping that is carried-out in a personal context (e.g., arguing with voices), while interpersonal coping refers to coping that occurs in an interpersonal context (e.g., discussing one's fear of voices with a friend). Other facets of the multifaceted coping model will, in part, determine the manner in which the personal or interpersonal context of a particular coping response is incorporated into the coping process.

As Skinner et al. (2003) pointed out, researchers have recently begun to appreciate the role that the social context plays in coping (Berg, Meegan, & Deviney, 1998). Nevertheless, most of the coping categories, which are included in the taxonomies of general coping, place a heavy emphasis on personal coping. For example, only one of the eight subscales of Folkman and Lazarus' (1988) popular Ways of Coping Questionnaire refers to seeking social support. Two of Skinner et al.'s (2003, Table 5) list of 13 potential higher-order families of coping might be characterized as having an interpersonal emphasis. One of these coping families, which bears the same "seeking social support" label as does Folkman and Lazarus' interpersonal coping subscale, is clearly interpersonal.

Designating the family of coping called "social withdrawal" as interpersonal is problematic because this type of coping is linked to the classification of coping by self-isolation. This form of coping may have a special significance for coping with a SMI such as schizophrenia. Social withdrawal is thought to be both one of the pre-illness impairments associated with schizophrenia (Willinger, Heiden, Meszaros, Formann, & Aschauer, 2001) and a coping strategy that individuals with schizophrenia use to avoid the stress of social interaction (Frese, 2000).

Social and interpersonal coping strategies are found in a number of taxonomies of coping with SMI. These include such coping strategies as social diversion (Cohen & Berk, 1985), asking for help (Thurm & Haefner, 1987), socialization (Carr, 1988), speaking to a close relative or friend (Kumar et al., 1989), increasing interpersonal contact (Dittmann & Schuttler, 1990), social change (Wahass & Kent, 1997), and social and non-social coping (Mueser et al., 1997).

Social Support Interventions

Training individuals with SMI to provide different forms of peer support is another example of the creation of an interpersonal context, which has the potential for empowering individuals to cope with the problems and challenges of a SMI (Gartner & Riessman, 1982). Yanos, Primsvera, and Knight (2001) found that individuals, who used consumer-run services, expressed greater social skills than those not enrolled in consumer services. They also showed that the relation between participation in consumer-run services and social functioning was partly mediated by the use of problem-focused coping. Another interpersonal psychosocial intervention for individuals with SMI is family psychoeducation (McFarlane, 2002). The focus of such an intervention is on the family of an individual with SMI, rather than the person him or herself.

There are a number of reasons for positing a personal-interpersonal context facet of coping in general, and of coping with SMI in particular. Baumeister, Faber, and Wallace (1999) argue that because interpersonal activity can serve both as intervention goal and as a means of achieving such goals, receiving various forms of social support could be an especially significant aid to coping. This factor is particularly pertinent for individuals with SMI, such as schizophrenia. Persistent and severe psychiatric disabilities have been shown to be associated with dysfunction and low levels of quality of life in the area of interpersonal relationships (Keefe et al., 1989).

Achieving control over the problems and consequences of SMI with the help of relationships with significant others can also have the negative connotations of dependency or secondary gain (i.e., eliciting benefits from one's illness). Accordingly, Smith et al. (2000) limit their findings of positive relations between interpersonal agency, perceived primary control, and psychosocial well-being with a question as to the "threshold point beyond which continued support leads to dependence, enmeshment, and decreased feelings of agency" (p. 466). In addition, social interactions can sometimes constitute a source of stress for individuals with SMI (Frese, 2000).

Because Figure 16.1 depicts Facet C as a dichotomous simplex, the context of coping with a SMI can theoretically vary from predominately personal to predominately impersonal. Therefore, specifying the extent to which context of coping is personal or interpersonal should be an essential aspect of descriptions of coping with SMI.

Implications of the Multifaceted Model of Coping with SMI for Research, Assessment, Intervention, and Recovery

Researching the Substance and Structure of Coping with SMI

As pointed-out above, Figure 16.1 presents a hypothetical structural model of coping with SMI that is based on this chapter's multifaceted theory of coping with SMI and the accompanying mapping sentence. The structural model and mapping sentence can play a two-fold heuristic role. It raises a number of theoretical and empirical questions, both substantive and structural, about coping with SMI. It also provides a framework for a critical examination of past and present research, assessment, and interventions related to coping with SMI.

Multidimensional methods exist for evaluating the validity of models, such as the multifaceted model of coping with SMI, as a whole (Borg & Shye, 1995; see Guttman & Levy, 1991 for an example of such an evalution). Quantitatively more-exact methods are available for assessing separate parts of this structural model. The circular ordering of elements of a facet, such as that which characterizes Facet A, has been termed a circumplex (Guttman & Greenbaum, 1998). There are number of quantitative ways of testing the circumplex structure of the ways of coping facet (Acton and Revelle, 2002; Tracey & Rounds, 1997). Inconsistencies between the findings of these assessments and the structural model presented in Figure 16.1 could serve as a basis for modifying the model.

The validity of other facets of coping with SMI can also be investigated. For example, Folkman and Moskovitz (2004) raise the possibility of a temporal facet for coping in general. Such a facet could differentiate between coping with past harm or loss (reactive passing), coping with critical events that are relatively certain to occur in the near future (reactive coping), coping with an uncertain potential in the distant future (preventive coping), and coping with future challenges that are opportunities for growth (proactive coping) (Schwarzer & Knoll, 2003). A temporal coping facet should be especially pertinent for SMI, because SMIs are conceptualized as having a definite course. Heinrichs, Cohen, and Carpenter (1985) found that over half of the participants in their retrospective study were able to identify and assess the onset of deterioration in their condition, and thus could seek help before their condition became worse. Consequently, for these individuals, outpatient care was feasible and effective.

While including temporal aspects of SMI was beyond the scope of this chapter, time may play an important role in the model that was proposed in this chapter. A structural model for each element of such a facet (i.e., past, near future, distant future) would have to be developed, in order to integrate a temporal facet into the model.

Developing and Assessing Coping-Focused Interventions for SMI

The structural model in Figure 16.1 presented in this chapter can also be used to examine critically efforts at developing and assessing interventions that focus on helping persons make effective use of strategies for coping with SMI. Much of the research into coping with SMI deals with a few elements of the problems and challenges facet (Facet B) of the multifaceted model of coping with SMI. These elements are the impairments and symptoms (e.g., Farhall & Gehrke, 1998; Wiedl, 1992; Yanos, Knight, & Bremer, 2003) and stress (e.g. Horan & Blanchard, 2003) that are associated with SMI.

Psychosocial interventions for individuals with SMI usually endorse the construct of coping specifically for symptoms and stress. Thus, the two modules of the Illness Management and Recovery intervention, *Coping with Stress* and *Coping with Problems and Symptoms* (Gingerich & Mueser, 2005), could be used to promote coping. Although the research and professional literature on social support and family psychoeducation relate to coping within an interpersonal context, the coping literature does not generally emphasize the importance of distinguishing between the personal and interpersonal context (Facet C) of coping with a SMI.

Garcelan and Rodriguez (2002) offer a number of related tentative conclusions, regarding the effectiveness of coping strategies, from their review of the research on coping with SMI. One conclusion is that the most effective ways of coping with impairments and symptoms, among individuals subject to high levels of stress and tension, are such strategies as acceptance of the disorder and non-confrontation. Acceptance of the disorder could be considered an example of accommodation, whereas non-confrontation could be a mild form of disengagement. Another conclusion is that the most effective ways of coping with impairments and symptoms, among individuals subject to low levels of stress and tension, is problem-focused coping. Problem-solving, which is aimed at changing the situation of the person with SMI, could be a form of assimilation and engagement. Assuming that these conclusions are valid for coping with the impairments and symptoms of SMI, they raise the question of whether they can be generalized to other elements of the problems and challenges facet (Facet C) of the multifaceted model.

One of the main goals of facet analysis is the development of a mapping sentence and structural model that can be used to systematically generate a comprehensive and representative set of items to measure a multifaceted universe of content. This deductive approach to measurement differs from an inductive approach, which most often is applied to develop measures of coping with SMI. As mentioned above, the latter approach usually formulates its pool of items from interviews with individuals with SMI (e.g., Yanos et al., 2003).

Garcelan and Rodriguez (2002) criticize intervention programs (e.g., Coping Strategy Enhancement; Tarrier et al., 1993) that identify the coping strategies, which are used naturally by individuals with a SMI, and then teach them to use these strategies systematically – because natural strategies may not necessarily be effective. This criticism can also be leveled against coping strategy assessment that is based solely on the spontaneous responses of individuals with SMI. A theory-based multifaceted model of coping with SMI can be used to produce a pool of coping strategies, which is representative of the facets' elements. This pool can be reviewed by a panel of service consumers and providers for comprehensibility and naturalness of language and then be used to construct coping measures, which can be applied toward evaluating the effectiveness of the coping strategies. Intervention programs can subsequently be formulated, which help individuals increase their coping efficacy by exposing them to a representative sample of relatively effective coping strategies.

Use of the questionnaire is the prevalent method of assessing of strategies for coping in general and of coping with SMI in particular. However, a multifaceted structural model of coping with SMI does not mandate the assessment of coping strategies by questionnaire. As this chapter's multifaceted structural model of coping reflects, coping strategies are complex phenomena. Skinner et al. (2003) designate such higher-order coping strategies as assimilation and accommodation as types of action that not only "incorporates behavior but also requires simultaneous consideration of individuals' emotions, attention, and goals" (p. 229). Thus, the difficulties with the classification of coping strategies, which were specified by Skinner et al. (2003), may not only be logical and semantic, but they also may stem from over-reliance on relatively simplistic questionnaire measures of complex phenomena.

The contextually rich narrative methods of assessment that have emerged from recent developments in narrative research and therapy may be more appropriate for the assessment of coping with SMI (Hardtke & Angus, 2004; Ridgway, 2001). Narrative research in the context of SMI suggests that individuals with SMI also construct life histories, in order to gain control over their lives and to create a sense of purpose in the face of serious life events (Lysaker & Lysaker, 2002; Roe & Ben Yishai, 1999; Roe & Kravetz, 2003). Folkman and Moskovitz (2004) provide a number of examples of the use of narratives to assess coping. Narrative assessment methods could be constructed and used to obtain nuanced evaluations of the different facets of coping with SMI.

Coping Interventions and Evidence-Based Practices

If coping is defined broadly, many psychosocial interventions for individuals with SMI would be expected to include significant reference to coping strategies. A review of evidence-based practices (EBP) (Drake, Merrens, & Lynde, 2005), also known as Empirically-Supported Treatments (EST) in mental health and psychiatry, indicates that the literature describing these practices frequently mentions coping. However, this literature does not systematically make use of the various facets of coping included in this chapter's model.

An EBP is an intervention that critical research has shown to be effective in assisting individuals with SMI to achieve desirable outcomes (Mueser et al., 2003). Because individuals with SMI, who are living in the community and receiving treatment and rehabilitation, often cannot be randomly assigned to different treatment groups, a levels-of-evidence approach has been suggested (Cook, Toprac, & Shore, 2004), which refers to levels of the quality of the evidence for a practice's effectiveness.

The strongest evidence usually consists of psychiatric rehabilitation practices, which are based on rigorously designed studies, using such scientific methods as randomized clinical trials, well-controlled, quasi-experimental designs, and multifaceted, multidimensional measures of outcomes. The weakest type of evidence refers to psychiatric rehabilitation practices that are supported by expert-panel recommendations that are based on controlled and non-controlled empirical research evidence.

The latter expert-panel approach includes research scientists and teams of multiple stakeholders, consisting of consumers, family members, researchers, clinicians and administrators, who review studies of psychiatric rehabilitation practices in order to develop their criteria for evaluating whether these practices are evidence-based (Cook et al., 2004; Drake et al., 2001). A recent application of the expert-panel approach has produced a list of EBPs. These EBPs are described in a series of papers in 2001 published in the journal, *Psychiatric Services*. These papers included the following six EBPs:

1) **Supported employment**, which uses job coaches to help individuals with SMI acquire and maintain competitive jobs in the community, while receiving the supports that they need, 2) **Illness Management and Recovery (IMR)**, which is a curriculum-based approach to helping consumers acquire the knowledge and skills that they need to manage their illnesses effectively and achieve personal recovery goals (Mueser et al., 2002), 3) **Collaborative psychopharmacology**, which includes a standard approach to documenting and monitoring symptoms and side effects, and guidelines for systematically making joint care-consumer and care-provider decisions about medication, 4) **Assertive Community Treatment (ACT)**, which centers on the active coordination and integration of services by a small professional staff for individuals with SMI (Rapp & Goscha, 2004), 5) **Family psychoeducation**, which focuses on improving the future functioning of all family members and strives to form a collaborative relationship between the treatment team and the family (Dixon et al., 2001), and 6) **Integrated Dual-Diagnosis Treatment**, which treat individuals with both a mental illness and a substance-abuse disorder.

Although a number of the above EBPs refer explicitly to coping, none of the interventions are guided by the kind of coping model that has been presented in this chapter. As pointed-out above, illness management and recovery includes two explicit coping modules. One module addresses coping with the impairments and symptoms of SMI, while the other presents strategies for coping with stress. By encouraging the consumer to assess her or his current modes of coping with SMI and exposing her or him to various other modes of coping, this intervention may also suggest ways of dealing with the mental illness diagnoses. The remaining interventions focus on the inter-personal context of the consumers' struggle with their SMI and emphasize such assimilative coping strategies as information-seeking and problem-solving. Supported employment involves assimilative attempts to increase the quality and meaning of life. However, it does not explicitly provide consumers with coping strategies.

Coping and Recovery

A decade ago, recovery, as an outcome, was given an ideological connotation by both consumers and providers of mental health and psychiatric services (Anthony, 1993; Deegan, 1988; Jacobson, 2004). Since then, the recovery movement has become a significant source of optimism for individuals with SMI. Before that, this term had been used to refer to mainly medical outcomes (i.e., the remission of symptoms), following mental health and psychiatric services.

However, a series of articles on mental health and psychiatric outcome-research spanning 40 years, indicated that, notwithstanding Kraeplin's initial pessimistic view of schizophrenia as following a deteriorating course, recovery from schizophrenia is achievable, with approximately 20–25% achieving complete recovery and with another 40–45% achieving social recovery (Warner, 2004). Jacobson (2004) describes two approaches to recovery, in terms of a serious disagreement between "consumers" with a reform agenda and "survivors" with a liberation agenda.

Using this chapters' multifaceted model of coping with SMI, it can be said that individuals in the recovery movement, whether they are consumers or survivors, have shifted from the traditional emphasis on assimilative, engaged coping with the impairments and symptoms of SMI to assimilative, engaged coping with the stigma, reduced quality of life, and meaning in life that accompany SMI. Yet, whereas consumers seem to accept their mental illness diagnosis and to engage in accommodative coping to deal with the consequences of this accep-tance, survivors appear to be engaged in assimilative coping with this diagnosis. Individuals in the survivor movement argue that the unequal power relations, which are inherent in mental-health systems, seriously limit their control of their lives. Therefore, they engage in negotiating the meaning and the implications of the experiences, which underlie their mental illness diagnosis, with their care-providers, so as to establish a more symmetric power relationship with them.

The coping with SMI model, proposed in this chapter, supports the holistic recovery viewpoint, because the model is multifaceted, comprehensive, and includes environmental influences. Hence, individuals, who take the recovery perspective, could utilize our non-linear model as a framework for research and interventions that focus on coping with SMI.

Illustrating the Model Using Schizophrenia as a Prototypical Severe Mental Illness

Schizophrenia demands the attention of rehabilitation professionals in the mental health field, due to its relatively high rate of prevalence, its variable course that is generally characterized by recurrent exacerbations and remissions of the illness, the stigma that it generates, and its dire consequences for quality of life and meaning in life. Due to the lack of a consensus regarding the etiology of schizophrenia, the diagnosis of schizophrenia is usually based on the manifestation of a specific set of symptoms with a specified duration and intensity.

Schizophrenia is considered a major psychosis, because individuals are given the diagnosis of schizophrenia when they exhibit symptoms indicating that they are having difficulty maintaining contact with reality. Although there are number of ways of classifying these symptoms, one of the most common classifications divides them into: (a) Positive symptoms, which consist of hallucinations and delusions; (b) negative symptoms, which include blunted affect, poverty of speech, anhedonia, and asociality; and (c) disorganized behavior and thought, manifested as inappropriate dress and conduct, and shifting from one topic to a completely unrelated topic during a conversation (Frith, 1992).

In addition to these symptoms, to receive a diagnosis of schizophrenia, a person must exhibit deterioration in functioning in such major areas of life as interpersonal relations, work, education, or self-care. According to the guidelines of the *DSM-IV-TR* (APA, 2000), a person should only be diagnosed with schizophrenia if the aforementioned symptoms are experienced for at least six months. During this period, that person must exhibit at least one month of such active phase symptoms as positive symptoms, negative symptoms, and/or disorganized behavior and thought.

A great deal of uncertainty and controversy surrounds the etiology of schizophrenia. The present understanding of schizophrenia generally attributes a major role to the central nervous system, in its etiology and treatment. Explanations of the development and/or course of schizophrenia encompass genetics, chemical imbalance of a variety of neurotransmitters, congenital viral infection, congenital subtle trauma to the central nervous system, and social stress (Warner, 2004). The stress-diathesis (i.e., innate vulnerability) model is a prevalent theory of the etiology of schizophrenia. According to this account, a chemical imbalance of a variety of neurotransmitters and/or various sources of congenital, subtle damage to the central nervous system create a propensity for the development of schizophrenia, which is awakened by the biopsychosocial stresses of late adolescence and early adulthood.

The approximate age of onset for men is between the late teens and the middle twenties. In contrast, the onset for women is typically between the mid-twenties and the mid-forties. The prevalence of schizophrenia has been estimated to be between 0.5% and 1.5%, with an annual incidence that range from 0.5 and 5.0 per 10,000 (APA, 2000). Although the course of schizophrenia is relatively heterogeneous, it is characterized for many individuals by a prodromal phase followed by exacerbations, remissions, and relapses. The term *prodromal* means the onset of symptoms, while the prodromal phase refers to both the period leading up to the first psychotic episode and to the period during a remission that precedes a relapse. During the prodromal phase, many of the individuals who eventually show the acute signs of schizophrenia manifest a gradual development of such symptoms as marked impairment in functioning, odd or bizarre ideation, magical thinking, and social withdrawal and isolation (McGorry, Mckenzie, Jackson, Waddel, & Curry, 2000). Identifying the signs that make-up the prodromal phase has been recommended as an important step in interventions, which can prevent either the onset of schizophrenia (McGorry et al., 2000) or relapse (Mendel, 1989).

The long-term outcomes of different types of schizophrenia are also quite variable. Retrospective (Stephens & Astrup, 1963; Vaillant, 1964) and prospective (Strauss & Carpenter, 1972) follow-up studies, some carried-out after considerably long-term follow-up periods (Harding, Brooks, Ashikaga, Strauss, & Breier, 1987a, 1987b; Huber, Gross, & Schuttler, 1975; Tsuang, Woolson, & Fleming, 1979), and meta-analytic studies (Hegarty, Baldessarini, Tohen, Waternaux, & Oepen, 1994) have challenged the once-widespread notion of uniformly poor outcomes for people with schizophrenia and related mental disorders. These studies have revealed their heterogeneous course, which often includes partial to full recovery (Warner, 2004).

Part of this more optimistic perspective on outcomes for individuals with SMI appears to be a function of changes in the manner in which an outcome is defined. Early research focused on assessing outcomes in terms of a reduction in symptom-severity (Overall & Gorham, 1962) and hospitalization (Bond & Resnick, 2000). Later research by Strauss and Carpenter (Strauss & Carpenter, 1972, 1974, 1977; Carpenter & Strauss, 1991) focused on broader outcome domains, including duration of hospitalization, quantity and quality of social relationships, severity of symptoms, and level of work-function.

Due to its effectiveness in reducing the positive symptoms and the disorganized behavior and thought of schizophrenia, antipsychotic medication, which act upon various neurotransmitters in the central nervous system (i.e., dopamine and serotonin), have become a major means of reducing symptoms and the chances of relapse. At present, two kinds of medication are used to treat schizophrenia: standard antipsychotics (once termed neuroleptics) and new antipsychotics (also termed atypical antipsychotics). From 10% to 45% of persons with schizophrenia who take standard antipsychotic drugs continue to experience prolonged moderate to severe disorganization and positive and/or negative symptoms along with poor social and vocational functioning (Meltzer, 1997).

When compared to new antipsychotics, standard antipsychotics are also thought to have less of an effect on the negative symptoms of schizophrenia and may result in serious side effects, such as sleepiness, muscle stiffness, tremors, weight gain, and tardive dyskinesia. Tardive dyskinesia is a particular disturbing involuntary movement disorder, which frequently includes puckering of the lips and tongue or writhing of the arms and legs. The newer antipsychotic medications are considered to elicit less-disturbing side effects, and some of them are thought to reduce both the positive and negative symptoms and cognitive impairment associated with schizophrenia (Julien, 2001).

At present, a broad spectrum of psychosocial and rehabilitation interventions are available to help individuals with schizophrenia manage and cope with the negative consequences of their illness. However, in comparison with these interventions, the pharmacotherapeutic interventions are considered the treatment of choice, which may possibly be due to remnants of the view of schizophrenia as an inevitably progressive and incurable illness (Roth & Fonagy, 1996).

Some of the psychosocial and rehabilitation interventions that have been used with individuals with schizophrenia include individual and group psychotherapy, vocational training, job acquisition and social skills training, social support, family education, and self-help groups (Bond & Resnick, 2000). Because antipsychotic medication does not ameliorate the symptoms, rejection, loss of social standing and self worth, unemployment, poverty, and homelessness that accompany schizophrenia for a significant percentage of persons with this condition (Warner, 2004), these psychosocial and rehabilitation interventions are especially important.

The model of coping with SMI presented in Figure 16.1 can serve as a guide for such interventions. This model is multifaceted and nonlinear. Therefore, it is especially appropriate for dealing with the heterogeneous courses of the illness that consumers with schizophrenia exhibit to the individuals and institutions, which are committed to providing them with the assistance that they may require to improve their lives.

Schizophrenia confronts both the care consumers and care providers with issues that are related to the facets and facet components of the multifaceted model of coping with SMI. Facet A concerns a central choice that consumers can make with regard to these issues. They can choose to accommodate these issues as expressions of a mental illness and engage in learning how best to live with this illness (see Frese, 2000, for an example of a care-provider and care-consumer, who accepts the medical model of schizophrenia) or they can assimilate these issues as part of their search for a self definition of identity and their examination of existential and/or spiritual issues (see Bassman, 2000, who treats schizophrenia as an existential and spiritual challenge).

Further, Facet B of the coping with SMI model focuses on such issues as the uncertain and controversial nature of the conditions, which give rise to the phenomena that is labeled diagnostically as schizophrenia, and the reduced quality of life and meaning in life, the stigma, the stress, the disabilities, the impairments and symptoms, and the side effects of the antipsychotic medications that are associated with this diagnosis.

Facet C pinpoints the intense ambivalence that consumers with schizophrenia often experience with regard to interpersonal relationships. Consumers often have to balance the benefits of interpersonal support against their special sensitivity to interpersonal stress. Thus, the model can facilitate the dialogue between the care-consumers and care-providers, as to the former person's choice of coping responses when faced with the challenge of schizophrenia.

Coping with SMI: Summary and Conclusions

As should be evident from this chapter, both coping and SMI refer to complex social and personal phenomena about which there is a great deal of controversy. A multifaceted approach to coping with SMI has been presented to clarify and integrate the conceptual, empirical, professional, and ideological issues that are the source of much of this complexity and controversy. According to this model, individuals who cope with SMI can decide how to answer three related major questions. As explained in this chapter, these questions concern the problems and challenges of SMI, ways of dealing with these problems and challenges, and the personal and interpersonal context of coping with these problems and challenges.

Figure 16.1 represents a way of framing possible answers to the above questions within areas of a three-dimensional, multifaceted coping model. This representation is intended to be sufficiently flexible, so as to incorporate the complexity and controversy surrounding coping with SMI, while, at the same time, providing guidelines for critical accumulative research, which could be used to modify significantly this putative model. Hopefully, this model could also serve as a map of a variety of coping strategies with the potential to help individuals with SMI make sense of and gain control over their lives.

References

Acton, G. S., & Revelle, W. (2002). Interpersonal personality measures show circumplex structure based on new psychometric criteria. *Journal of Personality Assessment, 79*(3), 446–471.

American Psychiatric Association. (2000). *Diagnostic and statistical manual of mental Disorders DSM IV-TR.* (4th ed., Text Revision). Washington, DC: American Psychiatric Association.

Andres K., Pfammatter, M., Fries A., & Brenner, H. D. (2003). The significance of coping as a therapeutic variable for the outcome of psychological therapy in schizophrenia. *European Psychiatry, 18,* 149–154.

Anthony, W. (1993). Recovery from mental illness: The guiding vision of the mental health system in the 1990s.*Psychosocial Rehabilitation Journal, 16*(4), 13–14.

Anthony, W., & Blanch, A. (1987). Supported employment for persons who are psychiatrically disabled: An historical and conceptual perspective. *Psychosocial Rehabilitation Journal, 11*(2), 5–23.

Anthony W. A., & Liberman, R. P. (1986). The practice of psychiatric rehabilitation: Historical, conceptual and research base. *Schizophrenia Bulletin, 12*, 542–558.

Bassman, R. (2000). Agents, not objects: Our fights to be. *Journal of Clinical Psychology, 56*, 1395–1411.

Baumeister, R. F., Farber, J. E., & Wallace, H. M. (1999). Coping and ego depletion: Recovery after the coping process. In C. R. Snyder (Ed.), *Coping: The psychology of what works* (pp. 50–69). New York: Oxford University Press.

Berg, C., Meegan, S., & Deviney, F. (1998). A social-contextual model of coping with every day problems across the life span. *International Journal of Behavioral Development, 22*, 239–261.

Boker, W., Brenner, H. D., & Wurgler, S. (1989). Vulnerability-linked deficiencies, psychopathology and coping behavior of schizophrenics and their relatives. *British Journal of Psychiatry, 155*(Suppl. 5), 128–135.

Bond, G. R., & Resnick, S. G. (2000). Psychiatric rehabilitation. In R. G. Frank & T. R. Elliot (Eds.), *Handbook of rehabilitation psychology* (pp. 235–258). Washington, DC: American Psychological Association.

Borg, I., & Shye, S. (1995). *Facet theory: Form and content*. Newbury Park, CA: Sage.

Boston University. (2006). *Reasonable accommodations for people with psychiatric disabilities: An online resource for employers and educators*. Retrieved on July 21, 2006, from http://www.bu.edu/cpr/reasaccom/

Brandstädter, J., & Greve, W. (1994). The aging self: Stabilizing and protective processes. *Developmental Review, 14*, 52–80.

Brandstädter, J., & Renner, G. (1990). Tenacious goal pursuit and flexible goal adjustment: Explication and age-related analysis of assimilative and accommodative strategies of coping. *Psychology and Aging, 5*, 58–67.

Byrne, P. (2000). Stigma of mental illness and ways of diminishing it. *Advances in Psychiatric Treatment, 6*, 65–72.

Canadian Mental Health Association. (1994). *Mental health stigma campaign public education strategy. Final report*. Toronto: Canadian Mental Health Association, Ontario Division.

Carpenter, W. T., & Strauss, J. S. (1991). The prediction of outcome in schizophrenia IV. Eleven-year follow-up of the Washington IPSS cohort. *Journal of Nervous and Mental Diseases, 179*, 517–525.

Carr, V. (1988). Patient's techniques for coping with schizophrenia: An exploratory study. *British Journal of Medical Psychology, 61*, 339–414.

Cohen, C. I., & Berk, L. A. (1985). Personal coping styles of schizophrenic outpatients. *Hospital and Community Psychiatry, 36*, 407–410.

Cook, J. A., Toprac, M., & Shore, S. E. (2004). Combining evidenced-based practice with stakeholder consensus to enhance psychosocial rehabilitation services in the Texas benefit design initiative. *Psychiatric Rehabilitation Journal, 27*(4), 308–318.

Corrigan, P. W. (1998). The impact of stigma on severe mental illness. *Cognitive and behavioral practice, 5*, 201–222.

Costa, P. T., Sommerfield, M. R., & McCrae, R. R. (1996). Personality and coping: A reconceptualization. In M. Zeidner & N. S. Endler (Eds.), *Handbook of coping: Theory Research, applications* (pp. 44–61). New York: Wiley.

Cresswell, C. M., Kuipers, L., & Power, M. J. (1992). Social networks and support in long term psychiatric patients. *Psychological Medicine, 22*(4), 1019–1026.

Crisp, A. H., Gelder, M. G., Rix, S., Meltzer, H. I., & Rowlands, O. J. (2000). Stigmatization of people with mental illnesses. *British Journal of Psychiatry, 177*, 4–7.

Deegan, P. E. (1988). Recovery: The lived experience of rehabilitation. *Psychosocial Rehabilitation Journal, 11*(4), 11–19.

Dicky, B. (2005). What is severe mental illness? In R. Drake, M. Merrens, & D. Lynde (Eds.), *Evidence-based mental health practice: A textbook* (pp. 1–18). New York: Norton.

Dittmann, J., & Schuttler, R. (1990). Disease consciousness and coping strategies of patients with schizophrenic psychosis. *Acta Psychiatrica Scandinavica, 82*, 318–322.

Dixon, L., McFarlane, W., Lefley, H., Luckstead, A., Cohen, M., Fallon, I., et al. (2001). Evidence based practices for services to family members of people with psychiatric disability. *Psychiatric Services, 52*, 903–910.

Drake, R. E., Howard, H. G., Leff, H. S., Lehman, A. F., Dixon, L., Mueser, K. T., et al. (2001). Implementing evidenced based practices in routine mental health service settings. *Psychiatric Services, 52*(2), 179–182.

Drake, R., Merrens, M., & Lynde, D. (Eds.). (2005). *Evidence-based mental health practice: A textbook*. New York: Norton.

Engel, G. L. (1977). The need for a new medical model: A challenge for biomedicine. *Science, 196*, 129–136.

Engel, G. L. (1980). The clinical application of the biopsychosocial model. *American Journal of Psychiatry, 137*, 535–544.

Epstein, J., Barker, P., Vorburger, M., & Murtha, C. (2002). *Serious mental illness and its co-occurrence with substance use disorders* (DHHS Publication No. SMA 04-3905, Analytic Series A-24). Rockville, MD: Substance Abuse and Mental Health Services Administration, Office of applied Studies.

Falloon, J. R., & Talbot, R. E. (1981). Persistent auditory hallucinations: Coping mechanism and implications for management. *Psychological Medicine, 11*, 329–339.

Farhall, J., & Gehrke, M. (1997). Coping with hallucinations: Exploring stress and coping framework. *British Journal Clinical Psychology, 36*, 259–261.

Fischler, G. L., & Booth, N. (1999). *Vocational impact of psychiatric disorders: A guide for rehabilitation professionals*. Gaithersburg, MD: Aspen Publishers.

Folkman, S., & Lazarus, R. S. (1988). *The ways of coping questionnaire*. Palo Alto, CA: Consulting Psychologists Press.

Folkman, S., & Moskowitz, J. T. (2004). Coping: Pitfalls and promise. *Annual Review of Psychology, 55*, 745–774.

Frese, F. J. (2000). Psychology practitioners and schizophrenia: A view from both sides. *Journal of Clinical Psychology, 56*, 1414–1426.

Frith, C. D. (1992). *The cognitive neuropsychology of schizophrenia*. Hove, UK: Erlbaum.

Garcelan, S. P., & Rodriguez, A. G. (2002). Coping strategies in psychotics: Conceptualizations and research results. *Psychology in Spain, 6*, 26–40.

Gartner, A., & Riessman, F. (1982). Self help and mental health. Hospital and community. *Psychiatry, 33*, 631–635.

Gingerich, S., & Mueser, K. T. (2005). Illness management and recovery. In R. E. Drake, M. R. Merrens, & D. W. Lynde (Eds.), *Evidence based mental health practices: A Textbook* (pp. 395–424). New York: Norton.

Gol, A. R., & Cook, S. W. (2004). Exploring the underlying dimensions of coping: A concept map approach. *Journal of Social and Clinical Psychology, 23*, 155–171.

Guttman, R., & Greenbaum, C. W. (1998). Facet theory: Its development and current status. *European Psychologist, 3*, 13–36.

Guttman, L., & Levy, S. (1991). Two structural laws for intelligence tests. *Intelligence, 15*, 79–103.

Harding, C. M., Brooks, G. W., Ashikaga, T., Strauss, J. S., & Breier, A. (1987a). The Vermont longitudinal study of persons with severe mental illness, II: Long-term outcome of subjects who retrospectively met DSM-III criteria for schizophrenia. *American Journal of Psychiatry, 144*, 727–735.

Harding, C. M., Brooks, G. W., Ashikaga, T., Strauss, J. S., & Breier, A. (1987b). The Vermont longitudinal study of persons with severe mental illness, I: Methodology, study sample, and overall status 32 years later. *American Journal of Psychiatry, 144*, 718–726.

Hardtke, K. K., & Angus, L. E. (2004). The narrative assessment interview: Assessing self-change in psychotherapy. In L. E. Angus & J. McLeod (Eds.), *The handbook of narrative and psychotherapy: Practice, theory, and research* (pp. 247–262). Thousand Oaks, CA: Sage.

Hegarty, J. D., Baldessarini, B. J., Tohen, M., Waternaux, C., & Oepen, G. (1994) One hundred years of schizophrenia: A meta-analysis of the outcome literature. *American Journal of Psychiatry, 151*, 1409–1416.

Heinrichs, D. W., Cohen B. P., & Carpenter, W. T., Jr. (1985). Early insight and the management of schizophrenic decompensation. *Journal of Nervous and Mental Disease, 173*, 133–138.

Horan, W. P., & Blanchard, J. J. (2003). Emotional responses to psychosocial stress in schizophrenia: the role of individual differences in affective traits and coping. *Schizophrenia Research, 60*(2), 271–283.

Horowitz, A. (2002). *Creating mental illness.* Chicago, IL: University of Chicago Press.

Huber, G., Gross, G., & Schuttler, R. (1975). A long-term follow-up study of schizophrenia: Psychiatric course of illness and prognosis. *Acta Psychiatrica Scandinavica, 52*, 49–57.

Jacobson, N. (2004). *In recovery: The making of mental health policy.* Nashville, TN: Vanderbilt University Press.

Julien, R. M. (2001). *A primer of drug action.* New York: Freeman.

Keefe, R. S. E., Mohs, R. C., Losonczt, M. F., Davidson, M., Silverman, J. M., Horvath, T. B., et al. (1989). Premorbid sociosexual functioning and long-term outcome in schizophrenia. *American Journal of Psychiatry, 146*(2), 206–211.

Kumar, S., Thara, R., & Rajkumar, S. (1989). Coping with symptoms of relapse in schizophrenia. *European Archives of Psychiatry and Neurological Sciences, 239*, 213–215.

Lackovic-Grgin, K., Grgin, T., Penezic, Z., & Soric, I. (2001). Some predictors of primary Control: Development in three transitional periods of life. *Journal of Adult Development, 8*, 149–160.

Leflley, H. P. (1996). *Family caregiving in mental illness.* Thousand Oaks, CA: Sage.

Lysaker, P. H., & Lysaker, J. T. (2002). Narrative structure in psychosis: Schizophrenia and the dialogical self. *Theory in Psychology, 12*, 207–220.

McFarlane, W. R. (2002). Family psychoeducation & schizophrenia: A review of the literature. In D. H. Sprenkle (Ed.), *Effectiveness research in marriage and family therapy* (pp. 255–288). Alexandria, VA: American Association for Marriage and Family Therapy.

McGorry, P. D., Mckenzie, D., Jackson, H. J., Waddel, F., & Curry, C. (2000). Can we improve the diagnostic efficiency and predictive power of prodromal symptoms for schizophrenia. *Schizophrenia Research, 42*, 91–100.

Meltzer, H. Y. (1997). Treatment resistant schizophrenia-the role of clozapine. *Current Medical Research Opinion, 14*(1), 1–20.

Mendel, W. M. (1989). *Treating schizophrenia.* San Francisco: Jossey-Bass.

Miles, A. (1987). *The mentally ill in contemporary society* (2nd ed.). Oxford, England: Basil Blackwell.

Mueser, K. T., Corrigan, P. W., Hilton, D. et al. (2002). Illness management and recovery for severe mental illness: A review of the research. *Psychiatric Services, 53*, 1272–1284.

Mueser, K. T., Valentine, D. P., & Agresta, J. (1997). Coping with negative symptoms of schizophrenia: Patient and family perspectives, *Schizophrenia Bulletin, 10*, 329–339.

Overall, J. E., & Gorham, D. R. (1962). The brief psychiatric rating scale. *Psychological Reports, 10*, 799–812.

Peck, M. C., & Scheffler, R. M. (2002). An analysis of the definitions of mental illness used in state parity laws. *Psychiatric Services, 53*, 1089–1095.

Rapp, C. A., & Goscha, R. J. (2004). The principles of effective case management of mental health services. *Psychiatric Rehabilitation Journal, 27*(4), 319–333.

Ridgway, P. (2001). Restorying psychiatric disability: Learning from first person recovery stories. *Psychiatric Rehabilitation Journal, 24*(4), 335–343.

Roe, D., & Ben Yishai, A. (1999). Exploring the relationship between the person and disorder among individuals hospitalized for psychotic disorder. *Psychiatry, 62*(4), 370–380.

Roe, D., & Kravetz, S. (2003). Different ways of being aware of a psychiatric disability: A multifunctional narrative approach to insight into mental disorder. *Journal of Nervous and Mental Disease, 191*(7), 417–424.

Romme, M. A. J., & Escher, A. D. M. A. C. (1996). Empowering people who hear voices. In G. Haddock & P. D. Slade (Eds.), *Cognitive-behavioural interventions with psychotic disorders* (pp. 137–167). London: Routeledge.

Rosenfeld, S. (1999). Factors contributing to the subjective quality of life of the chronic mentally ill. *Journal of Health and Social Behavior, 33*, 299–315.

Roth, A., & Fonagy, P. (1996). *What works for whom?* New York: Guilford Press.

Roth, M., & Krull, J. (1986). *The reality of mental illness.* New York: Cambridge University Press.

Schwazer, R. & Knoll, N. (2003). Positive coping: Mastering demands and searching for meaning. In S. I. Lopez & C. R. Snyder (Eds.), *Positive psychological assessment: A handbook of models and measures (pp 393–409)* Washington, DC: American Psychology Association.

Shepherd, G., Muijen, M., Dean, R., & Cooney, M. (1996). Residential care in hospital and in the community quality of care and quality of life. *British Journal of Psychiatry, 168*(4), 448–456.

Skinner, E. A., Edge, K., Altman, J., & Sherwood, H. (2003). Searching for the structure of coping: A review and critique of category systems for classifying ways of coping. *Psychological Bulletin, 129*, 216–269.

Smith, G. C., Kohn, S. I., Savage-Stevens, S. E., Finch, J. J., Ingate, R., & Yaon-Ok, L. (2000). The effects of personal and interpersonal agency on perceived control and psychological well-being in adulthood. *Gerontologist, 40*, 458–468.

Snyder, C. R. (1999). *Coping: The psychology of what works.* New York: Oxford University Press.

Stephens, J. H., & Astrup, C. (1963). Prognosis in "process" and "non-process" schizophrenia. *American Journal of Psychiatry, 119,* 945–953.

Strauss, J. S., & Carpenter, W. T., Jr. (1972). The predictions of outcome in schizophrenia. I. Characteristics of outcome. *Archive of General Psychiatry, 27,* 739–746.

Strauss, J. S., & Carpenter W. T., Jr. (1974). The prediction of outcome in Schizophrenia. II. Relationships between predictor and outcome variables. A report from the WHO international pilot study of schizophrenia. *Archives of General Psychiatry, 31,* 37–42.

Strauss, J. S., & Carpenter, W. T., Jr. (1977). The prediction of outcome in Schizophrenia. III. Five-year outcome and its predictors. *Archives of General Psychiatry, 34,* 159–163.

Susser, E., Struening, E., & Conover, S. (1989). Psychiatric problems in homeless men: Life time psychosis, substance use, and current distress in new arrivals at New York city shelters. *Archives of General Psychiatry, 46*(9), 845–850.

Takai, A., Uematsu, M., Kaiya, H., Inoue, M., & Ueki, H. (1990). Coping styles to basic disorders among schizophrenics. *Acta Psychiatica Scandinavica, 82,* 289–294.

Tarrier, N., Beckett, R., Harwood, S., Baker, A., Yusupoff, L., & Ugarteburu, I. (1993). A trail of two cognitive-behavioural methods of drug-resistant residual psychotic symptoms in schizophrenic patients: 1. Outcome. *British Journal of Psychology, 162,* 524–532.

Thurm, I., & Haefner, H. (1987). Perceived vulnerability, relapse risk, and coping in schizophrenia: An Exploratory study. *European Archives of Psychiatry and Neurological Sciences, 237,* 46–53.

Torrey, E. F., & Miller, J. (2001). *The invisible plague: The rise of mental illness from 1750 to the Present.* New Brunswick, NJ: Rutgers University Press.

Tracey, T. J. G., & Rounds, J. B. (1997). Circular structure of vocational interests. In H. E. Howe & H. R. Conte (Eds.), *Cicumplex models of personality and emotions* (pp. 183–201). Washington, DC: American Psychological Association.

Tsuang, M., Woolson, R., & Fleming, J. (1979). Long term outcome of major psychosis I: Schizophrenia and affective disorders compared with psychiatrically symptom-free Surgical conditions. *Archives of General Psychiatry, 36,* 1295–1301.

Vaillant, G. E. (1964) Prospective prediction of schizophrenia re-mission. *Archive of General Psychiatry, 11,* 509–518.

Wahass, S., & Kent, G. (1997). Coping with auditory hallucinations: A cross-cultural comparison between western (British) and non-western (Saudi Arabian) patients. *The Journal of Nervous and Mental Disease, 185*(11), 664–668.

Warner, R. (2004). *Recovery from schizophrenia: Psychiatry and political economy.* New York: Brunner-Routledge.

Wiedl, K. H. (1992). Assessment of coping with schizophrenia: Stressors, appraisals, and coping behavior. *Britsh Journal of Psychiatry, 161,* 114–122.

Willinger, U., Heiden, H. M., Meszaros, K., Formann, A. K., & Aschauer, H. N. (2001). Neurodevelopmental schizophrenia: Obstetric complications, birth weight, premorbid social withdrawal, and learning disabilities. *Neuropsychobiology, 43,* 163–169.

World Health Organization (1992). *International classification of diseases and related health problems* (10th ed.). Geneva, Switzerland: World Health Organization.

World Health Organization (2006a). *Mental health.* Retrived July 21, 2006, from http://www.who.int/mental_health/en/

World Health Organization (2006b). *Project Atlas: Resources for mental health and neurological disorders.* Retrieved July 21, 2006, from http://www.who.int/ global-atlas/default.asp

Yanos, P. T., Knight, E. L., & Bremer, L. (2003). A new measure of coping with symptoms for use with persons diagnosed with severe mental illness. *Psychiatric Rehabilitation Journal, 27*(2), 169–176.

Yanos, P. T., Primavera, E. L., & Knight, E. L. (2001). Consumer-run service participation, recovery of social functioning, the mediating role of psychological factors. *Psychiatric Services, 52,* 493–500.

Zhang, Q. (1998). Fuzziness-vagueness-generality-ambiguity. *Journal of Pragmatics, 11,* 3–31.

17
Coping with Spinal Cord Injuries: Wholeness Is a State of Mind

Erin Martz and Hanoch Livneh

Never to discover your own power and your own potential is to be mentally bedridden all of your life.

P. Starck (1981, p. 108)

Until the middle of the 20th century, individuals with spinal cord injuries (SCI) only survived a few weeks after injury in industrial countries (Kennedy, 2001). As medical and rehabilitation knowledge increased, the survival rate improved and life-spans increased after SCI. Nowadays, if proper medical care is accessible (as is usually common in high income, developed countries), an individual with SCI typically can survive the acute phases of the SCI and later become a participating and productive member of society.

Etiology

The spinal cord houses sensory, motor, and autonomic nerves of the central nervous system that extend to the extremities of the body. SCI occurs if the spinal is fractured, or if the spinal cord is compressed (by external force or by a tumor), lacerated, or stretched; if the disks of the spinal cord are displaced; or if the blood supply to the spinal cord is interrupted (Kennedy, 2001). Infectious diseases (e.g., a virus causing poliomyelitis) also can cause spinal injuries that lead to paralysis. Spinal injuries that do not cause neurological problems (e.g., some types of back injuries) are not included under the SCI label (Priebe, 1995).

The higher along the spinal cord that the injury occurs, the greater is the resulting loss of function. Thus, an injury to the vertebrae in the neck—the cervical section—can cause *quadriplegia* (also known as tetraplegia); whereas, an injury to a lower part of the spinal cord can cause *paraplegia*. SCI can be an incomplete or complete, which indicates whether all sensory and motor functions are lost (i.e., *complete* injury) or are partially impaired (i.e., *incomplete* injury) below the level of injury. According to the Centers for Disease Control (CDC; 2005), the two most common types of SCI injury in the United States are incomplete tetraplegia (34.5%) and complete paraplegia (23.1%).

Among 23,683 individuals with SCI in the U.S., the three top causes of SCI for both men and women were: Motor vehicle accidents (MVA, 34.6%), falls (19.7%), and gun-shot wounds (16.2%) (National Spinal Cord Injury Statistical Center, 2005). In developing countries, MVAs are a less frequent cause of SCI, while agriculturally-related injuries and falls that cause SCI are more frequent (Kennedy, 2001).

Incidence and Prevalence

The CDC (2005) reports that the annual incidence of SCI in the U.S. is about 11,000 individuals, while the prevalence is approximately 250,000. After compiling information from multiple international sources, the International Campaign for Cures of Spinal Cord Injury Paralysis (2004) stated that a conservative estimate of the world-wide prevalence of individuals with SCI-related paralysis is over 2.5 million, with the highest prevalence of SCI reported in China (420,000).

SCI is more common among men (81.1%; National Spinal Cord Injury Statistical Center, 2005) than women. Yet, the World Health Organization (2006) describes additional types of SCIs, which occur more often to women and children in developing countries when they are forced to walk long distances to obtain water. The carrying of heavily-weighted water, in addition to the risks present along unlit and unsafe paths or roads, may cause chronic or permanent damage to their spines.

Statistics from the National Spinal Cord Injury Statistical Center indicate that about half (52.6%) of SCI happen between the ages of 16 and 30 years and that the most common age of onset is 19 years old. The average age of onset reported by the CDC is 37.6 years, while the National Spinal Cord Injury Statistical Center (2005) stated that the average age of onset is 32.8 years. Both sources noted that the average age of SCI-onset has risen over the years, which may be partly due to increasing life-spans and older people who live a more active life.

The frequency of SCI, according to ethnicity, varies among databases, but the National Spinal Cord Injury Statistical Center (2005) reports that 67.4% of SCIs in the U.S. occurred among Caucasians. The National Spinal Cord Injury Statistical Center also indicates that there is a 70.5% cumulative survival rate (over 20 years) of individuals with SCI. The life expectancy of individuals, who are ventilator-dependent and who have any level of SCI, is almost 50% lower than those who are not ventilator-dependent. These data, of course, must be viewed as a trend, and must not be used to predict the life-span of specific individuals. However, the statistics do reflect an overall, increasing life-span of individuals with SCI in the U.S.

Medical Regimen

Acute Phase

The typical medical regimen for SCI depends on the type of injury. The acute care often involves stabilization of a fracture by means of external traction or surgery and postural reduction (i.e., bed-rest); this may last from three months to a year. Individuals with high-cord injuries (i.e., in the cervical area) may need a respirator to breathe. Other associated implications of SCI in the acute stage may include alterations in consciousness due to brain injury, pain medication, and a reduction of a person's sensory information, as a result of medical care needed for SCI (Kennedy, 2001).

The traumatic event that caused the SCI may cause cognitive impairments, because this trauma often involves rapid deceleration (e.g., MVA or falls) that can injure the brain; or the cognitive impairments may be related to pre-injury issues (Richards, Kewman, & Pierce, 2000). Other complications in the acute phase can include respiratory complications, deep venous thrombosis (i.e., blood clot in the legs), and issues arising from the quality of bladder, bowel, and skin care (Priebe, 1995).

Post-Acute Phase

The main post-acute medical treatment following SCI involves self-care or compliance with health maintenance, which can have important ramifications related to preventing secondary complications (i.e., problems that develop as a result of the existence of disability). For example, a failure to alternate positions while in a wheelchair can lead to pressure ulcers (i.e., decubitus ulcers or pressure sores), which may require re-hospitalization. The rate of pressure-ulcer development, according to 20 years of data from the U.S.'s Model Systems for SCI, was an average of 31.9% among individuals with SCI (Yarkony & Heinemann, 1995). Pressure ulcers during the acute care or rehabilitation phases are estimated to range between 30% and 40% of individuals with SCI, and 8% and 30% of individuals with SCI who reside in the community (Consortium for Spinal Cord Medicine, 2000).

Other secondary complications can include autonomic dysreflexia (for individuals with an injury in the 6th thoracic vertebrae or higher), spasticity, urinary tract infections, kidney and bladder stones, chronic pain, respiratory problems pneumonia(e.g.), fractures, and osteoporosis (Priebe, 1995). Allden (1992) reported that some individuals with SCI experience phantom sensations (e.g., tingling, burning) and spatial disturbances (e.g., thinking that one's limbs are in a certain position, but in reality, they are not). Muscle spasms can also cause pain for some individuals with SCI (Allden, 1992).

Secondary complications and illnesses are a serious issue following SCI, and are associated with the three leading causes of death, namely, respiratory system disease (21.9%), heart disease (12.4%), and infections (9.4%) (National

Spinal Cord Injury Statistical Center, 2005). A noteworthy point is related to the category of infections, because 94% of these deadly infections result from septicemia ("blood poisoning"), which is associated with pressure sores, urinary tract infections, or respiratory infections. Thus, lack of self-care can be dangerous to individuals with SCI, because a pressure ulcer (or other infections) may lead to septicemia, if the open wound allows harmful bacteria into the body (Boekamp, Overholser, & Schubert, 1996).

Hence, individuals with SCI need to be provided with appropriate education about possible SCI-related complications (e.g., the book by Senelick & Dougherty, 1998), so that they can monitor their condition, in order to prevent new health crises. Individuals with SCI also have to take responsibility for understanding and complying with self-care regimens, or seeking prompt medical attention at the onset of a secondary complication, because some of the possible medical complications in the post-acute phase are preventable or treatable with timely intervention.

Mental Health Issues

A controversy has persisted for decades about whether individuals with SCI experience depression after the onset of SCI. The Consortium for Spinal Cord Medicine (1998) noted that depression is not a single entity, because it includes several possible diagnoses. They also observed that individuals with SCI may not have confronted the full significance of the changes, which SCI imposes on them, while they are in the acute or rehabilitation phases. Hence, they may be more vulnerable to depression when returning home (or later in life), due a decrease of social and medical support, and the challenge of managing pain and spasticity (Consortium for Spinal Cord Medicine).

The Consortium for Spinal Cord Medicine (1998) emphasized that coping with SCI may involve forms of grieving (e.g., sadness, feelings of loss, longing for the past), and that these reactions must be distinguished from the more serious and extended depressive reactions (e.g., helplessness, hopelessness, feeling worthless, excessive guilt or self-reproach, thoughts about suicide). A variety of factors (e.g., reduced physical functioning, inaccessible environment, lack of social support, lack of a purpose or job) may heighten depression, as well as the risk of suicide after SCI.

According to different estimates, suicide after the onset of SCI ranges between 3.8% and 6% (Dijkers, Abela, Gans, & Gordon, 1995; National Spinal Cord Injury Statistical Center, 2005). Dijkers and colleagues suggested the 6% figure may be an underestimation, because some deaths appeared to be accidental or had unknown causes, which could have been suicidal in nature. Other sources suggest a possible association between the existence of a CID and suicide estimates, in view of some reports estimating that "35% to 40% of suicides have significant chronic physical illness or disability" (Consortium for Spinal Cord Medicine, 1998, p. 8).

Deaths through "indirect suicide," or "physiological suicide" by self-neglect, are also difficult to estimate. These statistics may be confounded by a lack of adequate medical and social services. Self-neglect or lack of medical care among individuals with SCI can result in pressure ulcers or muscle contractures, which can be equally as dangerous as direct attempts at suicide (Kennedy, 2001). Dijkers et al. (1995) noted a trend in the data, indicating that suicide is more likely to occur in the first few years after SCI, after which the suicide risk decreases. They suggested that individuals, who *cope unsuccessfully* with SCI, may be at risk for suicide, but noted that "after a stormy initial two to five years, most persons learn how to cope" (Dijkers et al., 1995, p. 209).

Coping with a Spinal Cord Injury

Coping is an important topic for SCI, in view of the permanency of the physical condition and the possibilities of secondary complications related to SCI. Coping includes cognitive, affective, and behavioral attempts to master events that are overwhelming to an individual or that an individual has not experienced previously and thus does not have automatic responses (Inglehart, 1991; Lazarus & Folkman, 1984; Livneh, 2000). Coping with disability can be described as a more immediate psychological reaction to disability (Bracken & Shepard, 1980), which is distinct from the long-term process of adaptation to a disability (Livneh, 1986; Livneh & Antonak, 1997). Frank, Elliott, Corcoran, and Wonderlich's (1987) review article on depression after SCI concluded with the suggestion that rather than focusing on whether or not an individual is experiencing depression, clinicians should evaluate and emphasize *"a person's previous coping abilities*, life experiences, *current coping resources*, social support systems, and interpersonal environments during and following rehabilitation" (p. 625; emphasis added).

The Structure of Coping with SCI

Frank, Umlauf, et al. (1987) examined the structure of coping strategies, as measured by the Ways of Coping (WOC), and health locus of control, as measured by the Multidimensional Health Locus of Control (MHLC), among SCI individuals. Their analysis yielded two clusters. Members of cluster one exhibited higher scores on all seven subscales of the WOC and the Powerful Others and Chance subscales of the MHLC. Members of cluster two had higher scores only on the Internal locus of control subscale. When the levels of depression, negative life stress, and general life stress for the two clusters were compared, individuals in cluster one showed higher scores on all of these three measures. Frank and colleagues noted that the individuals of cluster one adopted more coping strategies, while experiencing greater overall stress and depression. They suggested that this trend may indicate that the coping strategies used by members of cluster one were less effective, or that the greater use of coping strategies were a result of a higher level of perceived stress and depression.

Using a combined dataset (individuals with SCI and MS), Wineman, Durand, and McCulloch (1994) investigated the factor structure of the WOC. They suggested a three-factor solution, composed of Cognitive Reframing, Emotional Respite, and Direct Assistance. Wineman and colleagues emphasized that individuals with CID may have to deal with many more stressful situations than those without CID, and thus, may use a wider range of coping strategies.

McColl, Lei, and Skinner's (1995) research examined the factor structure of coping (as measured by WOC), as well as the factor structure of social support. Their work confirmed a three-factor solution of types of coping among individuals with SCI who were living in the community. These coping strategies included problem-oriented (e.g., planning, concrete action), perception-oriented (e.g., cognitive shift in perspective, positive growth), and emotion-oriented (e.g., expression of feelings, avoidance-type behavior) coping.

Chan, Lee, and Lieh-Mak (2000) investigated the use of coping strategies (as measured by the WOC), locus of control, and perceived social support among individuals with SCI in Hong Kong. Using cluster analysis, the researchers divided the sample into three clusters based upon these measures. They named the three groups externals, internals, and multi-controls. The group that exhibited the highest internal locus of control had the highest mean scores and displayed significant differences, compared to the other two groups, on the following coping strategies: Self-control, seeking social support, accepting responsibility, problem-solving, and positive reappraisal. This "internal" group also demonstrated significantly higher scores on the perceived family and friend support, as well as on life satisfaction, than the other two groups.

Descriptive/Longitudinal Studies on SCI

In a longitudinal study, Hanson, Buckelew, Hewett, and O'Neal (1993) studied coping and adjustment among individuals with SCI five years following release from a rehabilitation setting. They analyzed the associations between coping strategies (as measured by the WOC-Revised scale) and adjustment (as measured by multiple scales in two time periods). The results indicated that the coping strategies used in time one did not predict adjustment at time one. Further, repeated measures analyses demonstrated a trend of participants adopting more of the following three coping strategies over time: Threat minimization, information seeking, and cognitive restructuring. Coping strategies did not significantly predict three of the four measures of adjustment, but did predict acceptance of disability at time two. Individuals used cognitive restructuring strategies more often in time two than time one. The results of this study suggested that coping strategies, which were used early following injury, were different from the coping strategies that were used several years later. These findings also suggested, according to Hanson and colleagues, that situational factors may influence the choice of coping strategies.

In another longitudinal study, Hancock, Craig, Tennant, and Chang (1993) examined coping styles among a group of Australians with SCI and a control group without disabilities. Although these researchers did not choose an instrument that directly measured coping, they examined psychological responses after injury by the Locus of Control Behavior (LCB) scale, the Rosenberg Self-Esteem Scale, and the Mental Adjustment to Cancer (MAC) scale, which was adapted for SCI. They found significant differences between the group with SCI and the control group. The group with SCI reported more non-adaptive coping styles (e.g., higher helplessness, higher fatalism), along with lower self-esteem and a more external locus of control, than the control group.

Craig, Hancock, and Chang (1994) assessed whether coping styles (as measured by the Mental Adjustment to Cancer; in particular, the three subscales of Fighting Spirit, Helplessness/Hopelessness, and Fatalism) changed for individuals with SCI, as compared with a control group. The SCI group had significantly higher scores, only during the first year following SCI onset, on the helplessness and fatalistic coping scales. No significant changes were found in these three coping subscales over a two-year time period for the SCI group.

In a longitudinal study, Heinemann, Schmidt, and Semik (1994) examined if pre-injury drinking patterns and drinking expectancies influenced coping strategies (as measured by the WOC questionnaire) among individuals with SCI. Some of the most frequently used coping strategies in this sample included positive reappraisal, problem-solving, self-control, and support-seeking. The researchers found that even though the drinking rate declined over one year for individuals, who were identified as preinjury problem-drinkers, this group did not decrease the use of non-adaptive coping (e.g., escape-avoidance) and positive alcohol beliefs (e.g., the belief that alcohol will bolster social skills, sleep, mood, and reduce tension). Heinemann, Schmidt, and Semik suggested that the trends, which were observed among preinjury problem drinkers, may indicate that the coping processes had not changed and therefore, may put these individuals at risk for a resumption of heavy drinking as a form of coping. Heinemann (1995) noted elsewhere that substance abuse may be involved in the onset of SCI, may interfere with SCI rehabilitation, may cause higher rates of medical impairment or death, may reduce the ability to live independently, and may create a "dual disability".

In a study that examined life satisfaction and depression among three groups (individuals with post-polio, SCI, and a control group), Kemp and Krause (1999) focused on studying coping among the subsample with SCI. They found that of the two coping scales that were selected for their study (escape/avoidance and planful problem-solving, as measured by the WOC), only escape/avoidance had a significant inverse relationship with total life satisfaction, while depression had a significant positive association with escape/avoidance coping.

In a longitudinal study, Kennedy et al. (2000) examined coping strategies (as measured by the COPE scale), among individuals with SCI over nine assessment intervals. Repeated-measures analyses of variance indicated that there were no significant differences in the use of coping strategies over the nine time periods. The most frequently used coping strategy during all assessment points was acceptance, while other commonly used strategies included positive reinterpretation and growth, active coping, planning, and emotional social support. The least frequently used strategies were non-adaptive coping strategies, such as behavioral disengagement, denial, and alcohol and drug use. Kennedy and his colleagues also conducted an extensive series of stepwise multiple regressions to examine which coping strategies predicted depression and anxiety. The following coping strategies were found to significantly predict depression and anxiety: Acceptance (for depression), and behavioral disengagement, focus/venting emotions, and alcohol/drug use (for anxiety).

In a longitudinal study, Nielsen (2003) investigated whether coping (as measured by the Coping Style Questionnaire [CSQ]) predicted posttraumatic stress disorder (PTSD), beyond what crisis support predicted, among individuals with SCI in Denmark. She found that of the four types of coping styles measured by the CSQ, emotional coping at time one was the only strong predictor of PTSD.

Predictive Studies of Coping with SCI

Buckelew, Baumstark, Frank, and Hewett (1990) examined coping strategies used by individuals with tetraplegia and paraplegia. They found that coping scores (as measured by the WOC) significantly predicted psychological distress (as measured by the Global Severity Index of the Symptom Checklist 90-Revised), while age, time since injury, diagnosis, and health locus of control scores were not significant predictors of psychological distress. The coping strategy that was the strongest predictor of psychological distress was self-blame. After dividing their sample into three groups according to reported psychological distress, Buckelew and colleagues (1990) found that the group exhibiting the highest level of psychological distress relied more heavily on the following four coping strategies: Wish-fulfilling fantasy, emotional expressiveness, self-blame, and threat-minimization. This may indicate that a greater use of these types of coping strategies does not mitigate psychological distress, and therefore, could be considered ineffective coping.

Wineman, Durand, and Steiner (1994) compared coping behaviors of individuals with SCI and multiple sclerosis (MS), who lived in the community, using the WOC-Revised (Folkman & Lazarus, 1988). The researchers found that neither emotion-focused coping, nor problem-focused coping, predicted mood states in the SCI sample, after controlling for vulnerability (a composite variable of ethnicity, income, education, and functional ability) and perceived illness uncertainty. However, when the researchers examined levels of illness uncertainty (measured as no, low, moderate, and high uncertainty), and adjusted for the covariates of vulnerability and a time dimension (age and time since diagnosis), significant differences were found with the use of emotion-focused and problem-focused coping. Usage of problem-focused coping was highest at the no illness-uncertainty level, while usage of emotion-focused coping was highest at the high illness-uncertainty level.

Kennedy, Lowe, Grey, and Short (1995) collected data from individuals with SCI living in the United Kingdom, including information on coping strategies (as measured by the COPE scale), psychological distress, and depression. Two groups participated in the study: A short SCI duration and a long SCI duration. Significant differences in the use of coping strategies were found between the two groups for four of the coping scales: Emotional social support, instrumental social support, focusing/venting emotion, and behavioral disengagement. The two social support scales were significantly higher for the group with recent SCI, compared to the four to seven year post-injury group. Two coping scales (focus/venting emotion and behavioral disengagement) were significantly lower for the recent-onset group, than the group with the long-term SCI. Further, both the recent-onset group and the long-term SCI group demonstrated significant correlations between three of the COPE scales (acceptance, focusing/venting emotion, and behavioral disengagement) and both measures of psychological distress and depression.

Coping Strategies Used by Individuals with SCI

Engagement Strategies in Response to SCI

Engagement strategies include: (a) Problem-solving or problem-focusing; (b) seeking social support; (c) maintaining hope (in face of adversity); (d) goal-directed determination; (e) cognitive appraisal or restructuring; and (f) venting emotion. The following section briefly reviews findings from studies that report these strategies as fostering, in varying degrees, psychosocial adaptation to SCI.

Problem-Solving with SCI

Effective problem-solving was found to be predictive of lower levels of depression, lower psychosocial impairment, and higher degree of assertiveness among people with SCI (Elliott, Godshall, Herrick, Witty, & Spruell, 1991). As compared to those who relied more heavily on emotion-focused coping, individuals with SCI, who adopted problem-focused coping, exhibited higher scores on general coping effectiveness, and reported more positive mood and lower depression (Moore, Bombardier, Brown, & Patterson, 1993). One study, however, failed to find any relationship between emotion- or problem-focused coping and the respondents' emotional well-being (Wineman, Durand, & Steiner, 1994).

Seeking Social Support with SCI

The most widely researched engagement-type strategy among people with SCI has been that of seeking social support. Although researchers have utilized a number of conceptual and empirical approaches in measuring this coping strategy, these strategies will be discussed jointly. In general, the three factors of (a) the perceived availability and perceived quality of social support, (b) satisfaction with the support network and social integration, and (c) amount of social support, were all found to be associated with: (a) higher levels of psychological and physical well-being (Kennedy et al., 1995; Rintala, Young, Hart, Clearman, & Fuhrer, 1992; Schulz & Decker, 1985); (b) decreased depression (Elliott, Herrick, et al., 1991; Rintala et al., 1992; Whalley-Hammell, 1994); (c) general coping effectiveness (McNett, 1987); and (d) life satisfaction (Rintala et al., 1992).

Elliott and coworkers (Elliott, Herrick, Witty, Godshall, & Spruell, 1992a, 1992b) further elaborated upon the structure of social support as it relates to psychosocial adaptation to SCI. They concluded from their studies that: (a) Social relations, which reinforced the self-worth of the individual and that provided a sense of social integration, were linked to lower levels of depression and psychosocial impairment; and (b) those social relations, in which the person was responsible for the well-being of others (i.e., viewed by the authors as manifested by higher levels of nurturance and higher emotional support), were associated with higher levels of psychosocial impairment. Both of these studies and related research (e.g., McColl et al., 1995) implicated time since injury as an important interactive variable that influences the nature of the relationship between social support, coping, and psychosocial adaptation to SCI.

Other Engagement-Type Coping with SCI

Only sparse data are available on additional engagement-type coping strategies and they are, therefore, discussed jointly. In earlier clinical reports, Ray and West (1983, 1984) content-analyzed coping strategies of a small sample of individuals with SCI. Of the five coping strategies outlined (i.e., suppression, denial/repression, resignation/acceptance, positive thinking, and independence/ assertiveness), only the latter two are considered engagement-like strategies. The authors concluded, in their two studies, that no relationship was demonstrated between these strategies and successful adaptation to SCI, because adaptation is a function of the individual and his or her unique life circumstances.

In investigating the role of hope as a coping strategy associated with psychosocial adaptation to SCI, Elliott, Witty, Herrick and Hoffman (1991) reported that two components of hope, a sense of goal-directed determination and a sense of pathways (i.e., the ability to find ways to achieve goals), were both associated with lower levels of depression and psychosocial impairment. Additional coping strategies reported to be associated with psychosocial adaptation to SCI include: (a) Cognitive restructuring, which was related to higher scores on Linkowski's (1971) Acceptance of Disability Scale, but not to general psychological distress in a five-year follow-up study (Hanson et al., 1993); (b) acceptance, which was linked inversely to a number of indices of psychosocial adaptation including depression, hopelessness, anxiety, anger, and general psychological distress (Kennedy et al., 1995); and (c) venting emotions, which can arguably also be perceived as a disengagement-type coping modality, which was found to be associated with higher levels of psychosocial distress (Buckelew et al., 1990; Kennedy et al., 1995).

Disengagement Strategies in Response to SCI

This group of coping strategies commonly includes the following: (a) Denial, (b) wish-fulfilling fantasy, (c) self-blame, (d) other-blame, and (e) alcohol/drug abuse. The following section provides an overview of findings from studies that sought to investigate the association between disengagement coping strategies and psychosocial adaptation to SCI.

Denial of SCI

Surprisingly, the role of denial in adapting to SCI has been virtually left unexplored in the empirical literature. Bracken and Shepard (1980) provided a brief theoretical analysis of denial, but neglected to explore its role in fostering, or impeding, psychosocial adaptation to SCI. A subsequent study by Bracken and Bernstein (1980) reported that denial at one-year post-injury did correlate positively, but not significantly, with increased affective reactions (i.e., anger, anxiety, and depression) among persons with SCI. Martz, Livneh, Priebe, Wuermser, and Ottomanelli (2005) examined predictors of psychosocial adaptation among individuals with SCI and found that negative emotional responses (e.g., depression, anxiety), disengagement-type coping (e.g., disability denial, avoidance), and the severity and impact of disability were related to lower levels of adaptation.

Wish-Fulfilling Fantasy with SCI

Two studies, which examined the relationship between wish-fulfilling fantasy and psychosocial adaptation to SCI, concluded from their findings that this coping strategy was positively associated with higher level of psychological distress (Buckelew et al., 1990), and negatively related to acceptance of disability (Hanson et al., 1993). However, in a five-year follow-up study, wish-fulfilling fantasy was no longer related to severity of psychiatric symptomatology, or to vocational status (Hanson et al., 1993).

Self-Blame Related to SCI

The study of the relationship between self-attribution of blame and psychosocial adaptation to SCI has resulted in mixed findings. Most researchers (Buckelew et al., 1990; Hanson et al., 1993; Nielson & MacDonald, 1988; Reidy & Caplan, 1994) have reported positive associations between self-blame and higher levels of psychological distress, depression, and anxiety. However, some researchers (Bulman & Wortman, 1977; Schulz & Decker, 1985) have concluded from their research that self-blame was associated with better coping ability or effectiveness and with higher levels of perceived well-being. Other researchers failed to detect any relationship between self-blame and indices of psychosocial adaptation, including acceptance of disability (Heinemann, Bulka, & Smetak, 1988), depression during inpatient rehabilitation (Reidy & Caplan, 1994), and nurses' ratings of coping effectiveness (Sholomskas, Steil, & Plummer, 1990).

Other-Blame Related to SCI

Conflicting results were also reported when the relationship between blaming others for the occurrence of SCI and psychosocial adaptation was explored. While some researchers suggested that blaming others is associated with poorer coping ability (Bulman & Wortman, 1977; Sholomskas et al., 1990), other researchers (Nielson & MacDonald, 1988) reported that when compared to self-blamers, other-blamers demonstrated lower levels of pessimism, depression, anxiety, and hostility. Similarly, Reidy and Caplan (1994), reported that an increase of blaming chance (as another form of blaming "others") was associated with decreased level of depression.

Related literature on attribution of blame further suggests that: (a) Perceived avoidability of the accident is related to poorer coping ability (Bulman & Wortman, 1977; Van den Bout, Van Son-Schoones, Schipper, & Groffen, 1988); (b) individuals with SCI, who *do not* blame self or others, exhibit better coping effectiveness than those who blame either one (Sholomskas et al., 1990); (c) seeking an answer to "Why did this happen to me?" was associated with poorer coping behaviors among long-term individuals with disabilities, in one study (Van den Bout et al., 1988), but failed to be related to acceptance of disability in another study (Heinemann et al., 1988).

Using Alcohol and Other Drugs after SCI

Use of chemical substances is often regarded as a form of disengagement and non-adaptive coping (Carver, Scheier, & Weintraub, 1989; Heinemann, 1995; Wills & Hirky, 1996. Heinemann, Bulka, and Smetak (1988) reported that the absence of drinking was found to be a predictor of disability acceptance. Alcohol abuse was also found to be positively associated with other forms of disengagement and non-adaptive coping behaviors, such as self-blame (Sholomskas et al., 1990) and escape-avoidance (Heinemann et al., 1994), and inversely related to engagement coping strategies including positive reappraisal, problem-solving, and seeking social support (Heinemann et al., 1994). Finally, Schandler, Cohen, and Vulpe (1996) reported that a positive family history for alcoholism was associated with more use of coping strategies, which reflected acceptance of responsibility, problem-solving, and generally more problem-focused coping. These paradoxical findings were interpreted, by the authors, as suggesting a *preference* for more effective strategies among those with family history of alcoholism, but an *actual use* of less effective strategies as indicated by the increased frequency of their alcohol-related problems.

Other Disengagement-Type Coping with SCI

Only limited research findings are available on the relationship between other disengagement coping strategies and psychosocial adaptation to SCI. For instance, as compared to controls without disabilities, individuals with SCI reported higher levels of helpless/fatalistic coping, while scoring lower on a measure of self-esteem (Craig et al., 1994; Hancock et al., 1993). In another study, behavioral disengagement was inversely associated with feelings of vigor and positively with depression and general psychological distress (Kennedy et al., 1995). Finally, escape-avoidance coping was found to be negatively related to acceptance of disability, as well as to a variety of rehabilitation-outcome measures (Meyer, O'Leary, & Hagglund, 1999).

Coping with Secondary Complications

Pressure Ulcers

In a study that examined life adjustment among individuals with SCI, Krause (1998) found that 46% had at least one pressure ulcer. Krause also found that life adjustment was significantly correlated with pressure-ulcer severity and days impacted by pressure ulcers. In comparison to individuals with pressure ulcers, individuals with no pressures ulcers had higher scores on two subscales of the Life Situation Questionnaire-revised (LSQ-R)—Positive Engagement and Negative Emotions, which could be viewed as types of coping scales.

Elliott (1999) examined demographic and five social problem-solving variables as predictors of pressure-ulcer development among individuals with SCI. He found that only completeness of the SCI, and none of the problem-solving variables, significantly predicted a pressure-ulcer diagnosis. Individuals with a complete SCI had almost a ten-fold likelihood to have a pressure ulcer than individuals with an incomplete SCI.

In a longitudinal three-year study, Elliott, Bush, and Chen (2006) investigated the use of five forms of problem-solving (using the Social Problem-Solving Inventory-Revised [SPSI-R]) among individuals with SCI. They found that the use of rational problem-solving, at discharge from an inpatient rehabilitation unit, significantly predicted a lower likelihood of occurrence of pressure ulcers in the subsequent three years. A path analysis supported the inverse association between problem-solving abilities (a composite of all five subscales of the SPSI-R) and the occurrence of pressure ulcers.

SCI-Related Pain

The existence of daily pain concomitant with SCI may create additional coping challenges. Richards et al. (2000, p. 16) observed that individuals with SCI, who have to cope chronic pain, experience the pain as an "insult added to injury." Wilson, Richards, Klapow, DeVivo, and Greene (2005) noted that pain is a multidimensional problem that affects individuals on multiple levels, having physical, psychological, social, and environmental components. Wilson et al. (2005) summarized the literature on the prevalence of chronic (i.e., pain that exists for at least six months) SCI-related pain, as ranging between 11% and 94% of individuals with SCI.

Psychosocial reactions to chronic pain are "a function of the interplay between organic and learning factors including avoidance, social discomfort, absolution of responsibilities, negative prediction, and expectation of pain" (Allden, 1992, p. 457). Boekamp et al. (1996, p. 337) noted the possible association of depression and chronic, SCI-related pain:

[C]hronic pain may be associated with negative thinking, expectations of helplessness, restricted opportunities for pleasurable activities, and persistent taxing of behavioral and cognitive coping resources, all of which may heighten vulnerability for depression.

Kennedy, Frankel, Gardner, and Nuseibeh (1997) examined whether coping strategies (as measured by the COPE scale), among other variables, predicted pain intensity. They found that only anxiety, and not coping, was a significant predictor of pain at six weeks after SCI onset. Further, the only significant predictor of pain intensity at one year post-injury was the existence of pain at six weeks, not coping strategies or other psychological variables.

Turner, Jensen, Warms, and Cardenas (2002) examined coping with pain behaviors among community-based individuals with SCI, who reported chronic pain. Catastrophizing coping was the only coping strategy that significantly predicted pain intensity and pain-related disability (i.e., pain interference in daily activities), after controlling for demographics and pain intensity. Also, the coping strategies of catastrophizing, reinterpreting pain, coping self-statements, and ignoring pain significantly predicted levels of psychological distress among these respondents.

Giardino, Jensen, Turner, Ehde, and Cardenas (2003) examined the relationships among catastrophizing, pain intensity, social support, and depression among individuals with SCI. They found that catastrophizing was significant and positively related to all three of the other measures. Catastrophizing also significantly predicted the sensory pain score on the Short Form-McGill Pain Questionnaire. Further, social support was found to influence catastrophizing; individuals, who lived with a spouse or partner, tended to catastrophize more as they experienced greater pain.

Nielson, Jensen, and Kerns (2003) created a unique instrument to assess the self-management of pain, called the Multidimensional Pain Readiness to Change Questionnaire (MPRCQ), which assesses individuals' readiness to change their ways in nine different areas of coping with pain (e.g., exercise, relaxation, assertive communication, cognitive control). They first used the MPRCQ in a sample of individuals with fibromyalgia and then replicated the study among individuals with SCI and amputations. Two factors explained most of the variance of the coping scales: Active Coping (i.e., strategies to directly address problems) and Perservance (i.e., adaptive strategies to tolerate being in pain).

Henwood and Ellis (2004) examined reactions to neuropathic pain, defined as "pain that is initiated or caused by a primary lesion or dysfunction in the nervous system" (p. 39). Neuropathic pain was reported by focus-group participants with SCI to be the most difficult type of pain with which to cope. The participants reported the following as coping strategies for neuropathic pain: (a) Physical activities, such as swimming or bathing in warm or hot water; (b) massage; (c) stretching; (d) use of alternative therapies, such as acupuncture or hypnosis; and (e) cognitive coping strategies (e.g., information-seeking or positive thinking). Non-adaptive coping strategies (e.g., use of alcohol or illicit drugs) were also reported.

Summary on Coping Strategies

To summarize coping trends used by individuals with SCI, those who use engagement-type coping strategies, which include problem-solving, seeking social support, and other active measures that directly seek to defuse problems, generally have demonstrated better psychosocial adaptation. In contrast, individuals with SCI who use disengagement-type coping strategies, such as passive, avoidant-type behaviors that include drug and alcohol use, denial, fantasy, and blaming self and others, generally have manifested poorer psychosocial outcomes (Livneh, 2000).

Thus, it can be concluded that proactive coping, which focuses on addressing SCI-related issues, helps an individual maintain an adaptive psychosocial perspective. Such a view may also help to prevent or decrease the impact of secondary complications (e.g., pressure ulcers or pain), because—if viewed from a biopsychosocial perspective—one's coping and other psychological responses to SCI influence the complex web of health and stress (Sperry, 2006).

Physical and Psychosocial/Behavioral Interventions to Promote Coping.

Environmental Interventions

Upon completion of medical rehabilitation, individuals with SCI have to learn how to navigate in their former environments, such as their home and local communities. Although physically dependent for some level of assistance, individuals with SCI can control their circumstances by giving verbal directions to others (Priebe, 1995). Yet, often their homes need physical changes, in order to accommodate a wheelchair or other new equipment. Heinemann and Pape (2002) created an appendix of research studies on coping, adjustment, and use of assistive technology; many of these studies were conducted among samples of individuals with SCI. Assistive technology (e.g., orthoses, wheelchairs) can help individuals with SCI overcome barriers in the environment. Rehabilitation centers can help to transition a person with a recent-onset SCI back into the community by providing day and weekend passes, in order that the individual can be provided with additional support, training, or assistive technology equipment, as they discover new problems to solve or accommodations that are needed (Priebe, 1995).

There can be multiple physical or environmental barriers for an individual with SCI that require intervention. For example, transportation and buildings may be inaccessible, problems may arise with hiring personal assistants, others may demonstrate a negative attitude toward the person, or the individual with SCI may lack social support (Priebe, 1995). The Consortium for Spinal Cord Medicine (1998, p. 25) constructed a comprehensive list of interventions for 11 different areas of social support (e.g., housing, transportation, finances, employment). This list contains suggestions of agencies and resources, which can facilitate coping with SCI and functioning in the community. Robinson, West, and Woodworth (1995) compiled tables, one of which focused on spinal cord injuries (pp. 94–97), that detailed the needs, information needed, resources available, and goals related to navigating the environment and managing a life with CID. These tables were examples of ways in which individuals can learn how to determine what they need to better cope with a CID and how to obtain those resources.

The Job Accommodations Network of the U.S. Department of Education (2006) provides a wealth of suggestions about how to accommodate individuals with SCI in an office. These include permitting the individual to have: (a) A personal attendant and/or a service animal; (b) flexible scheduling and rest breaks for medically-related issues; (c) work-station modifications (related to desks, chairs, filing cabinets, office equipment, and shelves) that are adjusted to the height and reach of the individual; and (d) use low-tech (e.g., page-turners) and high-tech equipment (e.g., voice-activated phones and computers). Accommodations related to the space of the work-site include accessible parking, accessible doors to the building and office, accessible restrooms, and the ability to work from home if the workspace is not accessible.

Psychosocial Interventions

Kennedy (2001) discussed various types of psychosocial interventions, which are possible at different phases after SCI onset. Individuals with new SCI may be resistant to therapy during the acute phase, because "accepting psychological intervention may imply making plans for a future that could include a permanent disability" (Kennedy, 2001, p. 454). Richards et al. (2000) also described the initial resistance by many individuals with SCI to psychotherapy, which they surmised may be due to the primary focus on achieving physical independence.

Kennedy (2001) suggested that at the acute phase of rehabilitation, professionals should prioritize checking on how much medical and other types of information have been made available to the person, and discussing what can be expected from rehabilitation. When given permission by the person with SCI, the focus can shift to building rapport and normalizing the emotional reactions that are often experienced after the onset of SCI. Thus, according to Kennedy, the first step of therapy may be more of an "informal intervention" of supportive counseling. The next therapeutic step can focus on restructuring the cognitive elements and negative beliefs that are impeding self-efficacy, at the same time as acknowledging the chaos that has occurred in the person's life. Cognitive-behavioral interventions can be implemented, in order to facilititate better and more effective problem-solving.

Coping Effectiveness Training

Coping Effectiveness Training (CET) is a cognitive behavior therapy for groups, tailored by Kennedy and Duff (2001) and Kennedy, Taylor, and Duff (2005), for people with SCI. CET involves several facets. One is helping individuals appraise what is stressful to them, whether this stressor is global or specific, and whether the stressor is modifiable or unchangeable. Another aspect of CET is teaching a range of coping skills and encouraging the reduction of non-adaptive coping strategies. Finally, CET covers how to create and sustain social support.

According to Kennedy and Duff (2001), a stressor can be evaluated as global or specifc by asking four questions (in brief, who, what, where, and when questions, which can better identify the stressor). Because Kennedy and Duff view adaptive coping as finding an appropriate match between stressor and coping, then the appraisal of stressors becomes important. Further, CET encourages individuals to define their stressors and whether they represent a loss, threat, or challenge. "Loss or harm refers to issues that have already occurred, threat refers to potential things that may occur, whereas challenge reflects the opportunity for growth, mastery, or gain" (p. 9).

Kennedy and Duff (2001) defined the two major functions of coping as managing problems that are distressing and dealing with the emotional responses to distress; thus, coping strategies primarily focus on resolving an issue (i.e., problem-solving) or reframing one's thinking about the situation (i.e., emotion-focused). If the stressor is perceived to be alterable, then individuals are taught to use problem-solving coping techniques (i.e., identifying problems and possible solutions, choosing and implementing a solution, and evaluating outcomes) with the additional step of examining the consequences of the problem. If the stressor is not perceived as changeable, then emotion-focused coping techniques are used.

Kennedy and Duff (2001) also elaborated upon how the maintenance of negative cognitions influences unhelpful emotional reactions. Thus, in order to promote active coping, they suggested taking steps, such as engaging in pleasant activities and relaxation exercises, and identifying and challenging negative thoughts to help change the way a person thinks and behaves. They also described how to increase various types of social support by using assertiveness.

Kennedy, Duff, Evans, and Beedie (2003) compared a seven-session CET intervention with a SCI control group. Over the three assessment periods, the coping strategy of suppression of competing activities significantly decreased for both the intervention and the control group. Usage of alcohol was significantly lower for all three time periods among the intervention group. Kennedy, Taylor, and Duff (2005) analyzed the data from the 2003 study, focusing only on those who received the CET intervention. They split the group into those who benefited from the intervention and those who did not. No significant differences were found on the utilization of any of the coping strategies between the group that benefited from CET and the group that did not. A significant difference was found on time since injury: individuals, who benefited from the CET intervention, were more recently injured than those who did not profit from CET.

Cognitive Behavioral Therapy

Craig and Hancock (1994) described multiple facets of group cognitive-behavior therapy (CBT) for individuals with SCI. The focus of CBT is to provide skills to cope with problems in life, compared to therapies that aim to increase self-awareness. A therapy group, if composed only of individuals with SCI, can facilitate learning about perspectives on similar issues and problems, and can help bolster individuals' social skills and their ability to give and receive support.

Craig and Hancock (1994) noted several problems that may arise when implementing a CBT group with SCI. One is related to the fact that the typical percentage of SCI population is composed of 80% males, who may view therapy as an unneeded service. Individuals of either gender may not be accustomed to the verbal interaction and disclosure of therapy, due to their age or emphasis on risk-taking physical activities that may have led to the SCI. Denial of the permanency of the SCI may cause some people to decline CBT, because they may believe that they will walk again soon, and therefore, do not need coping skills that are geared toward overcoming SCI-related issues. Another challenge, related to providing a CBT group to individuals immediately following the onset of SCI, centers around the issue that these individuals have not spent time in the community and therefore, have little understanding of the types of problems that they may face once in the community. Consequently, they may minimize the need for learning specific coping skills during inpatient rehabilitation. Another possible difficulty in conducting CBT groups among individuals with SCI is due to the secondary complications that may accompany SCI, which may preclude individuals from participating in a regular CBT group. Thus, flexible scheduling and the involvement of the rehabilitation staff can help overcome fluctuating participation in a CBT group (Craig and Hancock, 1994).

Tirch and Radnitz (2000) described, from a cognitive-behavioral viewpoint, six types of cognitive distortions to which individuals with SCI may be particularly susceptible: a) An overriding negative perception of the world and that people will be prejudiced against a person with a disability; b) feeling personally worthless and of less value than others; c) expecting rejection by others; d) feeling hopeless and expecting continuous disappointment; e) believing that they are entitled to special treatment, due to their disability; and f) feeling vulnerable, especially because of their physical impairments. Tirch and Radnitz explained that these cognitive distortions may lead to non-adaptive coping (e.g., alcohol or drug use, self-neglect). The authors proposed treatment for such distortions by using cognitive-behavioral techniques, noting that a balance in the treatment should be made between confronting distorted thinking and acknowledging that many psychological reactions to the advent of SCI are normal. Tirch and Radnitz also noted that environmental factors, such as reactions of one's social group and family, will influence the coping of individuals with SCI to the drastic new changes in their lives.

Other Types of Psychotherapy

Starck (1981) conducted a study on the effectiveness of two forms of strategies (i.e., dereflection and paradoxical intention) from Frankl's logotherapy among individuals with SCI, who were at least one-year post-injury, unemployed, and living in the community. No significant differences were found between the treatment and control groups on several measures over a four-month period. Starck observed a trend, though non-significant, in the treatment group, of increased usage of dereflection and paradoxical intention over time.

Psychosocial interventions may need to include family members, as Steinglass, Temple, Lisman, and Reiss' (1982) case studies illustrated. They noted that some families may assume that the SCI is the *only* crisis issue, such that "all behavior [is] automatically interpreted in terms of the spinal cord injury" (p. 262), instead of viewing some family issues as developmental crises that are unrelated to the SCI existence. Hence, Steinglass and colleagues emphasized the need for a developmental perspective when working with families, in order to promote the long-term management of CID, and not merely using a crisis-intervention approach that is focused only on CID-related issues.

Peer counseling is an effective means of bolstering coping skills among individuals with recent onset SCI and can be done either on an individual basis or in a group format. Individuals with SCI, who are associated with an Independent Living Center (ILC), can provide this peer support, after they have received some training (Richards et al., 2000). Medical or psychological interventions by phone ("tele-health" or "tele-rehabilitation") may help to reach individuals with SCI, who lack transportation or who live in rural areas of a country, according to Richards and colleagues.

Livneh (2000) suggested that skill-training programs can enhance the coping abilities of individuals with SCI by focusing on areas such as: "Problem-solving, decision-making, goal-setting and implementation, assertiveness enhancement, self-monitoring, stress management, stress inoculation, and health-care resource utilization" (p. 7). Sharoff (2004) described numerous therapeutic techniques to facilitate coping with chronic illness, which can also be utilized for individuals with SCI.

Vocational and Social Implications

A spinal cord injury (SCI) is like a stone thrown in a pond: increasingly wider areas of the lives of the persons involved, and those around them, are affected

(Dijkers et al., 1995, p. 185).

The above quote illustrates the ripple effect of problems related to incurring SCI. Priebe (1995) noted that social reintegration starts in the smaller circle of one's immediate family, then proceeds to friends and the extended family, and finally extends to the larger community. Although 92.3% of individuals with SCI, according to the U.S.'s National Spinal Cord Injury Statistical Center database, are living in private residences after rehabilitation, social integration still may be a big challenge because of societal stigma and prejudicial practices.

Employment can be one of the best forms of social integration for individuals with CID. Thus, obtaining work after SCI onset is an important issue, besides the financial and psychological benefits of working. Statistics indicated that 64.1% of individuals were employed at the time of injury, while 13.6% were employed one year after SCI-onset (National Spinal Cord Injury Statistical Center, 2005). The same data source indicated that 22.8% were employed five years after SCI onset.

As previously mentioned, the Job Accommodations Network (2006) is a resource that can be utilized by individuals with SCI, as well as their employers, to help solve problems related to SCI and employment. This website provides ideas on modifying the work environment to provide greater access when mobility devices, such as when wheelchairs and other assistive technology are used. Other websites (Ability Hub, 2006; National Spinal Cord Injury Association, 2006; Paralyzed Veterans of America, 2006) can provide information about assistive technology and more resources that can facilitate returning to work and life. In addition, the World Health Organization (1996) has published an international manual about promoting independence after SCI, which was written for rehabilitation workers, yet includes practical information that would be useful for individuals with SCI and their friends and family. This manual also contains a brief section on coping with SCI and coping with reactions of others about the existence of SCI (see p. 3).

Conclusion

A spinal cord injury often occurs without warning, and therefore, simultaneously causes both physiological and psychological shock. As medical professionals work to stabilize the individual's system and reduce the physiological impact of the SCI, the psychological ramifications of the SCI start to develop. This chapter covered multiple aspects of coping with the onset of SCI, not only during the acute phase after injury, but during the long adjustment period, which may involve new challenges in the form of secondary complications or in the form of environmental and attitudinal barriers related to the SCI.

While different types of coping can be adaptive and are dependent on factors related to circumstances and timing, proactive coping (i.e., approach or problem-solving forms of coping) is typically related to better psychosocial outcomes. Avoidance or emotion-focused coping is, in general, related to poorer outcomes, such as those manifested by increased psychological stress and depression. Hence, interventions can be structured around helping individuals with SCI learn how to better integrate proactive forms of coping into their daily lives and choices. Proactive coping can help to decrease the possibility of further complications, which can result from a lack of proper self-care, and to address SCI-related issues and challenges that arise during every-day living.

References

Ability Hub. (2006). *Assistive technology.* Retrieved August 2, 2006, from http://www.abilityhub.com/

Allden, P. (1992). Psychological aspects of spinal cord injury. *Educational and Child Psychology, 9,* 34–48.

Boekamp, J. R., Overholser, J. C., & Schubert, D. S. P. (1996). Depression following a spinal cord injury. *International Journal of Psychiatry in Medicine, 26,* 329–349.

Bracken, M.B., & Bernstein, M. (1980). Adaptation to and coping with disability one year after spinal cord injury: An epidemiological study. *Social Psychiatry, 15,* 33–41.

Bracken, M.B., & Shepard, M.J. (1980). Coping and adaptation following acute spinal cord injury: A theoretical analysis. *Paraplegia, 18,* 74–85.

Buckelew, S. P., Baumstark, K. E., Frank, R. G., & Hewett, J. E. (1990). Adjustment following spinal cord injury. *Rehabilitation Psychology, 35*(2), 101–109.

Bulman, R. J., & Wortman, C. B. (1977). Attribution of blame and coping in the "real world": Severe accident victims react to their lot. *Journal of Personality and Social Psychology, 35,* 351–363.

Carver, C. S., Scheier, M., & Weintraub, K. (1989). Assessing coping strategies: A theoretically based approach. *Journal of Personality and Social Psychology, 56,* 267–283.

Centers for Disease Control (2005, June). Spinal cord injury information network. Retrieved December 30, 2005, from http://www.spinalcord.uab.edu/show.asp?durki=21446

Chan, R. C. K., Lee, P. W. H., & Lieh-Mak, F. (2000). The pattern of coping in persons with spinal cord injuries. *Disability and Rehabilitation, 22*(11), 501–507.

Consortium for Spinal Cord Medicine (1998). *Depression following spinal cord injury: A clinical practice guideline for primary care physicians.* Washington, DC: Paralyzed Veterans of America.

Consortium for Spinal Cord Medicine (2000). *Pressure ulcer prevention and treatment following spinal cord injury: A clinical practice guideline for health-care professionals.* Washington, DC: Paralyzed Veterans of American.

Craig, A., & Hancock, K. (1994). Difficulties in implementing group cognitive behaviour therapy for spinal cord injured persons: A clinical discussion. *Australian Psychologist, 29,* 98–102.

Craig, A. R., Hancock, K., & Chang, E. (1994). The influence of spinal cord injury on coping styles and self-perceptions two years after the injury. *Australian and New Zealand Journal of Psychiatry, 28,* 307–312.

Dijkers, M. P., Abela, M. B., Gans, B. M., & Gordon, W. A. (1995). The aftermath of spinal cord injury. In S. L. Stover, J. A. DeLisa, & G. G. Whiteneck (Eds.), *Spinal cord injury: Clinical outcomes from the model systems* (pp. 185–212). Gaithersburg, MD: Aspen Publishers.

Elliott, T. R. (1999). Social problem-solving abilities and adjustment to recent-onset spinal cord injury. *Rehabilitation Psychology, 44*(4), 315–332.

Elliott, T. R., Bush, B. A., & Chen, Y. (2006). Social problem-solving abilities predict pressure sore occurrence in the first 3 years of spinal cord injury. *Rehabilitation Psychology, 51*(1), 69–77.

Elliott, T. R., Godshall, F. J., Herrick, S. M., Witty, T. E., & Spruell, M. (1991). Problem-solving appraisal and psychological adjustment following spinal cord injury. *Cognitive Therapy and Research, 15*, 387–389.

Elliott, T. R., Herrick, S. M., Patti, A. M., Witty, T. E., Godshall, F. J., & Spruell, M. (1991). Assertiveness, social support, and psychological adjustment following spinal cord injury. *Behavior Research and Therapy, 29*, 485–493.

Elliott, T. R., Herrick, S. M., Witty, T. E., Godshall, F., & Spruell, M. (1992a). Social relationships and psychosocial impairment of persons with spinal cord injury. *Psychology and Health, 7*, 55–67.

Elliott, T. R., Herrick, S. M., Witty, T. E., Godshall, F., & Spruell, M. (1992b). Social support and depression following spinal cord injury. *Rehabilitation Psychology, 37*, 37–48.

Elliott, T. R., Witty, T. E., Herrick, S. M., & Hoffman, J. T. (1991). Negotiating reality after physical loss: Hope, depression, & disability. *Journal of Personality and Social Psychology, 61*, 608–613.

Folkman, S., & Lazarus, R. S. (1988). *Manual for the Ways of Coping Questionnaire.* Palo Alto: Consulting Psychologists Press.

Frank, R. G., Elliott, T. R., Corcoran, J. R., & Wonderlich, S. A. (1987). Depression after spinal cord injury: Is it necessary? *Clinical Psychology Review, 7*, 611–630.

Frank, R. G., Umlauf, R. L., Wonderlich, S. A., Askanazi, G. S., Buckelew, S. P., & Elliott, T. R. (1987). Differences in coping styles among persons with spinal cord injury: A cluster-analytic approach. *Journal of Consulting and Clinical Psychology, 55*, 727–731.

Giardino, N. D., Jensen, M. P., Turner, J. A., Ehde, D. A., & Cardenas, D. D. (2003). Social environment moderates the association between catastrophizing and pain among persons with a spinal cord injury. *Pain, 106*, 19–25.

Hancock, K., Craig, A., Tennant, C., & Chang, E. (1993). The influence of spinal cord injury on coping styles and self-perceptions: A controlled study. *Australian and New Zealand Journal of Psychiatry, 27*, 450–456.

Hanson, S., Buckelew, S. P., Hewett, J., & O'Neal, G. (1993). The relationship between coping and adjustment after spinal cord injury: A 5-year follow-up study. *Rehabilitation Psychology, 38*(1), 41–51.

Heinemann, A. W. (1995). Spinal cord injury. In A. J. Goreczny (Ed.), *Handbook of Health and Rehabilitation Psychology* (pp. 341–360). New York: Plenum Press.

Heinemann, A. W., Bulka, M., & Smetak, S. (1988). Attributions and disability acceptance following traumatic injury: A replication and extension. *Rehabilitation Psychology, 33*, 195–205.

Heinemann, A. W., & Pape, T. L. (2002). Coping and adjustment. In M. J. Scherer (Ed.), *Assistive technology: Matching device and consumer for successful rehabilitation.* Washington, DC: American Psychological Association, 123–141.

Heinemann, A. W., Schmidt, M. F., & Semik, P. (1994). Drinking patterns, drinking expectancies, and coping after spinal cord injury. *Rehabilitation Counseling Bulletin, 38*, 134–153.

Henwood, P., & Ellis, J. A. (2004). Chronic neuropathic pain in spinal cord injury: The patient's perspective. *Pain Research Management, 9*, 39–45.

Inglehart, M. R. (1991). *Reactions to critical life events: A social psychological analysis.* New York: Praeger.

International Campaign for Cures of Spinal Cord Injury Paralysis (2004). *Global summary of spinal cord injury, incidence and economic impact.* Retrieved July 28, 2006, from http://www.campaignforcure.org/globalsum.htm

Job Accommodations Network (2006). Accommodations ideas for wheelchair use. Retrieved July 26, 2006, from http://www.jan.wvu.edu/media/whee.htm

Kemp, B. J., & Krause, S. (1999). Depression and life satisfaction among people ageing with post-polio and spinal cord injury. *Disability and Rehabilitation, 21*, 241–249.

Kennedy, P. (2001). Spinal cord injuries. In M. Johnston & D. Johnston (Eds.), *Coping and Spinal Cord Injury* (pp. 445–462). Netherlands: Elsevier Science Publishers.

Kennedy, P., & Duff, J. (2001). *Coping effectively with spinal cord injury.* United Kingdom: Stoke Mandeville Hospital NHS Trust.

Kennedy, P., Duff, J., Evans, M., & Beedie, A. (2003). Coping effectiveness training reduces depression and anxiety following traumatic spinal cord injuries, *British Journal of Clinical Psychology, 42*, 41–52.

Kennedy, P., Frankel, H., Gardner, B., & Nuseibeh, I. (1997). Factors associated with acute and chronic pain following traumatic spinal cord injuries. *Spinal Cord, 35*, 814–817.

Kennedy, P., Lowe, R., Grey, N., & Short, E. (1995). Traumatic spinal cord injury and psychological impact: A cross-sectional analysis of coping strategies. *British Journal of Clinical Psychology, 34*, 627–639.

Kennedy, P., Marsh, N., Lowe, R., Grey, N., Short, E., & Rogers, B. (2000). A longitudinal analysis of psychological impact and coping strategies following spinal cord injury. *British Journal of Health Psychology, 5*, 157–172.

Kennedy, P., Taylor, N., & Duff, J. (2005). Characteristics predicting effective outcomes after coping effectiveness training for patients with spinal cord injuries. *Journal of Clinical Psychology in Medical Settings, 12*, 93–98.

Krause, J. S. (1998). Skin sores after spinal cord injury : Relationship to life adjustment. *Spinal Cord, 36*, 51–56.

Lazarus, R. S., & Folkman, S. (1984). *Stress, appraisal, and coping.* New York: Springer.

Linkowski, D. (1971). A scale to measure acceptance of disability. *Rehabilitation Counseling Bulletin, 14*(4), 236–244.

Livneh, H. (1986). A unified approach to existing models of adaptation to disability: Part Ia model of adaptation. *Journal of Applied Rehabilitation Counseling, 17*(1), 5–17, 56.

Livneh, H. (2000). Psychosocial adaptation to spinal cord injury: The role of coping strategies. *Journal of Applied Rehabilitation Counseling, 31*(2), 3–10.

Livneh, H., & Antonak, R. F. (1997). *Psychosocial adaptation to chronic illness and disability.* Gaithersburg, MD: Aspen Publishers.

Martz, E., Livneh, H., Priebe, M., Wuermser, L., & Ottomanelli, L. (2005). Predictors of psychosocial adaptation among individuals with spinal cord injury/disorder.*Archives of Physical Medicine and Rehabilitation, 86*, 1182–1192.

McColl, M.A., Lei, H., & Skinner, H. (1995). Structural relationships between social support and coping. *Social Science and Medicine, 41*, 395–407.

McNett, S.C. (1987). Social support, threat, and coping responses and effectiveness in the functionally disabled. *Nursing Research, 36*, 98–103.

Meyer, T.M., O'Leary, V., & Hagglund, K.J. (1999). *Coping and adjustment during acute rehabilitation for spinal cord injury.* Paper presented at the APA annual convention, Boston, MA.

Moore, A. D., Bombardier, C. H., Brown, P. D., & Patterson, D. R. (1993). *Coping and emotional attributions over inpatient rehabilitation stay following spinal cord injury.* Paper presented at the APA annual convention, Toronto, Ontario.

National Spinal Cord Injury Statistical Center (2005). *Annual report for the Model Spinal Cord Injury Care Systems* (public version). Birmingham, AL: Author.

National Spinal Cord Injury Association (2006). *Resource center*. Retrieved August 2, 2006, from http://www.spinalcord.org/resources/

Nielsen, M. S. (2003). Crisis support and coping as mediators of well-being in persons with spinal cord lesion. *Journal of Clinical Psychology in Medical Settings, 10*, 91–99.

Nielson, W. R., Jensen, M. P., & Kerns, R. D. (2003). Initial development and validation of a multidimensional pain readiness to change questionnaire. *The Journal of Pain, 4*, 148–158.

Nielson, W. R., & MacDonald, M. R. (1988). Attributions of blame and coping following spinal cord injury: Is self-blame adaptive? *Journal of Social and Clinical Psychology, 7*, 163–175.

Paralyzed Veterans of America (2006). *Other PVA publications*. Retrieved August 2, 2006, from http://www.pva.org/cgi-bin/pvastore/products.cgi?id=2

Priebe, M. (1995). Spinal cord injury. In A. E. Dell Orto & R. P. Marinelli (Eds.), *Encyclopedia of Disability and Rehabilitation* (pp. 688–695). New York: Simon and Schuster Macmillan.

Ray, C., & West, J. (1983). Spinal cord injury: The nature of its implications and ways of coping. *International Journal of Rehabilitation Research, 6*, 364–365.

Ray, C., & West, J. (1984). Coping with spinal cord injury. *Paraplegia, 22*, 249–259.

Reidy, K., & Caplan, B. (1994). Causal factors in spinal cord injury: Patients' evolving perceptions and association with depression. *Archives of Physical Medicine and Rehabilitation, 75*, 837–842.

Richards, J. S., Kewman, D. G., & Pierce, C. A. (2000). Spinal cord injury. In R. G. Frank & T. R. Elliott (Eds.), *Handbook of Rehabilitation Psychology* (pp. 11–27). Washington, DC: American Psychological Association.

Rintala, D. H., Young, M. E., Hart, K. A., Clearman, R. R., & Fuhrer, M. J. (1992). Social support and the well-being of persons with spinal cord injury living in the community. *Rehabilitation Psychology, 37*, 155–163.

Robinson, F. M., West, D., & Woodworth, D. (1995). *Coping + Plus: Dimensions of disability*. Westport, CT: Praeger.

Schandler, S. L., Cohen, M. J., & Vulpe, M. (1996). Problem-solving and coping strategies in persons with spinal cord injury who have and do not have a family history of alcoholism. *Journal of Spinal Cord Medicine, 19*, 78–86.

Schulz, R., & Decker, S. (1985). Long-term adjustment to physical disability: The role of social support, perceived control, and self-blame. *Journal of Personality and Social Psychology, 48*, 1162–1172.

Senelick, R. C., & Dougherty, K. (1998). *The spinal cord injury handbook for patients and their families*. Birmingham, AL: Healthsouth Press.

Sharoff, K. (2004). *Coping skills therapy for managing chronic and terminal illness*. New York: Springer Publishing Co.

Sholomskas, D. E., Steil, J. M., & Plummer, J. K. (1990). The spinal cord injured revisited: The relationship between self-blame, other-blame and coping. *Journal of Applied Social Psychology, 20*, 548–574.

Sperry, L. (2006). *Psychological treatment of chronic illness: The biopsychosocial therapy approach*. Washington, DC: American Psychological Association.

Starck, P. L. (1981). Rehabilitative nursing and logotherapy: A study of spinal cord injured clients. *International Forum for Logotherapy, 4*, 101–109.

Steinglass, P., Temple, S., Lisman, S. A., & Reiss, D. (1982). Coping with spinal cord injury: The family perspective. *General Hospital Psychiatry, 4*, 259–264.

Tirch, D. D., & Radnitz, C. L. (2000). Spinal cord injury. In C. L. Radnitz (Ed.), *Cognitive-behavioral therapy for persons with disabilities* (pp. 39–57). Northvale, NJ: Jason Aronson, Inc.

Turner, J. A., Jensen, M. P., Warms, C. A., & Cardenas, D. D. (2002). Catastrophizing is associated with pain intensity, psychological distress, and pain-related disability among individuals with chronic pain after spinal cord injury. *Pain, 98*, 127–134.

Van den Bout, J., Van Son-Schoones, N., Schipper, J., & Groffen, C. (1988). Attributional cognitions, coping behavior, and self-esteem in inpatients with severe spinal cord injuries. *Journal of Clinical Psychology, 44*, 17–22.

Whalley-Hammell, K. R. (1994). Psychosocial outcome following spinal cord injury. *Paraplegia, 32*, 771–779.

Wilson, M. W., Richards, J. S., Klapow, J. C., DeVivo, M. J., and Greene, P. (2005). Cluster analysis and chronic pain: An empirical classification of pain subgroups in a spinal cord injury sample. *Rehabilitation Psychology, 50*(4), 381–388.

Wineman, N. M., Durand, E. J., & McCulloch, B. J. (1994). Examination of the factor structure of the ways of coping questionnaire with clinical populations. *Nursing Research, 43*, 268–273.

Wineman, N. M., Durand, E. J., & Steiner, R. P. (1994). A comparative analysis of coping behaviors in persons with multiple sclerosis or a spinal cord injury. *Research in Nursing & Health, 17*, 185–194.

World Health Organization (1996). *Promoting independence following a spinal cord injury: A manual for mid-level rehabilitation workers.* Retrieved July 28, 2006, from http://whqlibdoc.who.int/hq/1996/WHO_RHB_96.4.pdf

World Health Organization (2006). *Water-related diseases: Spinal injury.* Retrieved July 26, 2006, from http://www.who.int/water_sanitation_health/diseases/spinal/en/

Yarkony, G. M., & Heinemann, A. W. (1995). Pressure ulcers. In S. L. Stover, J. A. DeLisa, & G. G. Whiteneck (Eds.), *Spinal cord injury: Clinical outcomes from the model systems* (pp. 100–119). Gaithersburg, MD: Aspen Publishers.

18
Coping with Traumatic Brain Injury: Existential Challenges and Managing Hope

Joseph H. Hinkebein and Renee C. Stucky

Introduction

Traumatic brain injury (TBI) is among the most challenging and potentially catastrophic of disabling conditions. The centrality of the brain for the effective production and regulation of essentially every critical human attribute, faculty, and capacity contributes to the exquisite psychosocial vulnerability of individuals who sustain TBI. Following TBI, the individual often finds that the very personal skills and resources necessary to cope with disability are the ones most undermined by their injury.

Further, the prevalence of this disabling condition is almost staggering in proportion, yet it may be one of the most unrecognized disabling conditions to the general public, as it is often "invisible" to the uninformed observer. Ironically, because of the stealth quality of this disability, society is dreadfully unaware of the epidemic proportions of the problem. If a new contagious disease or cancer was discovered that occurred with the frequency and life-disrupting potential of TBI, it would be considered a national emergency, warranting huge expenditure for prevention and treatment. Yet expenditures for research into TBI prevention and treatment lag far behind other illnesses and disabilities, largely because of the public's lack of awareness, and also because survivors of brain injury are infrequently capable of being effective advocates for their own cause, secondary to the nature of the disabling consequences arising from TBI.

TBI Prevalence, Etiology, and Demographics

The extent of the problem posed by TBI is illustrated by the most recent data on the prevalence and etiology. In the U.S. alone, it is estimated that 1.5 million sustain a TBI each year, with up to 50,000 deaths, 230,000 hospitalizations, and 80,000–90,000 experiencing long-term disability that is associated with TBI (Thurman, Alverson, Dunn, Guerrero, & Sniezek, 1999). These estimates are likely low, given the reality that many people with milder TBI are seen in emergency rooms and then released without hospitalization, and possibly, without a formal diagnosis of TBI.

Traumatic Brain Injury is defined by the TBI Model Systems National Data Base as "damage to brain tissue caused by an external mechanical force, as evidenced by loss of consciousness due to brain trauma, posttraumatic amnesia (PTA), skull fracture, or objective neurological findings that can reasonably be attributed to TBI on physical examination or mental status examinations" (Harrison-Felix, Newton, Hall, & Kreutzer, 1996, p. 2).

Demographically, TBI is most prevalent in two age-groups, with those 15–24 years of age have a 176.7 per 100,000 rate of TBI occurrence, while those over 75 years have a 186.2 per 100,000 rate (Centers for Disease Control, 1997). Motor vehicle crashes are the most common cause in the younger group, with falls constituting the primary cause in the elderly. Other common etiologies include assaults and sports/recreation-related injuries (Rosenthal & Ricker, 2000). Alcohol is a common contributing factor in TBI (Kraus, Morgenstern, Fife, Conroy, and Nourjah, 1989). Lower SES and a history of legal problems are also demonstrated risk factors (Collins, 1993; Kreutzer, Marwitz, & Witol, 1995).

TBI Presentation and Course

A lengthy discussion of TBI presentation and course is beyond the scope and purpose of this chapter, but a brief description is warranted before discussing the literature on coping with TBI. It should be noted that a great variability in TBI presentation and course is common, although it is possible to offer a cautious description of a "typical" clinical pathway for moderate to severe TBI injuries. Most individuals with TBI will first receive medical attention at the scene of the injury from emergency medical technicians. Stabilization of vital functions (e.g., respiration, blood pressure, oxygen supply) is the goal at this stage, both to prevent secondary injury (anoxia) and to allow for safe transport to the emergency room.

Stabilization and evaluation at the emergency room will focus on assessing neurological status (level of consciousness and responsiveness) and ruling out life-threatening complications, such as uncontrolled hemorrhaging and edema. This evaluation will include neuroimaging such as CT scanning, but will also include qualitative measurements such as the Glasgow Coma Scale, which rates the individual's highest level of response with respect to eye-opening, motor function, and verbalization. Emergent interventions may be necessary (neurosurgery to control bleeding, intracranial pressure monitoring/treatment), and general attempts to minimize secondary neurological injury will be implemented. Most severely-injured individuals will then be monitored in a neurological intensive care unit, with eventual transfer to a neurological medical bed, with the goal of ongoing medical stabilization, prevention of medical complications, and hopefully increasing responsiveness.

Ideally, most individuals of moderate to severe TBI will eventually be transferred to an acute inpatient rehabilitation medicine-setting, where the gradual and challenging work of regaining functions and increasing independence can begin. The multidisciplinary rehabilitation team assesses and treats those domains that support independence. Assessment of mobility, basic activities of daily living, cognition, memory, speech/language, behavior and emotional functioning ensues. Intra-individual, familial, and community resources and supports are also identified, with the goal of planning for eventual return to the community in the least restrictive environment, which permits the highest functioning.

It is during this stage that most (but not all) individuals with TBI first begin to develop an awareness of what has transpired. Yet, often this awareness is quite limited, and for some unfortunate individuals, full awareness may never be achieved. As awareness of the environment and circumstances slowly develops, the long and often painful process of coping with disability will begin for the individual with TBI, his or her family, and friends.

Optimally, the process of community integration following hospital discharge will be facilitated by the receipt of comprehensive and integrated multidisciplinary, outpatient, rehabilitation services. The involvement of rehabilitation psychology and neuropsychology services at the acute and post-acute stages is essential, in order to begin addressing the difficult emotional and behavioral challenges that many individuals will encounter.

Unfortunately, many individuals with TBI do not receive these critical specialized outpatient rehabilitation services, secondary to financial constraints and/or because of lack of geographic access to such programs. The well-known health-care crisis of the uninsured exerts a particularly heavy toll with respect to accessing rehabilitation services, given the earlier discussed reality of low SES as a risk factor for TBI (with consequent higher rates of uninsured status). The challenge of learning to live and cope with TBI is magnified and exacerbated for those individuals who are unable to access specialized TBI rehabilitation services.

Coping and Traumatic Brain Injury

It is a substantial understatement to report that the challenge of coping with and adjusting to the often catastrophic consequences of TBI will persist for years, if not for the rest of the individual's life. Consequently, it is important to consider the individual's stage in rehabilitation when addressing the question of coping and adaptation. The challenges encountered at the acute stage of rehabilitation often differ in quality and severity from those encountered at the post-acute and long-term stages of rehabilitation. The authors find the metaphor of a river useful. The Mississippi River extends from Minnesota to the Gulf of Mexico near New Orleans. Yet, a person, who is only familiar with this river in Minneapolis, Memphis, or New Orleans, does not fully understand the nature of the river. It is optimal to have familiarity of the topography and features of the river's entire length. Similarly, those seeking to understand the coping and adaptation process after TBI should strive for familiarity with issues encountered at all stages of the rehabilitation process.

A review of the scientific literature, pertaining to adaptation and coping with TBI, is complicated by the reality that the experience of sustaining and living with TBI is highly individualized and influenced by factors such as injury severity, pre-injury capacities, access to specialized rehabilitation service, and the presence of familial and community supports. To simplify the task of reviewing the TBI coping literature, this chapter will primarily focus on the coping and adjustment of adults who have suffered moderate to severe injuries. Regrettably, space constraints preclude a discussion of coping with pediatric TBI, which is a topic that merits its own chapter, given the unique challenges faced by this population and their families. Similarly, the extensive coping literature that considers the impact of TBI on the individual's support network (family and friends) will not be covered. Finally, there is a large literature dedicated to mild TBI. It is widely recognized that the issues encountered by those with "mild" TBI may have qualitative and quantitative differences, relative to the more severely injured individual. The reader is referred to *Neuropsychological Management of Mild Traumatic Brain Injury* by Raskin and Mateer (2000) for an excellent discussion of these issues.

It may be illustrative to imagine the subjective experience of sustaining TBI, as difficult as this might be for those who have been fortunate enough to avoid such a traumatic event. Imagine gradually awakening in an environment that is unfamiliar. There are strangers entering and exiting the room without asking permission. You are lying in a bed with a mesh veil that prevents your exiting. A tube protrudes from your throat, and other tubes enter your stomach and arm. You do not know how you got here; further, your perceptions seem distorted and surreal. The strangers who are entering your room speak; but their words frequently do not make sense. You are frightened, but unable to find the words to express your fear or to demand explanation. Further, a dull roar or "static" seems to be coming from within that makes it very difficult to be still. Your inability to interpret the motives of those around you and your confusion regarding your circumstances lead you to resist the actions of the people around you. Your attempts to pull the tubes from your body are vigorously resisted, resulting in your hands being restrained to prevent your efforts to manipulate your environment.

The above exercise in imagination is offered to provide an imperfect insight into what an individual emerging from coma after TBI might experience. Imagine the fear, perhaps even terror, which would naturally be evoked by such an experience. Yet, this is often the first subjective experience that individuals with TBI encounter in the Herculean task of recreating their life after brain injury.

TBI as an Existential Crisis

Traumatic brain injury is an existential crisis. It radically disrupts the topography of a person's life, eliminating or altering landmarks that have served to guide one's efforts and activities, and often leaves the individual feeling alienated and lost. Rollo May coined the vivid phrase "dissolutions of self" to describe how disability can challenge an individual's sense of meaning, sense of self, and basic human integrity (May, 1977).

The challenge of adapting to TBI is also existential in nature. It is the process of separating what has been lost from what has not been lost, and re-establishing a sense of meaning and purpose in life. Existential psychologists, such as Viktor Frankl and Rollo May, have observed that without a sense of meaning and purpose, individuals may lose the will to live. It is therefore obvious that effective rehabilitation services, with integrated and sustained psychotherapeutic input, are critical in helping the individual with TBI navigate this crisis, and again establish a sense of meaning and purpose in their lives. This is a process that can take years, if not the rest of the individual's life, to achieve.

As the rehabilitation course progresses, and with appropriate care and interventions, the individual with TBI moves through the early stages of rehabilitation, and gradually begins to more reliably retain information about time, place, and circumstances. However, this ability is often fragmented, and the individual may become quite frustrated by the difficulty of reliably processing and retaining information. With the help of repetition, the individual eventually learns and is able to retain the fact that he or she suffered a traumatic injury, although it seems unreal – because he or she has no recollection of the event and is forced to rely on others for information.

As the protracted process of developing awareness of how this event has disrupted the person's life begins and develops, strong emotional reactions often occur, including grief, self-reproach, anger, depression, and anxiety. Further, medical and rehabilitation specialists are unable to provide clear and tangible answers to questions about how soon the individual will be "back to normal." In fact, questions about regaining normalcy seem to yield answers that are frightening in their ambiguity and equivocation. Coping with ambiguity about the future may be one of the biggest challenges that individuals with TBI and their families encounter.

Stages of thought w/ TBI

Challenges of Coping with TBI

There is an inherent paradox when considering the topic of coping with TBI. Most disabling injuries and illnesses, which do not involve the brain, allow the individual access to their personal repertoire of coping strategies that have developed as a consequence of earlier life challenges and events. These strategies may include cognitive and emotional resources, personality characteristics, interpersonal skills, and personal philosophies and beliefs. Complicating the coping

We draw on our coping mechanisms to get us through however, if you can remember what they are it makes it very frustrating.

process is the reality that these resources are often lost or damaged, leaving the individual with TBI feeling adrift and frustrated. The individual often needs to learn new strategies for coping before substantial traction is achieved on the road to adaptation.

Common cognitive deficits after TBI may involve impairment in sensory-perceptual abilities, attention, memory, language, reduced capacity for processing information, and limited executive skills (initiation, task-persistence, planning, organization, and problem-solving). Emotional and behavioral disruption, as a direct result of an injured brain, may also seriously impede the adaptation process. Impaired impulse-control, an inability to effectively regulate emotion, an inability to take the perspective of others, or an inability to detect non-verbal nuances can all challenge the individual's ability to cope. Individuals with TBI often have difficulty accurately assessing their own strengths and weaknesses following injury. The injured brain may be incapable of recognizing its own injury and weaknesses.

Problems that occur

Other challenges created by a TBI are related to an individual's social network. The aftermath of TBI can exert a heavy toll on the individual's friends and families. Sadly, it is not uncommon for friends and families to be unable to cope with the changes in the individual, and to consequently detach emotionally and socially, further exacerbating the sense of alienation.

Social network. Problems

Despite the grim picture painted in the preceding paragraphs, it should be noted that this seemingly insurmountable challenge of coping and adapting to TBI is being met on a daily basis by hundreds of thousands of individuals with TBI. While almost always a life-changing event, TBI does not have to be a life sentence of despair and depression. However, much work needs to be done, in order to educate policy-makers and the general public about TBI, and about how to optimally facilitate the rehabilitation, reintegration, and adjustment of people with TBI back to meaningful and productive societal roles.

TBI and Psychosocial Outcome: The Scope of the Problem

There is an appalling level of misconceptions about TBI in the general public; this reality serves as an obstacle to psychosocial and community reintegration (Willer, Johnson, Rempel & Linn, 1993). It seems likely that much of the misunderstanding, related to TBI and its long-term consequences, is tied to inaccurate and almost caricatured depictions of TBI in the popular media. While it is true that some individuals of TBI make incredible, indeed miraculous recoveries, the majority of individuals with TBI are left with often radically altered life-courses, capabilities, and self-images. It is not uncommon for individuals of TBI to encounter assumptions that their level of motivation or determination must have been inadequate, if they did not achieve the types of recoveries typically depicted in the popular media. Hopefully, this review of the psychosocial outcome literature will offer the reader a more accurate and realistic framework for appreciating the challenges that are faced by those living with TBI.

Tate, Lulham, Broe, Strettles, and Pfaff (1989) examined psychosocial outcomes in 100 individuals, who suffered severe blunt head injury an average of six years prior to the study. Only 24% of the individuals experienced "good" psychosocial reintegration, while psychosocial integration was rated as "substantially limited" or "poor" for 42.5% and 33.3% of the remaining individuals respectively. Perhaps not surprisingly, individuals who were rated as having a good recovery, as measured by the Glasgow Outcome Scale (GOS), were more likely to have experienced a good psychosocial outcome; although well over half of the people falling in this group still received "substantially limited" psychosocial ratings. By contrast, of those receiving severe disability GOS ratings, 100% received "poor" psychosocial reintegration ratings. Those with moderate disability ratings predominately fell in the "substantially limited" and "poor" categories of psychosocial reintegration.

Tate and colleagues (1989) offered a "good news-bad news" analysis of their findings. Specifically, it was encouraging that in a sample, which was characterized as having "severe" blunt head injury, fully one-quarter of the individuals achieved a rating of "good" psychosocial reintegration. However, even those falling in this one-quarter experienced psychosocial challenges and adversity, including an increased need for emotional support to live independently, a decline in work skills and occupational status, and social isolation. In essence, having a "good" psychosocial outcome does not equate with a full resumption of a pre-injury lifestyle (Tate et al., 1989). This is contrasted with the severe disability group, in which none of the individuals were capable of independent living. The psychosocial challenges of this group included very limited social contact, social isolation, and absence of meaningful leisure-activity (despite ample "spare time"). The authors recommended that rehabilitation targets psychosocial outcomes by addressing independent living skills, relational skills (i.e., how to establish and maintain friendships), and leisure-skill development that takes into account ones' interests and impairments. A strong argument is also made for ongoing community-supports to maintain optimal levels of psychosocial integration.

In a more recent study examining psychosocial outcomes in three domains (occupational activities, interpersonal relationships, and independent living skills), Tate and Broe (1999) found that in a sample of 70 individuals with varying levels of disability after severe TBI (average length since injury: six years), psychosocial outcomes were predicted by degree of neurophysical impairment, neuropsychological impairment, chronicity, and level of self-esteem. Within the neuropsychological domain, behavioral-regulation difficulties were more significantly related to psychosocial outcomes than cognitive capacities. Self-ratings of handicap/disability were unrelated to psychosocial outcomes.

Some researchers interested in psychosocial outcomes have focused on the construct known as "quality of life" (QOL) . The literature related to QOL following TBI is, like many other constructs, plagued by varying conceptual and methodological strategies for defining QOL. In a review of the literature examining QOL (broadly defined) following neurological illness, Murrell (1999)

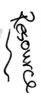

notes that the multidimensional nature of the QOL construct contributes to the difficulty that is associated in studying QOL related to health status. Specific to neurological illnesses and injuries, QOL can be difficult to measure, because of the impact of neurological injuries on cognition and emotions. The authors stressed that the search for objective indicators of QOL is fraught with difficulty, and that essentially a more subjective approach may be necessary for neurological populations.

It perhaps should be obvious that an injury which damages the very circuitry that gives rise to the sense of self should have a substantial impact on quality of life and coping with TBI. In an effort to better understand this relationship, Vickery, Gontkovsky, and Caroselli (2005) examined a relatively small sample of individuals ($N = 19$), who sustained acquired brain injury (ABI). The authors found that disrupted or negative self-concept had a greater impact on quality of life than demographic variables. These authors also stress that research in this area is also limited by conceptual and measurement limitations.

Emotional/Psychological Disruption and TBI

Given the potential magnitude of disruption to a person's capabilities, sense of self, and life pursuits that result from a TBI, it is not surprising that strong emotional and psychological reactions to this disruption are common. In fact, some experts state that the emotional, psychological and behavioral difficulties may contribute more to disability than do the cognitive or physical sequalae of TBI (Lezak, 1987). For many, these difficulties create the primary obstacles in developing and maintaining meaningful relationships, family life, work, and other life activities.

Further, the presence of pre-injury psychiatric disorders appears to predispose individuals with TBI to even greater coping challenges, and often to more enduring and complicated psychosocial difficulties (Ponsford et al., 2000). Estimates of the rate of psychological disorders following TBI are somewhat nebulous; reported rates of psychiatric disorders, such as major depression and anxiety-spectrum disorders, vary greatly in the literature.

There are several factors complicating the diagnostic picture following TBI. Variability in how psychological distress is assessed, an inadequate understanding of the relationship of emotional distress and TBI, and the complex interactive relationship between symptoms of psychological distress and TBI may result in underdiagnosis or misdiagnosis by uninformed practioners (Ownsworth & Oei, 1998). In addition, the severity of emotional distress and the availability of coping resources typically fluctuate over time, creating a vacillating and unpredictable course for both the individual and the family.

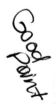

Very commonly, emotional distress increases as insight improves regarding the circumstances and difficulties caused by the injury. Unfortunately, this generally occurs prior to regaining the requisite coping skills that are necessary to manage and work through this distress. Thus, individuals with TBI may be stuck in an "emotional desert," in which they are bombarded by an often overwhelming level of distress, with absent or inadequate coping capacities. Grief, depression, and anxiety/posttraumatic stress are common recovery issues. Given the potential for emotional complications to negatively effect recovery and achieving an optimal outcome, appropriately diagnosing and treating psychological distress is critical.

Grief is a common human response to any type of substantial loss, and the loss occasioned by TBI is usually profound and far-reaching. Some of these losses are immediately evident, although it is common for the individual and family to struggle with the ambiguity regarding whether the losses will be transient and partial, versus permanent and extensive. Tangible losses may include aspects of physical functioning, cognitive abilities, relationships, financial resources, and vocational and educational pursuits. Equally devastating, but less easily quantified, is the loss of independence and freedom, the sense of normalcy and predictability, and the loss of a sense of knowing one's self. Most individuals with TBI feel the "loss of self" in an extremely painful and poignant manner. Grief following TBI is phenomenologically quite similar to the grieving process experienced after losing a loved one (Haynes, 1994).

The interaction between depression and TBI is complex, and believed to be the result of a diverse, complex, and dynamic array of interrelated factors, which complicate treatment of depression following TBI (Ownsworth & Oei, 1998). Depression may occur as a direct consequence of the injury (with a certain lesion-location within the brain being more likely to cause depression), or may arise as a psychological reaction to the impact of the injury. Frequently, depression after TBI is synergistically related to both the actual injury to the brain, and the psychological reaction to its impact on life.

There are additional factors that impose a greater risk of developing depression following TBI. As previously noted, individuals with pre-existing psychiatric difficulties are more susceptible to depression following TBI. Furthermore, post-TBI depression has been linked to persistent negative ruminations, frustration, and confusion (Prigatano, 1999), decreased self-esteem (Morton & Wehman, 1995), and poor insight into deficits, which results in unrealistic expectations and failure (Fleming, Strong, & Ashton, 1996; Prigatano, 2005). Research has also revealed an increased risk for suicide following brain injury, exceeding the risk that is associated with pre-injury personality characteristics (Teasdale & Engberg, 2001).

Depression, in and of itself, often results in significant disability. When occurring as a complication of TBI, depression may substantially exacerbate the TBI-related disability, and may seriously complicate rehabilitation, adaptation, and coping. Unfortunately, depression may be obscured or masked by other symptoms that arise from the brain injury (e.g., apathy/abulia). Consequently, depression is frequently undiagnosed and untreated, resulting in less than optimal rehabilitation outcomes.

In an attempt to improve upon methodological shortcomings of previous research seeking to understand the relationship between depression and TBI, Seel and colleagues (2003) completed a prospective, nationwide, multi-center study as part of the Traumatic Brain Injury Model Systems program. The study revealed that fatigue, distractibility, anger/irritability, and rumination were the most commonly reported depressive symptoms. Further, they found that the three symptoms which most effectively differentiated depressed from non-depressed individuals were feelings of worthlessness, feelings of hopelessness, and difficulty enjoying activities.

As with depressive disorders, there are a myriad of factors that contribute to the development of anxiety and anxiety-spectrum disorders following a brain injury. A controversy exists in the TBI literature as to whether an event, which is not consciously processed or recalled, can be "traumatic" and can result in acute stress disorder (ASD) or posttraumatic stress disorder (PTSD).

Harvey and Bryant (1998) examined predictors of ASD following mild traumatic brain injury, which was defined in this study as a period of posttraumatic amnesia (PTA) of less than 24 hours. These authors found significant levels of ASD (14.6% meeting full criteria) in their population of individuals with mild traumatic brain injury, suggesting that stress reactions do occur in individuals with TBI. They also found that depression and an avoidant coping style significantly predicted acute stress reactions, which is also consistent with findings in non-TBI populations. The authors concluded that, although a number of acute stress symptoms overlap with TBI symptoms and that further research is needed to distinguish these symptomatic reactions, traumatic stress reactions are present in a substantial percentage of individuals who sustain a mild TBI. Being able to provide early identification and specific treatment for individuals at risk could enhance overall recovery and adjustment.

While TBI often results in disruption of emotional functioning, it is not clear whether cognitive factors may predispose individuals to a greater susceptibility to poor emotional adaptation following injury. Skeel, Johnstone, Schopp, Shaw, and Petroski (2000) evaluated the relationships between the absolute level of cognitive functioning, the estimated decline in cognitive functioning, and emotional distress following injury. In contrast to previous assumptions that greater cognitive decline would be associated with more emotional distress, the authors found that estimated level of pre-injury functioning was the best cognitive predictor of distress level following TBI. The authors surmised that individuals with higher pre-injury functioning may also have a wider array of psychosocial and cognitive resources available, which may allow for a more effective coping with TBI.

Coping Strategies and TBI

Moore, Stambrook, and Peters (1989) utilized a cluster-analytic approach for identifying coping strategies, used by a group of 69 individuals with closed head injury, in order to better understand how coping mechanisms serve as moderators of psychosocial and emotional adjustment after brain injury. Three coping "clusters" were identified. The first cluster was characterized by a low use of coping strategies and low endorsement of psychosocial distress. The second cluster was characterized by a wide and relatively indiscriminate use of coping strategies with subsequent higher endorsements of psychosocial distress. Finally, the third cluster represented a group that used a combination of specific coping strategies, which focused on the external environment, as well as positive reappraisal and seeking social-support. Clusters one and three were both associated with less endorsement of depression, psychosocial difficulties, and physical difficulties. The authors speculated that the first cluster may have reflected people who were using denial or lacked insight into the extent of their difficulties, and who were subsequently shielding themselves from emotional distress.

In a similar study that examined both coping strategies and locus of control (LOC) in relationship to long-term outcomes after TBI, Moore and Stambrook (1992) again used a cluster-analytic approach to study these variables in a group of 53 males with TBI. Results showed that different patterns of coping strategies and locus of control were associated with different quality of life outcomes after TBI. The findings also indicated that age played a role in the type of coping strategies and LOC beliefs that were adopted by participants. Better outcomes were associated with a group of respondents who used self-controlling and positive-reappraisal coping strategies, in combination with having a lower external LOC. Further, this pattern of findings was associated with higher self-esteem. In this study, external LOC was related to poorer outcomes; higher external LOC scores were more commonly observed in older individuals with less severe TBI. In their interpretation of the results, the authors suggested that chronological age may play an important role in influencing the individual's coping efforts and LOC beliefs.

Finset and Andersson (2000) examined a sample of 70 individuals approximately one year following the onset of an acquired brain injury. Of these, 27 had a TBI, 30 incurred a Cerebral Vascular Accident (CVA), and 13 experienced Hypoxic Brain Injury (HBI). The authors correctly noted that surprisingly little research has specifically addressed coping strategies and coping processes after brain injury. Using a two-dimensional taxonomy of coping strategies, including *active* or *approach-oriented coping* (planning, positive reinterpretation, growth, acceptance, seeking social support) and *avoidant coping* (mental avoidance, behavioral disengagement, and denial), the researchers found that individuals with brain injury reported less use of approach-oriented or active coping strategies relative to a non-injured comparison group, as well as greater reliance on a restricted set of coping strategies.

Further, Finset and Andersson (2000) found that individuals with greater apathy (a common symptom associated with disruption of medial frontal cortical systems) were less likely to use approach-oriented strategies. The use of avoidant coping strategies was highest among brain-injured individuals with positive symptoms of depression. Interestingly, preferred coping strategies were largely unrelated to identifiable brain-lesion location, except for those individuals with apathy arising from demonstrable right hemisphere and sub-cortical lesions. The authors suggested that psychological factors, such as pre-injury personality and coping repertoire, are more relevant than lesion location within the brain.

Bryant, Margosszeky, Crooks, Baguley, and Gurka (2000) found that an avoidant coping style was a predictor of PTSD severity in individuals who have suffered severe TBI. As noted above, there is no consensus regarding the occurrence of PTSD in individuals who have sustained moderate to severe TBI – because, almost always, there is no personal memory of the injury/event. Neither is there consensus about whether PTSD-like symptoms are more accurately attributed to the TBI itself.

Bryant et al. (2000) cited studies supporting the possibility that PTSD and TBI can co-occur and speculated that cognitive deficits arising from severe TBI limit the individuals' problem-solving repertoire and result in an over-reliance on avoidant and emotion-focused strategies. Consequently, the individual never confronts the aversive emotion, nor has the opportunity to habituate to the associated anxiety or to modify cognitions related to the trauma. Whether one accepts or rejects the premise that PTSD can occur after a TBI, Bryant and colleagues' study provides support for the premise that avoidant coping strategies after TBI are associated with greater levels of distress.

While not specific to predefined coping strategies, Wilson (2000) found that the ability of individuals with TBI to utilize compensatory strategies for cognitive/neuropsychological deficits related to TBI is in part linked to the number of impaired cognitive domains. Individuals experiencing impairment primarily in memory domains were better able to utilize compensatory strategies than individuals with memory deficits that were accompanied by other cognitive impairments. This raises an interesting question as to whether the extent and severity of cognitive impairment is also related to the ability to utilize coping strategies following brain injury.

When comparing coping strategies that are used by individuals with TBI versus by individuals with other type of neurological illness (brain tumor, stroke, Parkinson's Disease), Herrmann et al. (2000) found that coping styles largely did not differ across different types of acquired brain dysfunction, although demographic variables, such as age and social factors, did account for some of the differences in coping strategies. The authors utilized a five-factor model of coping, including: Depressive coping; active, problem-oriented coping; distraction and self-reorganization; religious belief/quest for sense; and minimization/wishful thinking. For all neurological patient groups, active/problem-oriented coping strategies tended to be most commonly utilized, although some of the disability groups (specifically stroke individuals) tended to rely less on these strategies and more on religious/quest for sense strategies, which was thought to likely be related to chronological age and chronicity of disability.

Interestingly, Herrmann and colleagues (2000) did not find coping behavior to be associated with severity of neurological symptoms. The authors concluded that illness/injury-specific variables contributed little to choice of coping strategies; most of the variance could be explained by cultural and socio-demographic variables. It was thought that pre-injury personality traits had more to do with coping than the illness/injury-specific psychological reactions.

TBI and Self-Awareness

TBI, by definition, affects the very organ that gives rise to the phenomenon of consciousness and awareness, in essence, "the mind." Consequently, TBI often damages structures and functions that are highly involved in how individuals adapt and cope with crisis. For example, a common difficulty encountered after brain injury is an incomplete or even absent awareness of how the injury has affected ones' abilities. It is not uncommon to encounter individuals who insist that they are no different or less capable than prior to TBI, despite extensive feedback and evidence to the contrary. Disturbances in self-awareness have been found to be common in severe TBI, although less so with mild or moderate TBI (Leathem, Murphy, & Flett, 1998). It stands to reason that an individual, who lacks insight into the reality of their circumstances and the nature of their strengths and limitations, is likely to be challenged in their ability to cope with the consequences of this reality.

While the ego defense-mechanisms of denial, repression, minimizing, and rationalization may contribute to the phenomenon of limited insight, neuropsychological research suggests that the problem is caused by cognitive deficits, rather than reflecting a conscious or unconscious choice to use non-adaptive coping strategies. Not surprisingly, deficits of awareness pose challenges in the rehabilitation and coping process. In essence, the individual who lacks awareness or insight may adhere to the belief "if it's not broken... it doesn't need fixing." Also, as discussed above, the limited awareness of problems frequently leads to unrealistic expectations for recovery and resumption of pre-injury life-roles and activities, often resulting in failure.

Self-awareness deficits following TBI have been well studied phenomenon. A number of roughly-synonymous constructs may be used to describe this capacity, including cognitive appraisal accuracy (Kervick & Kaemingk, 2005), metacognitive skills (Ownsworth & Fleming, 2005), and anosognosia. Rather than embarking on a lengthy neuropsychological explanation of the phenomenon, the authors will focus on studies that have examined the role of self-awareness in emotional adaptation and coping with TBI. For readers, who are interested in a more in depth exploration of the phenomenon of disturbed self-awareness, the authors recommend an excellent review article of the TBI self-awareness literature by Prigatano (2005).

Wallace and Bogner (2000) studied the implications of awareness deficits on emotional status following TBI. Fifty individuals with at least moderately severe TBI and their significant others completed Patient Competency Rating Scales (PCRS), for which difference scores (between the individual with TBI ratings and these of the significant other) were used as a measure of deficit awareness. Study results yielded support for the premise that an awareness of deficits is at least partially related to the endorsement of distress on measures such as the Beck Depression Inventory (BDI) and the Beck Anxiety Inventory (BAI). Individuals who endorsed fewer deficits than reported by their significant other were less likely to endorse emotional distress on the BDI and BAI. Potential confounds, which were discussed by the authors, include the possibility that those endorsing more depression may also be more likely to endorse deficits on the PCRS.

Interestingly, PCRS difference scores in the Wallace and Bogner study were not related to the emotional well-being of significant others, although length of time since injury was associated with less emotional symptom endorsement. However, Prigatano, Borgaro, Baker, and Wethe (2005) found that the level of distress endorsed by family members of individuals with TBI was significantly correlated with their rating of the individual's lack of awareness (particularly lack of awareness regarding socially inappropriate behaviors and difficulties controlling emotions). This finding, which is related to family coping, underscores one of the limitations of this type of research: specifically, outcomes may be affected by how lack of awareness is conceptualized psychometrically. As discussed in the Prigatano literature review (2005), no "gold standard" has been established for the measurement of self-awareness deficits.

In another study focusing on a component of awareness, the discrepancies between 103 individuals with TBI and family-member ratings of cognitive function were examined by Kervick & Kaemingk (2005). These researchers found that cognitive-appraisal deficits were predictive of injury severity and outcomes. Yet, cognitive appraisal accuracy did not solely account for psychosocial outcomes; instead, it acted as a moderating variable between injury severity and occupational and independent living. However, appraisal accuracy did not moderate the relationship between injury severity and interpersonal outcomes. Severe TBI was associated with lower social functioning, regardless of appraisal accuracy.

Vocational Reintegration after TBI

The centrality of vocational activity to one's sense of identity and self-worth is often overlooked and taken for granted until threatened or lost. Upon first meeting a person, usually the second question (after name) is "What do you do for a living?" Vocational activity provides a source of pride, prestige, meaning and purpose, and optimally provides economic independence and financial well-being. In short, vocational activity plays a critical role in quality of life.

Traumatic brain injury often has a devastating impact on vocational status, and the consequent economic impact usually further impedes the coping process. Individuals who sustain TBI may lose the requisite capacities for maintaining competitive employment; or if they are able to work, may only be able to do so at a much reduced capacity. A full explication of the extensive literature related to vocational adjustment after TBI is beyond the scope of this chapter. In the interest of offering a glimpse of the importance of this domain, some select research will be discussed.

In an interview-based study of individuals with TBI, Power and Hershenson (2003) found several salient themes to be associated with TBI that occurs in mid-career. They found that in almost all cases, TBI resulted in a "major blow to self-concept, manifested by a dramatic drop in self-image" (p.1025). Those who possessed strong work ethics encountered a loss of a sense of value as a person. The extent of these self-esteem losses was mediated by a number of factors, including age and prior work history, the nature of the disability associated with TBI, the effectiveness of coping resources, and whether or not the individual was participating in post-TBI employment or related activities (such as retraining for alternate employment).

In the clinical experience of the authors, those individuals who histori-cally placed the greatest value on intellectual capacities, or whose employment clearly was more associated with intellectual versus physical endeavors, usually will suffer an even greater blow to self-esteem and coping. Power and Hershenson (2003) provide validation for this anecdotal observation, in that self-concept was more dramatically affected when TBI resulted in serious deficits in cognitive capacities that were essential in the performance of pre-injury vocations. The resultant grief and depression can become obstacles to the consid-eration of other vocational directions, an effect that is exacerbated when an individual is older and perceives that his or her age is an additional obstacle to re-training.

Promoting Coping after TBI

As has been discussed, the aftermath of TBI creates an overwhelming challenge to coping and adaptation, not just for the individual with TBI, but also for families and health-care providers. Given the complexity of the challenge, the rehabili-tation of an individual with TBI requires a multidisciplinary approach with an integrated purpose: an amelioration and/or minimization of deficits to allow for community re-integration and a return-to-life activities and responsibilities at the highest possible level.

While great strides have been made in protocols and technologies that save and prolong life after trauma, particularly trauma to the brain, our knowledge and skill in being able to ameliorate the multi-faceted TBI sequelae lag far behind. This reality is resulting in a tremendous crisis in our health-care system: a chasm between our medical-technological, life-sustaining capabilities, contrasted with society's ability to meet the health-care and psychosocial needs of this population. There is much still to learn about how to effectively intervene in order to improve the quality of life of individuals living with TBI.

A full exploration of the literature pertaining to intervention practices after TBI is beyond the scope of this chapter. However, some general discussion related to the TBI-intervention literature is pertinent to this chapter on coping with TBI. The lion's share of TBI intervention research has targeted the remediation of neurocognitive deficits. Certainly, improving neurocognitive function and teaching compensatory strategies to individuals with TBI are critical and necessary components of learning to live and cope after TBI. However, the focus on deficit remediation and compensation is rarely sufficient, in and of itself, for teaching individuals with TBI how to cope and achieve a sense that life is again worth living.

Intervention research which focuses specifically on coping strategies that are utilized by individuals with TBI seems to have lagged behind research into cognitive interventions. Mental-health practitioners who provide services to individuals with TBI often find that educational and cognitive-behavioral therapeutic approaches are most practical and useful. This is perhaps because of the obvious and substantial need for the person living with TBI to have reality-based, normative data about their injury, to help them maintain accurate self-appraisals and attributions, and to help with their consequent efforts to have this self-knowledge guide behavior. The individual with TBI often needs direct and tangible feedback as to how he or she may need to approach certain situations (e.g., interpersonal, social, and vocational) in a manner that differs from pre-injury approaches. Often such interventions need to be reiterated given the difficulty that many individuals have with new learning, particularly when the new learning is changing long-held beliefs and behavioral patterns.

However, it is essential to stress that the practitioner, who only addresses the behavioral component of the brain-injury experience without exploring the phenomenological and existential reality of the injury for the individual, is probably doing the individual a disservice. The challenge of helping individuals with TBI understand and integrate the reality of the injury and its consequences, while facilitating the grief process and promoting a positive orientation to the future, is great but rewarding for those who have dedicated their professional efforts to helping this population.

Family and Social Support

Rehabilitation interventions are often targeted at the family and the community-level. Families generally provide the primary context of social and emotional support following an injury. Just as with individual coping resources, the degree of effectiveness of this support is determined in a large part by the pre-injury characteristics, emotional/coping health, and basic resources of the family system.

Given the increased rates of survival following TBI, as well as changes in the health-care system (i.e., decreased funding for longer-term care), the caregiver burden on families continues to expand. There is a tremendous mismatch between the needs of people living with disabilities, including brain injury, and available societal resources. Given that so many family members are functioning as care providers, and that these are the individuals that promote or undermine the health of the individual, it is vital to consider the family context and family needs in interventions for individuals with brain injury.

Not uncommonly, family members of individuals with TBI have encountered the uncomfortable challenge of persuading the person with TBI to refrain from an activity that has been rendered dangerous by TBI-related deficits (e.g., driving a vehicle, when there are clear visual or attention deficits that the individual does not recognize). Conversely, families of persons with TBI may be struck by the absence of an appropriate emotional response from the individual, who is unable to appreciate the gravity and implications of the injury and deficits. Clearly, the presence or absence of self-awareness after TBI is an important variable to examine when addressing the question of how individuals with TBI and their families cope.

Psychosocial adjustment and outcomes appear to be related to social supports. Kaplan (1991) found that ratings of family cohesion and available perceived social support were related to the three-year psychosocial and vocational status in 25 individuals with severe TBI. Specifically, families, who were rated as having high levels of organization were associated with better temperaments and social behavior among individuals with TBI. The author suggested that such environments impose more optimal structure and organization in the lives of individuals with TBI, with consequent psychosocial and emotional benefits. Also, higher degrees of shared familial religious values, a familial recreational orientation, and the degree of encouragement and expressiveness that is manifested in the family unit were related to better psychosocial outcomes.

Discussion and Summary

Traumatic brain injury is a life-changing event. While there has been extensive research on the impact of TBI on psychosocial adjustment, there is much that is still unknown about the process by which individuals cope with this event. Perhaps this is not surprising, when one considers the myriad of variables at play. There is vast individual variability with regard to demographic variables, pre-injury experiences, personality, coping strategies, community resources, familial resources, and spiritual resources. Further complicating the scenario is the reality that while all brain injuries share some similarities, no two brain injuries are exactly alike. The complexity of the brain and the almost infinite number of ways that the structural and functional architecture of the brain can be altered by trauma suggest that every person with TBI has a unique path to follow in their attempt to reconstruct their life.

It may be instructive to consider an anecdotal case from the authors' clinical experience. This is the case of a successful middle-aged man, who sustained a severe TBI when he was struck by a vehicle that was driven by an intoxicated driver. During a prolonged rehabilitation course, this individual (we will call him "Jim") continued to experience loss that was related to the initial injury. While Jim had been successfully employed in a prestigious occupation that afforded a very good living, he was no longer capable of competitive employment, as a result of cognitive impairment. Even more tragically, Jim's spouse was not able to cope with the emotional and behavioral changes wrought by the TBI, and divorced Jim, which also resulted in the loss of close contact with his children. While achieving independence in basic activities of daily living, Jim needed to return to the home of his parents. Not surprisingly, around two years post-injury, Jim was referred for psychotherapy, due to depression and anger-control problems.

The predominant tone of Jim's presentation was anger that was fueled by bitterness. The enormous unfairness of all that transpired overwhelmed Jim, who could not understand or accept how a person, who had "played by the rules" and who had been responsible in all spheres of life, could experience such enormous loss as a result of another person's irresponsibility. The precipitating event (the motor-vehicle collision that he was unable to remember) was an obsessive fixation, with an equally obsessive, ruminative anger toward the person who caused the accident. Unfortunately, Jim's anger was all-consuming and poorly directed, and his supportive but beleaguered parents were the lightning rods for Jim's outrage.

In the process of psychotherapy, it became clear that Jim had a belief in a "just-world," and was unable to accept that sometimes bad things happen to people who are striving to "play by the rules." The injury clearly created an immense existential crisis for Jim, who had lost everything that had given his life a sense of meaning (i.e., his role as a father and husband; the respect, life-style and prestige afforded by his occupation; his independence). He continued to intensely grieve these losses and struggled to maintain a belief that life was still worth living. Of course, his anger and bitterness were understandable; it would unreasonable to assert that he should feel otherwise. However, his inability to grapple with this loss, because of the far-reaching nature of the loss and the functional consequence of his brain injury, was clearly an obstacle to re-establishing a sense of purpose and direction in life.

While acknowledging the validity of Jim's anger and bitterness, an attempt was made to help him understand that "living in anger" was consuming all of his energies and preventing him from having any chance of learning how to be happy again. The metaphor of "walking backwards into his future while fixing his gaze on the past trauma" was used to help Jim understand that he was erroneously hoping to find some answer or solution for his pain in the past. Jim was challenged to "turn around" psychologically, and start walking "face forward" into the future, where he had at least a chance to identify opportunities that may exist. This was a very difficult challenge, and Jim needed to understand that he was not being asked to forget the trauma or his losses, but to recognize that his exclusive focus on both was preventing him from learning how to live again.

Efforts were made to help Jim separate what had been lost from what had not been lost. While he suffered definite cognitive losses (particularly in the realm of memory and processing speed), he was helped to understand that he still had numerous strengths that could be utilized to help him achieve a sense of direction and accomplishment, perhaps in a volunteer position. Further, the need to start reaching out again to the community was identified as a goal.

This individual was able to eventually make an essential transition, in which the existential crisis imposed by his TBI was identified and the long and difficult struggle of learning to enjoy life again was engaged. His challenge became one of "embracing the full catastrophe" (Kabat-Zinn, 1990), learning to reconnect with what is good in life and live in the present, rather than allow the catastrophe to become an all-consuming focus. Such an existential struggle, faced by individuals with brain injuries, is one that can be facilitated by knowledgeable and supportive mental-health professionals. Yet, ultimately this challenge is one that can only be met by the individual with TBI. As authors of this chapter and as psychologists who work with individuals learning to live with TBI, it is gratifying to report that the challenge is being met on a daily basis by thousands of individuals with TBI.

It is customary at the end of such a chapter to discuss directions for further research. The authors would instead prefer to issue a different type of challenge. While research to better understand and promote coping with TBI is clearly needed, perhaps even more critically needed at this stage are efforts to increase public awareness of the epidemic that TBI truly is, and to help change the many misconceptions and prejudices held by the public about TBI.

It is human nature to fear what is not understood, and that lack of understanding relating to TBI and its consequences can only portend additional and unnecessary challenges for those living with TBI. An accurate understanding of the nature and scope of the problem is absolutely critical, if public policy and the medical-industrial complex are ever to adequately meet the challenge of providing comprehensive prevention, treatment, rehabilitative, and long-term living assistance to the many "invisibly-injured" individuals who are living with TBI.

References

Bryant, R. A., Margosszeky, J. E., Crooks, J., Baguley, I., & Gurka, J. (2000). Coping style and post-traumatic stress disorder following severe traumatic brain injury. *Brain Injury, 14*(2), 175–180.

Centers for Disease Control. (1997, January 10). Traumatic brain injury – Colorado, Missouri, Oklahoma, and Utah, 1990–1993. *Morbidity and Mortality Weekly Report, 48*(1), 8–11.

Collins, J. G. (1993). Types of injuries by selected characteristics: United States. 1986–1988. National Center for Health Statistics. *Vital Health Statistics, 2*(182), 1–87.

Finset, A., & Andersson, S. (2000). Coping strategies in patients with acquired brain injury: Relationships between coping, apathy, depression and lesion location. *Brain Injury, 14*(10), 887–905.

Fleming, J. M., Strong, J., & Ashton, R. (1996). Self-awareness of deficits in adults with traumatic brain injury. How best to measure? *Brain Injury, 10*, 1–15.

Harrison-Felix, C., Newton, C. N., Hall, K. M., & Kreutzer, J. S. (1996). Descriptive findings from the traumatic brain injury model systems national data base. *Journal of Head Trauma Rehabilitation, 11*(5), 1–14.

Harvey, A. G., & Bryant, R. A. (1998). Predictors of acute stress following mild traumatic brain injury. *Brain Injury, 12*(2), 147–154.

Haynes, S. D. (1994). The experience of grief in the head-injured adult. *Archives of Clinical Neuropsychology, 9*(4), 323–336.

Herrmann, M., Curio, N., Petz, T., Synowitz, H., Wagner, S., Bartels, C., et al. (2000). Coping with illness after brain diseases – A comparison between patients with malignant brain tumors, stroke, Parkinson's disease and traumatic brain injury. *Disability and Rehabilitation, 22*(12), 539–546.

Kabat-Zinn, J. (1990). *Full catastrophe living: Using the wisdom of your body and mind to face stress, pain, and illness.* New York: Delacorte Press.

Kaplan, S. P. (1991). Psychosocial adjustment three years after traumatic brain injury. *The Clinical Neuropsychologist, 5*(4), 360–369.

Kervick, R. B., & Kaemingk, K. L. (2005). Cognitive appraisal accuracy moderates the relationship between injury severity and psychosocial outcomes in traumatic brain injury. *Brain Injury, 19*(11), 881–889.

Kraus, J., Morgenstern, H., Fife, D., Conroy, C., & Nourjah, P. (1989). Blood alcohol tests, prevalence of involvement, and outcomes following brain injury. *American Journal of Public Health, 79*(3), 294–299.

Kreutzer, J. S., Marwitz, J. H., & Witol, A.D. (1995). Interrelationships between crime, substance abuse and aggressive behaviours among persons with traumatic brain injury. *Brain Injury, 9*(8) 757–768.

Leathem, J. M., Murphy, L. J., & Flett, R. A. (1998). Self- and informant-ratings on the patient competency rating scale in patients with traumatic brain injury. *Journal of Clinical and Experimental Neuropsychology, 20*(5), 694–705.

Lezak, M. D. (1987). Relationships between personality disorders, social disturbances, and physical disability following traumatic brain injury. *Journal of Head Trauma Rehabilitation, 2*, 57–69.

May, R. (1977). *The meaning of anxiety.* New York: Norton.

Moore, A. D., & Stambrook, M. (1992). Coping strategies and locus of control following traumatic brain injury: Relationship to long-term outcome. *Brain Injury, 6*(1), 89–94.

Moore, A. D., Stambrook, M., & Peters, L.C. (1989). Coping strategies and adjustment after closed-head injury: A cluster analytical approach. *Brain Injury, 3*(2), 171–175.

Morton, M. V., & Wehman, P. (1995). Psychosocial and emotional sequelae of individuals with traumatic brain injury: A literature review and recommendations. *Brain Injury, 9*, 81–92.

Murrell, R. (1999). Quality of life and neurological illness: A review of the literature. *Neuropsychology Review, 9*(4), 209–229.

Ownsworth, T. L., & Fleming, J. (2005). The relative importance of metacognitive skills, emotional status, and executive function in psychosocial adjustment following acquired brain injury. *Journal of Head Trauma Rehabilitation, 20*(4), 315–332.

Ownsworth, T. L., & Oei, T. P. S. (1998). Depression after traumatic brain injury: Conceptualization and treatment considerations. *Brain Injury, 12*(9), 735–751.

Ponsford, J., Willmont, C., Rothwell, A., Cameron, P., Kelly, A., Nelms, R., et al. (2000). Factors influencing outcome following mild traumatic brain injury in adults. *Journal of International Neuropsychological Society, 6*(5), 568–579.

Power, P. W., & Hershenson, D. B. (2003). Work adjustment and readjustment of persons with mid-career onset traumatic brain injury. *Brain Injury, 17*(12), 1021–1034.

Prigatano, G. P. (1999). *Principles of neuropsychological rehabilitation.* New York: Oxford University Press.

Prigatano, G. P. (2005). Disturbance of self-awareness and rehabilitation of patients with traumatic brain injury: A twenty year perspective. *Journal of Head Trauma Rehabilitation, 20*(1), 19–29.

Prigatano, G. P., Borgaro, S., Baker, J., & Wethe, J. (2005) Awareness and distress after traumatic brain injury: A relative's perspective. *Journal of Head Trauma Rehabilitation, 20*(4), 359–367.

Raskin, S. A., & Mateer, C. A. (2000). *Neuropsychological management of mild traumatic brain injury.* New York: Oxford University Press.

Rosenthal, M., & Ricker, J. (2000). Traumatic brain injury. In R. G. Frank & T. R. Elliot (Eds.), *Handbook of Rehabilitation Psychology* (pp. 49–74). Washington DC: American Psychological Association.

Seel, R. T., Kreutzer, J. S., Rosenthal, M., Hammond, F. M., Corrigan, J. D., & Black, K. (2003): Depression after traumatic brain injury: A National Institute on Disability and Rehabiltation Research model systems multicenter investigation. *Archives of Physical Medicine & Rehabilitation, 84*(2), 177–184.

Skeel, R. L., Johnstone, B., Schopp, L., Shaw, J., & Petroski, G. F. (2000). Neuropsychological predictors of distress following traumatic brain injury. *Brain Injury, 14*(8), 705–712.

Tate, R. L., & Broe, G. A. (1999). Psychosocial adjustment after traumatic brain injury: What are the important variables? *Psychological Medicine, 29,* 713–725.

Tate, R. L, Lulham, J. M., Broe, G. A., Strettles, B., & Pfaff, A. (1989). Psychosocial outcome for the survivors of severe blunt head injury: The results from a consecutive series of 100 patients. *Journal of Neurology, Neurosurgery, and Psychiatry, 52,* 1128–1134.

Teasdale, T. W., & Engberg, A. W. (2001). Suicide after traumatic brain injury: A population study. *Journal of Neurology, Neurosurgery, and Psychiatry, 71,* 436–440.

Thurman, D. J., Alverson, C., Dunn, K. A., Guerrero, J. & Sniezek, J. H. (1999). Traumatic brain injury in the United States: A Public Health Perspective. *Journal of Head Trauma Rehabilitation, 14*(6), 602–615.

Vickery, C. D., Gontkovsky, S. T., & Caroselli, J. S. (2005). Self concept and quality of life following acquired brain injury: A pilot investigation. *Brain Injury, 19*(9), 657–665.

Wallace, C. A., & Bogner, J. (2000). Awareness of deficits: Emotional implications for persons with brain injury and their significant others. *Brain Injury, 14*(6), 549–562.

Willer, B., Johnson, W. E., Rempel, R. G., & Linn, R. (1993). A note concerning misconceptions of the general public about brain injury. *Archives of Clinical Neuropsychology, 8,* 461–465.

Wilson, B. A. (2000). Compensating for cognitive deficits following brain injury. *Neuropsychology Review, 10*(4), 233–243.

Appendix of Commonly Used Coping Instruments

Instrument	Authors/Publication year	Type	Subscales	Psychometric properties
Ways of Coping Checklist (WCC)	Folkman and Lazarus (1980)	A 68-item self-report inventory that uses a "yes"/"no" response format to measure problem-solving and emotion-regulation coping functions.	• Problem-focused coping • Emotion-focused coping	Cronbach's alpha reliabilities for the problem-focused and emotion-focused coping were .80 and .81, respectively. Most factor-analytic studies failed to support the checklist's hypothesized 2-factor structure. Limited validation data are available.
Ways of Coping Questionnaire (WCQ)	Folkman and Lazarus (1985, 1988); Folkman, Lazarus, Dunkel-Schetter, DeLongis, and Gruen (1986)	A 66-item (50 rated items and 16 "fill in" items) self-report inventory composed of 8 subscales. The inventory uses a 4-point frequency-of-use rating format. Respondents are asked to direct their ratings of real-life stresses experienced during the past 7 days.	• Confrontation coping • Distancing • Self-controlling • Seeking social support • Accepting responsibility • Escape-avoidance • Planful problem-solving • Positive reappraisal	Cronbach's alpha reliabilities, for the 8 subscales, ranged from .56 to .85. Inter-scale correlations ranged from −.04 to +.39. Several factor-analytic studies failed to replicate the proposed 8-factor structure.

(Continued)

(Continued)

Instrument	Authors/Publication year	Type	Subscales	Psychometric properties
Coping Strategies Questionnaire (CSQ)	Rosentiel and Keefe (1983)	A 44-item self-report inventory that measures coping strategies of pain patients, composed of (a) 6 cognitive strategies, (b) 2 behavioral strategies, and (c) 2 effectiveness ratings. Items are rated on a 7-point frequency format.	*Coping Strategies* • Diverting attention • Reinterpreting pain • Coping self-statements • Ignoring pain • Praying/hoping • Catastrophizing *Behavioral Strategies* • Increasing activity level • Increasing pain behavior *Effectiveness Ratings* • Control over pain • Ability to decrease pain	Cronbach's alpha reliabilities range from .71 to .85 (except "increasing pain behaviors"). Factor analysis yielded 3 main factors: (a) Cognitive coping and suppression, (b) helplessness, and (c) diverting attention and praying. Construct validity: The empirically-derived factors predicted criterion measures of average pain, depression, state anxiety, and functional capacity.
Coping Strategies Inventory (CSI)	Tobin, Holroyd, Reynolds, and Wigal (1989); Tobin, Holroyd, and Reynolds (1984)	A 72-item self-report inventory that uses a 5-point frequency rating and is composed of 15 scales (8 primary, 4 secondary, and 2 tertiary scales).	*Primary Scales* • Problem-solving • Cognitive restructuring • Suppressing emotions • Social support • Problem-avoidance • Wishful thinking • Social withdrawal • Self-criticism	A hierarchically structured coping inventory. Factor analysis supported inventory's structure. Scale test-retest reliabilities ranged from .67 to .83. Cronbach's alpha reliabilities ranged from .72 to .94.

Instrument	Description	Scales	Psychometric properties
		Secondary Scales	Coefficients of congruence across 2 samples ranged from .85 to .97 for the 14 scales. Construct validity: Adequate correlations with measures of depression and self-efficacy.
		• Problem-engagement • Emotion-engagement • Problem-disengagement • Emotion- disengagement	
		Tertiary Scales	
		• Engagement • Disengagement	
Measure of Daily Coping (MDC) Stone and Neale (1984)	A 55-item (originally 87-item) self-report check list to measure daily coping (with a recent problem). Items are rated as "yes" (coping strategy is used), "might," or left unchecked ("no"). In this situation-specific instrument, respondents specify a problem, describe it, appraise it, and then indicate which of the 8 coping strategies they have used.	• Distraction • Situation redefinition • Direct action • Catharsis • Acceptance • Social support • Relaxation • Religion	Cronbach's alpha reliabilities ranged from .36 to .78 ($M = .57$). Inter-scale correlations ranged from $-.28$ to $+.18$. Construct validity: The Catharsis and Acceptance scales correlated with decreased levels of perceived control. No other supportive validation data have been provided.
Life Situations Inventory (LSI) Feifel and Strack (1989)	A 28-item (later reduced to 21-item) self-report inventory addressing 5 conflict areas (i.e., decision-making, defeat in competition, frustrating situation, difficulty with authority, and general disagreement with a peer). The inventory is rated on a 4-point response format and is represented by 3 types of coping.	• Problem-solving • Avoidance • Resignation	Cronbach'a alpha reliabilities ranged from .75 to .82. Inter-scale conditions ranged from .01 to .51. No supportive validation data are provided.

(Continued)

Instrument	Authors/Publication year	Type	Subscales	Psychometric properties
COPE Inventory	Carver, Scheier, and Weintraub (1989)	*Version I* A 53-item self-report inventory, using a 4-point frequency scale, composed of 13 4-item scales, and a 1-item Alcohol and Drug Use scale. *Version II* A 60-item self-report inventory composed of 15 scales (adding a Humor scale and increasing the Alcohol and Drug Use scale to 4 items).	Designed originally as a coping disposition inventory. Dimensions and their associated scales include: • *Emotion-focused* (seeking social support- emotional, venting emotions). • *Problem-solving* (active coping, planning, suppression, restraint, seeking social support- instrumental). • *Dysfunctional coping* (behavioral disengagement, mental disengagement, substance use). • *Other strategies* (positive reinterpretation/growth, denial, acceptance, turning to religion).	Scales' test-retest reliabilities ranged from .42 to .89. Cronbach's alpha reliabilities ranged from .45 to .92. Inter-scale correlations ranged from −.28 to +.69. Construct validity: Adequate scale correlations with measures of optimism, control, self-esteem, hardiness, and anxiety. Fit indices from an independent confirmatory factor analysis supported the full 15-factor model structure (Clark, Bormann, Cropanzano, and James, 1995).

Brief COPE Inventory	Carver (1997)	A brief version of COPE. A 28-item self-report inventory using a 4-point frequency format, composed of 14 2-item scales (13 of the original 15 scales and a new scale).	• Suppression and Restraint scales deleted • A Self-blame scale added • The Mental Disengagement scale renamed Self-distraction.	Cronbach's alpha reliabilities for the 14 scales ranged from .50 to .90. No validity data are available.
Coping Strategy Indicator (CSI)	Amirkhan (1990, 1994)	A 33-item self-report of 3 subscales (rated on a 3-point scale). Each subscale is composed of 11 items.	• Problem-solving • Seeking support • Avoidance	Factor analytic studies supported the 3-scale solution. Cronbach's alpha reliabilities for the 3 scales ranged from .84 to .93. Test-retest reliabilities ranged from .77 to .86. Construct validity: adequate convergent validity correlations with the WCC (problem-solving, seeking support, avoidance), but also an unexpected significant correlation between the problem-solving subscale and the WCC seeking social support scale. Appropriate correlations with measures of locus of control and depression. Fit indices from a confirmatory factor analysis supported the 3-factor model structure (Clark et al., 1995).

(Continued)

(Continued)

Instrument	Authors/Publication year	Type	Subscales	Psychometric properties
Coping Inventory for Stressful Situations (CISS)	Endler and Parker (1990a, 1990b, 1994)	A 24-item self-report inventory using a 5-point Likert-type format and measuring 3 primary coping strategies.	• Task-oriented • Emotion-oriented • Avoidance-oriented (addressing both distraction and social diversion)	Construct validity: Adequate correlations with the WCQ and with several measures of personality traits (depression, anxiety, neuroticism, extraversion). Also, supportive correlations with the Coping Strategy Indicator and measures of psychiatric symptomatology from the MMPI-2. Factor analysis supported the 3-coping dimensions structure.

References

Amirkhan, J. H. (1990). A factor analytically derived measure of coping: The coping strategy indicator. *Journal of Personality and Social Psychology, 59*, 1066–1074.

Amirkhan, J. H. (1994). Criterion validity of a coping measure. *Journal of Personality Assessment, 62*, 242–261.

Carver, C. S. (1997). You want to measure coping but your protocol's too long: Consider the Brief COPE. *International Journal of Behavioral Medicine, 4*, 92–100.

Carver, C. S., Scheier, M. F., & Weintraub, J. K. (1989). Assessing coping strategies: A theoretically based approach. *Journal of Personality and Social Psychology, 56*, 267–283.

Clark, K. K., Bormann, C. A., Cropanzano, R. S., & James, K. (1995). Validation evidence for three coping measures. *Journal of Personality Assessment, 65*, 434–455.

Endler, N. S., & Parker, J. D. A. (1990a). *Coping Inventory for Stressful Situations (CISS): Manual.* Toronto: Multi Health Systems.

Endler, N. S., & Parker, J. D. A. (1990b). Multidimensional assessment of coping: A critical evaluation.*Journal of Personality and Social Psychology, 58*, 844–854.

Endler, N. S., & Parker, J. D. A. (1994). Assessment of multidimensional coping: Task, emotion, and avoidance strategies. *Psychological Assessment, 6*, 50–60.

Feifel, H., & Strack, S. (1989). Coping with conflict situations: Middle-aged and elderly men. *Psychology and Aging, 4*, 26–33.

Folkman, S., & Lazarus, R. S. (1980). An analysis of coping in a middle-aged community sample. *Journal of Health and Social Behavior, 21*, 219–239.

Folkman, S., & Lazarus, R. S. (1985). If it changes it must be a process: A study of emotion and coping during three stages of a college examination. *Journal of Personality and Social Psychology, 48*, 150–170.

Folkman, S., & Lazarus, R. S. (1988). *Manual for the Ways of Coping Questionnaire.* Palo Alto, CA: Consulting Psychologist Press.

Folkman, S., Lazarus, R. S., Dunkel-Schetter, C., DeLongis, A., & Gruen, R. J. (1986). Dynamics of a stressful encounter: Cognitive appraisal, coping, and encounter outcomes. *Journal of Personality and Social Psychology, 50*, 992–1003.

Rosenstiel, A. K., & Keefe, F. J. (1983). The use of coping strategies in chronic low back pain patients: Relationship to patient characteristics and current adjustment. *Pain, 17*, 33–44.

Stone, A., & Neale, J. (1984). New measure of daily coping: Development and preliminary results. *Journal of Social Psychology and Personality, 62*, 892–906.

Tobin, D. L., Holroyd, K. A., & Reynolds, R. V. (1984). *User's manual for the Coping Strategies Inventory.* Athens, OH: Ohio University, Department of Psychology.

Tobin, D. L., Holroyd, K. A., Reynolds, R. V., & Wigal, J. K. (1989). The hierarchical factor structure of the coping strategies inventory. *Cognitive Therapy and Research, 13*, 343–361.

Index

Made in the USA
Lexington, KY
22 August 2012